Baillière's
CLINICAL
GASTROENTEROLOGY
INTERNATIONAL PRACTICE AND RESEARCH

Baillière's

CLINICAL

GASTROENTEROLOGY

INTERNATIONAL PRACTICE AND RESEARCH

Volume 11/Number 2
June 1997

Portal Hypertension

J. BOSCH MD
Guest Editor

Baillière Tindall
London Philadelphia Sydney Tokyo Toronto

This book is printed on acid-free paper.

Baillière Tindall   24–28 Oval Road
W.B. Saunders   London NW1 7DX, UK
Company Ltd

The Curtis Center, Independence Square West,
Philadelphia, PA 19106–3399, USA

55 Horner Avenue
Toronto, Ontario M8Z 4X6, Canada

Harcourt Brace & Company
Australia
30–52 Smidmore Street, Marrickville, NSW 2204, Australia

Harcourt Brace & Company
Japan Inc
Ichibancho Central Building,
22–1 Ichibancho, Chiyoda-ku, Tokyo 102, Japan

Whilst great care has been taken to maintain the accuracy of the information contained in this issue, the authors, editor, owners and publishers cannot accept any responsibility for any loss or damage arising from actions or decisions based on information contained in this publication; ultimate responsibility for the treatment of patients and interpretation of published material lies with the medical practitioner. The opinions expressed are those of the authors and the inclusion in this publication of material relating to a particular product, method or technique does not amount to an endorsement of its value or quality, or of the claims made by its manufacturer.

ISSN 0950–3528

ISBN 0–7020–2339–6 (single copy)

Baillière's Clinical Gastroenterology is published four times each year by Baillière Tindall. Prices for Volume 11 (1997) are:

TERRITORY	ANNUAL SUBSCRIPTION	SINGLE ISSUE
Europe including UK	£108.00 (Institutional) post free	£30.00 post free
	£90.00 (Individual) post free	
All other countries	Consult your local Harcourt Brace & Company office	

The editor of this publication is Ian Bramley, Baillière Tindall, 24–28 Oval Road, London NW1 7DX, UK.

Baillière's Clinical Gastroenterology is covered in Index Medicus, Current Contents/Clinical Medicine, Current Contents/Life Sciences, the Science Citation Index, SciSearch, Research Alert and Excerpta Medica.

Baillière's Clinical Gastroenterology was published from 1972 to 1986 as *Clinics in Gastroenterology*

Typeset by Phoenix Photosetting, Chatham.
Printed and bound in Great Britain by the University Printing House, Cambridge, UK.

Contributors to this issue

GENNARO D'AMICO MD, Professor on Tenure of Gastroenterology, Divisione di Medicina, Ospedale V Cervello, Via Trabucco 180, 90146 Palermo, Italy.

VICENTE ARROYO MD, Professor of Medicine, University of Barcelona School of Medicine, Liver Unit, Hospital Clínic i Provincial, Villarroel 170, 08036 Barcelona, Spain.

JAUME BOSCH MD, Professor of Medicine, Hepatic Haemodynamic Laboratory, Liver Unit, Department of Medicine, Hospital Clínic i Provincial, University of Barcelona, Villarroel 170, 08036 Barcelona, Spain.

A. K. BURROUGHS MBChB(Hons), FRCP, Consultant Physician and Hepatologist, Department of Liver Transplantation and Hepato-Biliary Medicine, The Royal Free Hampstead NHS Trust, Pond Street, Hampstead, London NW3 2QG, UK.

LISA CHEN MD, Post-doctoral Fellow, Yale University School of Medicine and Hepatic Hemodynamic Laboratory (111J), VA Medical Center, 950 Campbell Avenue, West Haven, CT 06516, USA.

GLÒRIA FERNÁNDEZ-ESPARRACH MD, Research Fellow, Liver Unit, Hospital Clínic i Provincial, Villarroel 170, 08036 Barcelona, Spain.

ROBERTO DE FRANCHIS MD, Associate Professor of Medicine and Head of Department, Gastroenterology and Gastrointestinal Endoscopy Service, Istituto di Medicina Interna, University of Milan, IRCCS Ospedale Policlinico, Via Pace 9, 20122 Milan, Italy.

JOAN CARLES GARCÍA-PAGÁN MD, Staff Member, Hepatic Haemodynamic Laboratory, Liver Unit, Department of Medicine, Hospital Clínic i Provincial, University of Barcelona, Villarroel 170, 08036 Barcelona, Spain.

PERE GINÈS MD, Faculty Member, Liver Unit, Hospital Clínic i Provincial, Villarroel 170, 08036 Barcelona, Spain.

ROBERTO J. GROSZMANN MD, FRCP, Professor of Medicine and Chief, Digestive Diseases, Yale University School of Medicine and VA Medical Center, Digestive Disease Section (111H), 950 Campbell Avenue, West Haven, CT 06516, USA.

TARUN K. GUPTA MD, Assistant Adjunct Professor, Yale University School of Medicine and Bridgeport Hospital, Bridgeport, CT; Hepatic Hemodynamic Laboratory (111J), VA Medical Center, 950 Campbell Avenue, West Haven, CT 06516, USA.

J. MICHAEL HENDERSON MD, ChB, FRCS, FACS, Chairman, Department of General Surgery A8-146, The Cleveland Clinic Foundation, 9500 Euclid Avenue, Cleveland, OH 44195, USA.

DAVID A. IANITTI MD, Fellow in Pancreatic and Hepatobiliary Surgery, Department of General Surgery A8-418, The Cleveland Clinic Foundation, 9500 Euclid Avenue, Cleveland, OH 44195, USA.

Editorial Note

The presentation of material in *Baillière's Clinical Gastroenterology* has been updated, and we hope that the changes will make the information in the series more accessible to readers.

Each chapter is now preceded by a short abstract summarizing the content and by keywords that will be used for indexing and abstracting purposes.

Where the author has identified the most important references cited in the chapter, these have been indicated in the reference list with asterisks.

PATRICK S. KAMATH MD, Assistant Professor of Medicine and Consultant, Department of Gastroenterology and Internal Medicine, Mayo Clinic and Mayo Medical School, 200 First Street Southwest, Rochester, MN 55905, USA.

DIDIER LEBREC MD, FRCP, Director of Research, Splanchnic Haemodynamic and Vascular Laboratory, INSERM U-24 and Department of Hepatology, Hôpital Beaujon, 100 Blvd du General Lecler, 92118 Clichy, France.

ANGELO LUCA MD, Research Fellow in Clinical Radiology, Divisione di Medicina, Ospedale V Cervello, Via Trabucco 180, 90146, Palermo, Italy.

MICHAEL A. McKUSICK MD, Assistant Professor of Medicine and Consultant, Department of Diagnostic Radiology, Mayo Clinic and Mayo Medical School, 200 First Street Southwest, Rochester, MN 55905, USA.

D. PATCH MBBS, MRCP, Senior Registrar, Department of Liver Transplantation and Hepato-Biliary Medicine, The Royal Free Hampstead NHS Trust, Pond Street, Hampstead, London NW3 2QG, UK.

JOSEP M. PIQUÉ MD, Chief, Gastroenterology Department, Hospital Clínic i Provincial, University of Barcelona, Villarroel 170, 08036 Barcelona, Spain.

MASSIMO PRIMIGNANI MD, Senior Lecturer, Gastroenterology and Gastrointestinal Endoscopy Service, Istituto di Medicina Interna, University of Milan, IRCCS Ospedale Policlinico, Via Pace 9, 20122 Milan, Italy.

JOSEP ROCA MD, Associate Professor of Medicine; Chief of Section and Consultant, Servei de Pneumologia i Al·lèrgia Respiratòria, Departament de Medicina, Hospital Clínic, Universitat de Barcelona, Barcelona, Spain.

ROBERT RODRIGUEZ-ROISIN MD, FRCPE, Professor of Medicine, Chief of Service and Senior Consultant, Servei de Pneumologia i Al·lèrgia Respiratòria, Departament de Medicina, Hospital Clínic, Universitat de Barcelona, Barcelona, Spain.

PHILIPPE SOGNI MD, Praticien Hospitalier Universitaire, Department of Hepatology and Gastroenterology, Hôpital Cochin, 75674 Paris, France.

VALERIE VILGRAIN MD, Professor of Radiology, Department of Radiology, Hôpital Beaujon, 100 Blvd du General Lecler, 92118 Clichy, France.

Table of contents

Preface/J. BOSCH ix

1 Pathophysiology of portal hypertension 203
T. K. GUPTA, L. CHEN & R. J. GROSZMANN

2 Evaluation of patients with portal hypertension 221
D. LEBREC, P. SOGNI & V. VILGRAIN

3 Natural history. Clinical–haemodynamic correlations.
Prediction of the risk of bleeding 243
G. D'AMICO & A. LUCA

4 Portal hypertensive gastropathy 257
J. M. PIQUÉ

5 Pharmacological prevention of variceal bleeding.
New developments 271
J. C. GARCÍA-PAGÁN & J. BOSCH

6 Endoscopic treatments for portal hypertension 289
R. DE FRANCHIS & M. PRIMIGNANI

7 Advances in drug therapy for acute variceal haemorrhage 311
D. PATCH & A. K. BURROUGHS

8 Transjugular intrahepatic portosystemic shunts (TIPS) 327
P. S. KAMATH & M. A. McKUSICK

9 Surgery in portal hypertension 351
D. A. IANNITTI & J. M. HENDERSON

10 Ascites and renal functional abnormalities in cirrhosis.
Pathogenesis and treatment 365
P. GINÈS, G. FERNÁNDEZ-ESPARRACH & V. ARROYO

11 Hepatopulmonary syndrome: the paradigm of
liver-induced hypoxaemia 387
R. RODRIGUEZ-ROISIN & J. ROCA

Index 407

PREVIOUS ISSUES

Vol. 8, No. 4 1994
Diagnostic Imaging of the Gastrointestinal Tract: Part I
G. N. J. Tytgat & J. W. A. J. Reeders

Vol. 9, No. 1 1995
Diagnostic Imaging of the Gastrointestinal Tract: Part II
G. N. J. Tytgat & J. W. A. J. Reeders

Vol. 9, No. 2 1995
Coeliac Disease
P. D. Howdle

Vol. 9, No. 3 1995
Helicobacter pylori
J. Calam

Vol. 9, No. 4 1995
Investigations in Hepatology
P. C. Hayes

Vol. 10, No. 1 1996
Cytokines and Growth Factors in Gastroenterology
R. A. Goodlad & N. A. Wright

Vol. 10, No. 2 1996
Viral Hepatitis
A. Alberti

Vol. 10, No. 3 1996
Liver and Gastrointestinal Immunology
M. P. Manns

Vol. 10, No. 4 1996
Gastrointestinal Endocrine Tumours
D. O'Shea & S. R. Bloom

Vol. 11, No. 1 1997
Ulcerative Colitis
P. R. Gibson

FORTHCOMING ISSUE

Vol. 11, No. 3 1997
Paediatric Gastroenterology
J. A. Walker-Smith

Preface

Portal hypertension is a common clinical syndrome and a severe complication in chronic liver disease such as cirrhosis of the liver. It affects millions of patients the world over. Its treatment has experienced a marked progress over the past few years, largely as a result of a better understanding of the mechanisms involved in its pathogenesis in experimental models, the new and useful methods for the clinical evaluation of the portal hypertensive patient, and finally, owing to the introduction of new and effective medical treatments to prevent and correct the major complications of portal hypertension.

Owing to these advances an updated review on portal hypertension is timely. As Guest Editor, I have striven to evaluate and focus on the areas that have undergone major advancement, and to introduce innovative pathogenetic knowledge, along with its clinical applications. The contributors to this issue include some of the leading experts in the field who have been involved in the development of new approaches to the understanding and treatment of portal hypertension.

The contents of this issue of *Baillière's Clinical Gastroenterology* have been divided into 11 chapters. The majority address the most common complication of portal hypertension, bleeding from ruptured gastroesophageal varices, and encompass the major advances in pathophysiology, clinical evaluation and pharmacological treatment, with regard to both the prevention of variceal haemorrhage and the treatment of acute bleeding episodes. Additional chapters review the innovations of endoscopic treatment, surgery and transjugular intrahepatic portosystemic shunts (TIPS), and their use for the optimal management of the portal hypertensive patient. Finally, I have included the chapters that review the pathophysiological and therapeutic aspects of three distinct complications of portal hypertension: ascites and renal dysfunction, portal hypertensive gastropathy and the hepatopulmonary syndrome.

It is hoped that this issue will help to bring into practice new concepts that have been emerging in the last few years, and thus be useful to clinicians caring for patients with portal hypertension, as well as stimulating interest in this field. I would like to thank all the contributors whose effort and co-operation in compiling this issue have been exceptional. I would also like to thank Diana Bird for her excellent assistance throughout this project.

J. BOSCH

1

Pathophysiology of portal hypertension

TARUN K. GUPTA MD

Assistant Adjunct Professor
Hepatic Hemodynamic Laboratory, VA Medical Center, West Haven, CT 06516; Yale University School of Medicine, New Haven, CT 06510 and Bridgeport Hospital, Bridgeport, CT 06610, USA

LISA CHEN MD

Post-doctoral Fellow
Hepatic Hemodynamic Laboratory, VA Medical Center, 9 West Haven, CT 06516 and Yale University School of Medicine, New Haven, CT 06510, USA

ROBERTO J. GROSZMANN* MD, FRCP

Professor of Medicine and Chief, Digestive Diseases
Hepatic Hemodynamic Laboratory, VA Medical Center, West Haven, CT 06516 and Yale University School of Medicine, New Haven, CT 06510, USA

Portal hypertension is a common clinical syndrome associated with chronic liver diseases and is characterized by a pathological increase in portal pressure. Increase in portal pressure is because of an increase in vascular resistance and an elevated portal blood flow. The site of increased intrahepatic resistance is variable and is dependent on the disease process. The site of obstruction may be: pre-hepatic, hepatic, and/or post-hepatic. In addition, part of the increased intrahepatic resistance is because of increased vascular tone. Another important factor contributing to increased portal pressure is elevated blood flow. Peripheral vasodilatation initiates the classical profile of decreased systemic resistance, expanded plasma volume, elevated splanchnic blood flow and elevated cardiac index. The elevated portal pressure leads to formation of portosystemic collaterals and oesophageal varices. Pharmacotherapy for portal hypertension is aimed at reducing both intrahepatic vascular tone and elevated splanchnic blood flow.

Key words: portal hypertension; porto-systemic collaterals; hyperdynamic circulation; vasodilators; vasoconstrictors; oesophageal varices; variceal haemorrhage; plasma volume; intrahepatic resistance; pharmacotherapy.

Portal hypertension is a common clinical syndrome associated with chronic liver diseases and is characterized by a pathological increase in portal pressure. Elevated portal pressure results in extensive formation of porto-

* Address for correspondence: R. J. Groszmann Yale University School of Medicine, Hepatic Hemodynamic Laboratories/111H, VA Connecticut Healthcare System, 950 Campbell Avenue, West Haven, CT 06516, USA.

Baillière's Clinical Gastroenterology—
Vol. 11, No. 2, June 1997
ISBN 0–7020–2339–6
0950–3528/97/020203 + 17 $12.00/00

systemic collaterals that divert portal blood to the systemic circulation. This causes many haemodynamic disturbances, which result in complications of portal hypertension. The major consequences of portal hypertension are gastrointestinal bleeding from ruptured oesophageal varices, ascites formation and hepatic encephalopathy. A grasp of the biological mechanisms involved in the pathogenesis of portal hypertension is essential to an understanding of the complications of chronic liver disease and to the development of rational therapies. This chapter is an overview of the basic pathophysiological mechanisms of the splanchnic and systemic circulatory derangements that lead to portal hypertension and cause the portosystemic collaterals to develop.

Some recapitulation of general principles is essential to the understanding of the pathophysiology of portal hypertension. When Ohm's law is applied to the vascular system, the pressure gradient between two points $(P1 - P2)$ in a blood vessel can be described as the product of blood flow (Q) and resistance to flow (R)

$$P1 - P2 = Q \times R$$

Unlike pressure and flow, resistance can not be directly measured, but it can be derived from pressure and flow. However, resistance to the flow of blood in a vessel is best understood when expressed according to Pouseuille's law:

$$R = \frac{8\eta L}{\pi r^4}$$

in which
η = coefficient of viscosity
L = length of vessel
r = radius of vessel

Expressed in these terms, substitution of resistance (R) into Ohm's equation yields

$$P1 - P2 = \frac{Q \times 8\eta L}{\pi r^4}$$

Under physiological conditions, the length of blood vessel (L) can be assumed to be constant. Similarly, unless there are large changes in haematocrit, the viscosity (η) is taken as constant. Hence, the changes in the pressure $(P1 - P2)$ are largely accounted for by changes in flow (Q) and are inversely related to the changes in the radius (r) of the vessel. The contribution of these factors to the portal hypertensive syndrome will be discussed in the subsequent sections (Figure 1).

INCREASED RESISTANCE

Portal hypertension is associated with increased resistance to portal blood flow. Increased vascular resistance is because of an increase in both intra-

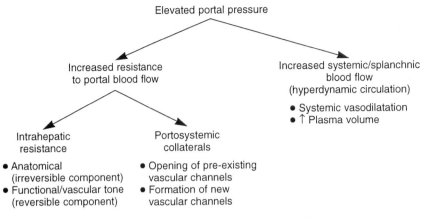

Figure 1. Contributing factors to portal hypertension.

hepatic and portosystemic collateral resistance in comparison with the low resistance of the normal liver.

Intrahepatic resistance

The normal liver is a very compliant organ. Hence, the intrahepatic resistance decreases with increase in blood flow because of distension of the vascular tree in response to increased inflow. This compensatory mechanism maintains the portal pressure within normal limits with a wide range of portal flow in normal livers (Greenway and Stark, 1971). This phenomenon is not seen in the portal hypertensive states in which the intrahepatic resistance becomes fixed due to fibrosis and mechanical distortion of the vascular tree and the hepatic vascular compliance is greatly reduced. Moreover, the splanchnic flow is increased as discussed in the subsequent sections. Decreased compliance and increased blood flow are probably instrumental in initiating and perpetuating the portal hypertension.

As stated above, there is little resistance in the normal liver, and the portal pressure remains low (4–8 mmHg) over a wide range of portal flows. The main site of resistance in normal livers is somewhat controversial. The hepatic sinusoids (where stellate cells are present), terminal hepatic venules and also portal venules have been suggested as possible sites of resistance. However, in view of the minimal contribution of intrahepatic resistance to portal pressure in the normal liver, this issue is of little importance. The flow into the portal system is actively regulated by changes in vascular resistance at the level of splanchnic arterioles and not by the liver itself (Greenway and Stark, 1971). In portal hypertensive syndromes, increased resistance to portal venous flow may be localized to pre-hepatic, post-hepatic, or intrahepatic (pre-sinusoidal, sinusoidal or post-sinusoidal) sites (Genecin and Groszmann, 1993). In pre-hepatic and post-hepatic portal hypertension, increased resistance is secondary to obstruction of portal venous inflow or hepatic venous outflow, respectively. Unlike pre- and post-hepatic portal hypertension, the intrahepatic syndromes are more complex and rarely can be classified according to a single site of resistance.

An early view of vascular resistance in cirrhotic livers hypothesized that portal hypertension is the consequence of a vascular obliterative process with scar tissue and regenerative nodules, both occluding and compressing vascular structures (Popper, 1958; Baldus and Hoffbauer, 1963). Thus earlier understanding of intrahepatic portal hypertension emphasized the role of anatomical alterations leading to mechanical obstruction (irreversible component) in the increased intrahepatic resistance. However, recently it has been shown that there is also an increased vascular tone in the cirrhotic liver (reversible component) (Bhathal, 1985).

In intrahepatic portal hypertension, there may be several areas of obstruction, and as the disease progresses, new sites may become involved. For example, in hepatic schistosomiasis, the increased intrahepatic resistance results from granulomas located in the presinusoidal areas (Beker and Valencia-Parparcen, 1968). However, in late stages, an elevated hepatic wedge venous pressure gradient may be observed, reflecting increased sinusoidal resistance. Chronic hepatitis seems to have both pre-sinusoidal and sinusoidal abnormalities, which increasingly contribute to vascular resistance as the lesion progresses towards cirrhosis (van Leeuwen et al, 1991). In ethanol-induced liver disease, the resistance is increased because of lesions in sinusoidal and post-sinusoidal sites. The terminal hepatic vein fibrosis (or sclerosis), encroachment on sinusoids by enlarged hepatocytes, collagen deposition in the perisinusoidal region or the space of Disse, result in elevated portal pressure even in a pre-cirrhotic stage (Schaffner and Popper, 1963; Reynolds et al, 1969; Lieber et al, 1976). However, in advanced stage or cirrhosis, regenerating nodules and pruning of the vascular tree contribute to increased vascular resistance. A variety of other non-alcoholic liver diseases cause portal hypertension because of increased sinusoidal vascular resistance. In hepatic amyloidosis, resistance is increased due to deposition of amyloid in the space of Disse (Brion et al, 1991). The capillarization process and occlusion of the fenestrae are postulated to increase the resistance of passage of fluid across the endothelium, but the extent of their effect on resistance to blood flow is unknown.

The morphological changes that occur in chronic liver diseases are undoubtedly the most important factor involved in the increased intrahepatic resistance. However, recent data also suggest a role of functional factors that lead to increased vascular tone, similar to that which is seen in the arterial hypertension. In chronic liver disease and also during acute liver injury, hepatic stellate cells acquire contractile properties and may contribute to the dynamic modulation of intrahepatic resistance (Pinzani et al, 1992). These cells may act as pericytes, a type of cell that has been shown to regulate blood flow in other organs. The hepatic stellate cells, which are also the main source of collagen synthesis, may contribute to the regulation of hepatic blood flow at the microcirculatory level. Stellate cells are strategically located in the sinusoids with perisinusoidal and inter-hepatocellular branching processes that contain actin-like filaments. They also express the alpha smooth-muscle actin gene, which is characteristic of vascular smooth muscle cells. The characteristics of these cells make them similar to myofibroblast. Myofibroblasts are intermediate in structure between smooth muscle cells and fibroblasts. Myofibroblast-like cells have been shown to exist in fibrous septa around the sinusoids and terminal hepatic venules in cirrhotic livers (Rudolph et al, 1979). These cells are postulated to play a role in the regulation of vascular resistance in the cirrhotic rat liver (Bhathal and Grossman, 1985).

The vascular endothelium synthesizes vasodilators such as nitric oxide, prostacyclins, hyperpolarizing factor and vasoconstrictors such as endothelins and prostanoids (Rubnayi, 1990; Vane et al, 1990). These vasoactive substances act in a paracrine fashion on the underlying vascular smooth muscle and modulate vascular tone. Normal vascular tone is maintained by a delicate balance between these vasodilatory and vasoconstrictive substances. Perturbation of this balance leads to abnormal vascular tone. Increased vascular tone seen in cirrhotic livers could be because of a deficit of endothelial vasodilators or an increase in the vasoconstrictors, or combination of both. Nitric oxide is a potent endothelial vasodilator that has been shown to play an important role in the modulation of intrahepatic vascular tone in normal livers (Mittal et al, 1994). Preliminary evidence from our laboratory suggest that there may be deficit of nitric oxide in the cirrhotic intrahepatic microcirculation as seen in other hypertensive regional microcirculations (Gupta and Groszmann, 1994). Using an isolated rat liver perfusion model, we have demonstrated that there is endothelial dysfunction in the intrahepatic microcirculation of cirrhotic livers (Gupta et al, 1995). Endothelial dysfunction leads to impaired release of endothelial vasodilators which, in part, may be responsible for the increased vascular tone observed in cirrhotic livers. More recently, it has been shown that the stellate cells (myofibroblasts) from cirrhotic livers exhibit an enhanced response to endothelins (Rockey and Weisiger, 1996). An imbalance between endothelial vasodilators and vasoconstrictors can affect the activated stellate cells (myofibroblasts), which modulate intrahepatic vascular tone. It is possible that both a deficit of vasodilators and an increase in vasoconstrictors may be responsible for the increased vascular tone.

In summary, there are multiple factors that may lead to increased resistance to portal blood flow. Some of these are irreversible, such as fibrosis, capillarization, regenerating nodules, and some are quite dynamic, such as the imbalance between endothelial factors that leads to increased vascular tone.

Portosystemic collateral resistance

Although the collateral circulation begins as a consequence of portal hypertension, it evolves into an important mediator of the circulatory derangements of portal hypertension in its own right. The portosytemic collaterals provide a route to decompress the hypertensive portal system; however, the vascular resistance of this collateral bed is still greater than the resistance of the normal liver. Hence, portosystemic collaterals do not permit a complete portal decompression. Development of portosystemic collaterals is discussed in detail later.

HYPERDYNAMIC CIRCULATION IN PORTAL HYPERTENSION

Chronic elevations in systemic and splanchnic blood flow have been documented as key elements of the hyperdynamic circulatory state (HCS) of portal hypertensive animals and humans. Peripheral vasodilatation initiates the development of the classic profile of decreased systemic vascular resistance and mean arterial pressure, plasma volume expansion, elevated splanchnic blood flow, and elevated cardiac index that characterizes this state (Colombato et al, 1991).

Systemic vasodilatation

At least three mechanisms are thought to contribute to this peripheral vasodilation: (i) increased concentrations of circulating vasodilators; (ii) increased endothelial production of local vasodilators; and (iii) decreased vascular responsiveness to endogenous vasoconstrictors. The last mechanism is probably because of the effect of the first two components. The relative importance of each of these potential causes of peripheral vasodilation is unknown.

Increased circulating vasodilators

In portal hypertensive states, there is increase in both endothelium-dependent and independent vasodilators. Possible aetiologies for increased circulatory concentrations of vasodilatory substances include increased production, decreased catabolism secondary to impaired hepatic function, and portosystemic shunting.

Circulating bile acids and glucagon increase splanchnic flow. Circulating bile acids, routinely cleared by the liver, are present in elevated concentrations when liver function is impaired. Bile acid depletion has been shown to be associated with decrease in splanchnic hyperaemia. Experimental evidence, however, suggests that an increase in circulating bile acids is not essential for maintaining the HCS in portal hypertension. More specifically, cholestyramine-induced reduction of bile acids to concentrations seen in placebo-treated controls did not ameliorate the haemodynamic changes of the HCS in portal hypertensive animals (Genecin et al, 1990b)

Elevated concentrations of circulating glucagon also have been documented in both animals and humans with portal hypertension. Rats with portal hypertension induced experimentally by either partial portal vein-ligation (PVL) or carbon tetrachloride inhalation had significantly higher glucagon and insulin concentrations compared with control rats (Gomis et al, 1994; Pizcueta et al, 1995). In addition, pancreatic islet isolates from these animals exhibited significantly higher glucagon secretion in response to glucose and arginine administration compared with controls, although insulin secretion appeared to be impaired. Of note, this heightened pancreatic alpha cell glucagon secretion was not inhibited by increasing the glucose concentration in the incubation medium. Intraoperative glucagon concentrations measured from the portal vein and inferior vena cava increased significantly after surgical portosystemic shunting in Budd-Chiari patients and slightly, but not significantly, in cirrhotic patients (Sitzmann et al, 1993). Glucagon concentrations in this study, however, did not correlate with portal pressure. By infusing glucagon into normal rats to achieve levels seen in portal hypertensive rats, Benoit and co-workers demonstrated that glucagon significantly reduces splanchnic vascular resistance (Benoit et al, 1984).

Pizcueta and co-workers (1991) have demonstrated in PVL rats that the administration of somatostatin, which inhibits glucagon secretion, was associated with a marked decrease in glucagon secretion, a significant decrease in portal pressure and portal venous inflow. They postulated that this decrease in portal inflow was secondary to increased splanchnic vasoconstriction (Pizcueta et al, 1991). Administration of glucagon and somatostatin in these animals abolishes the above effects of somatostatin suggesting that somatostatin's haemodynamic effects, probably, are elicited via inhibition of glucagon secretion. In an earlier study, we found no correlation between glucagon levels and portal venous inflow, thus questioning a major role for glucagon in mediating the hyperdynamic circulation (Sikuler and Groszmann, 1986). A recent study from our laboratory has not found increased levels of glucagon in cirrhotic patients, nor could a correlation be demonstrated between changes in their levels and changes in forearm haemodynamics (Rodriguez-Perez et al, 1993). Therefore, whether glucagon plays a role in the production of the HCS remains unclear.

Increased endothelial production of vasodilators

Recently, increasing evidence has pointed towards a major role for the endothelium in the maintenance of basal vascular tone and the development of local and generalized vasodilatation in portal hypertension. The endothelium produces at least two substances that are known to contribute to the development of systemic and splanchnic vasodilatation in portal hypertension: nitric oxide (NO) and prostaglandins (Casadevall et al, 1993).

Nitric oxide. Nitric oxide, previously known as endothelial derived relaxing factor, is synthesized from L-arginine by the enzyme nitric oxide synthase (NOS), which has constitutive and inducible forms in different cell types. Nitric oxide mediates its potent vasodilatory action on smooth muscle cells through soluble guanylate cyclase. Evidence exists that elevated production of NO is essential to the development of portal hypertension; treatment with N-nitro-L-arginine (L-NNA), a competitive inhibitor of NOS, prevented the development of peripheral vasodilatation, decreased systemic arterial pressure, and plasma volume expansion in PVL rats (Lee et al, 1993b). Similarly, chronic continuous administration of N-nitro-L-arginine (L-NAME), another inhibitor of NOS, recently has been shown to delay splanchnic vasodilatation, increase splanchnic blood flow and the development of collaterals in PVL rats (Garcia-Pagan et al, 1994a). The vasodilatory effects of NO in portal hypertension are not limited to the splanchnic circulation. In PVL rats, isolated aortic rings demonstrated increased relaxation to acetylcholine, an endothelial agonist, compared with sham controls. This increased response to acetylcholine was partly reversed with L-NAME (Karatapanis et al, 1994).

Whether production of NO is a primary stimulus in the development of vasodilatation or a subsequent phenomenon that results from shear, and secondarily contributes to increased flow, has yet to be determined. Vallance and co-workers hypothesized that chronic endotoxaemia in portal hypertension and cirrhosis may upregulate inducible NOS, thus causing the increased NO production that leads to splanchnic vasodilation (Vallance and Moncada, 1991). Tumour necrosis factor (TNF)-α may play an important role in the vasodilatation by upregulating the inducible NOS. Treatment with anti-TNFα polyclonal antibodies and thalidomide have been shown to ameliorate the hyperdynamic circulation (Lopez-Talavera et al, 1995, 1996). The relative contributions of the constitutive and inducible forms of NOS are still under investigation. Although NO plays a definite role in vasodilation in portal hypertension, clearly other factors are also involved.

Prostaglandins. Several studies in animals and humans have implicated increased endothelial production of prostaglandins as a cause of splanchnic vasodilatation in portal hypertensive states. Portal vein concentrations of prostacyclin (PGI$_2$), for example, have been found to be elevated in PVL rabbits and rats, as well as in patients with cirrhosis and Budd-Chiari syndrome. These PGI$_2$ concentrations have correlated with portal pressure (Wu et al, 1993). In addition, increased concentrations of the prostaglandin metabolite 2,3-dinor-6 keto PGF$_{1\alpha}$ have been observed in cirrhotic patients, and elevated gastric PGE$_2$ synthesis has been seen in cirrhotic humans with severe portal hypertensive gastropathy (Casadevall et al, 1993).

In the PVL animal model of portal hypertension, increased prostaglandin production appears to have a more prominent role in rabbits than in rats. Inhibition of prostaglandin synthesis through pharmacological cyclo-oxygenase blockade has been shown to prevent development of the HCS in portal hypertensive rabbits. Wu and co-workers (1993) measured splanchnic flow and portal pressure in PVL rabbits in the presence and absence of the respective inhibitors of cyclo-oxygenase and NO synthase, indomethacin and L-NAME; their results were consistent with mediation of splanchnic hyperaemia predominantly by a prostaglandin, possibly prostacyclin, with a limited role for NO as a mediator of basal vascular tone. In addition, the effects of NO blockade with the NO synthase competitive inhibitor L-NAME, and reversal of that blockade with the naturally occurring substrate for NO synthase, L-arginine, were not significantly different between normal and PVL rabbits, thus implying that, at least in rabbits, increased NO production may not be responsible for the HCS associated with portal hypertension.

Similar studies performed in PVL rats, however, suggest that both NO and prostaglandins contribute to gastric hyperaemia. In PVL rats, haemo-dynamic measurements in the presence and absence of indomethacin and L-NAME demonstrated that prostaglandins and NO do not appear to act synergistically. In addition, an in vitro endothelial study suggested that prostacyclin release may be markedly suppressed by NO (Doni et al, 1988), and other researchers have found that NO inhibition may be associated with increased prostacyclin production (Claria et al, 1993).

Thus, both NO and prostaglandins appear to act through separate path-ways to contribute to the vasodilatation that leads to increased splanchnic flow in portal hypertension, although the relative contribution of each may vary among different species. Although prostaglandins appear to have a more prominent role than NO in the rabbit model of portal hypertension, both of these endothelial-derived vasodilators appear to play central roles in the development of the HCS in portal hypertensive humans and rats.

Decreased response to vasoconstrictors

Basal vascular tone is regulated by the complex balance between endogenous vasodilators and vasoconstrictors. A blunted response to vaso-constrictors, therefore, should also contribute to vasodilatation and, sub-sequently, hyperdynamic flow. In portal hypertensive states, in vitro hyporesponsiveness to the endogenous vasopressors norepinephrine, arginine vasopressin, and angiotensin II has been reported to contribute to the HCS (Sieber and Groszmann, 1992a).

This hyporeactivity to vasopressors appears to be mediated largely by NO. In portal hypertensive rats, inhibition of NO in isolated, perfused superior mesenteric artery beds has been shown to prevent the development of vascular hyperreactivity to the endogenous vasoconstrictors norepi-nephrine, and vasopressin (Sieber and Groszmann, 1992a), the exogenous alpha-agonist methoxamine, and the receptor-independent vasoconstrictor potassium chloride (Sieber and Groszmann, 1992b). These observations are consistent with the previous hypothesis that the decreased response to vaso-constrictors in portal hypertension is mediated by receptor-independent mechanisms.

In portal hypertensive rats, a role for prostaglandins in hyporesponsive-ness to vasoconstrictors has not been substantiated. In fact, cyclo-oxygenase inhibition with indomethacin did not ameliorate vascular hyporeactivity in superior mesenteric artery preparations in partial portal vein ligated rats (Sieber and Groszmann, 1992b). Therefore, at least in the rat model of portal hypertension, NO appears to cause the vascular hypo-reactivity to endogenous and exogenous vasoconstrictors that contributes to the generalized vasodilation seen in the HCS.

Plasma volume

The hyperdynamic circulation is mediated in part by vasodilatation, but this alone is not sufficient to cause the circulation to become hyperdynamic.

Plasma volume expansion has been recognized in portal hypertension for many years (Liebermann and Reynolds, 1967). In the PVL rat model of portal hypertension, plasma volume failed to expand in animals on sodium restricted diet as compared with those on normal diet. Moreover, the fully developed hyperdynamic circulation is found to be nearly reversible by sodium restriction (Genecin et al, 1990a). Subsequent studies have demonstrated that in the PVL rats, vasodilatation, expansion of plasma volume by sodium retention, and development of the hyperdynamic circulation follow each other in a stepwise fashion (Albillos et al, 1992: Colombato et al, 1992). Vascular resistance in the systemic circulation dropped significantly within 1 day of partial portal vein ligation, followed on day 2 by parallel increases in plasma volume and a progressive increase in systemic and regional blood flows. The fully expanded plasma volume was observed on day 4 and coincided with maximally hyperkinetic cardiac index. These studies provided important evidence for the existence of several events in the pathogenesis of hyperdynamic circulation. These include initial vasodilatation (induced by humoral and local endothelial factors) and subsequently, plasma volume expansion. Our laboratory have demonstrated that both octreotide, which suppresses the secretion of vasodilatory peptides, and nitric oxide blockers decrease renal sodium retention and plasma volume expansion by diminishing vasodilatation, thereby preventing the full expression of the hyperdynamic circulation (Albillos et al, 1993; Lee et al, 1993b).

The studies that examine the role of vasodilatation and plasma volume expansion in the hyperdynamic circulation provide support for the peripheral vasodilatation hypothesis. According to this hypothesis, portal hypertension leads to a relative hypovolaemia induced by the dilatation of the systemic and splanchnic circulation. This results in underfilling of the systemic vascular space with the consequent decrease in central blood volume. This in turn leads to activation of the sympathetic nervous system, renin–angiotensin system and release of anti-diuretic hormone. Mediators from these systems result in sodium and water retention by the kidneys, which results in increased plasma volume. Peripheral vasodilatation and increased plasma volume result in a hyperdynamic circulatory state (Figure 2).

DEVELOPMENT OF PORTOSYSTEMIC COLLATERALS AND OESOPHAGEAL VARICES

Portosystemic collaterals develop as a result of portal hypertension. The development of collaterals is the central pathophysiological event that leads to variceal bleeding and portosystemic encephalopathy in patients with portal hypertension.

The exact nature of the physiological stimuli responsible for initiating the collateral formation remains controversial. Propranolol and clonidine have been shown to ameliorate the development of the collateralization of the portal system thus implicating increased portal pressure in the pathophysiology of collateral formation (Halvorsen and Myking, 1974). Lee et al (1993a) however, demonstrated that collateral formation could be

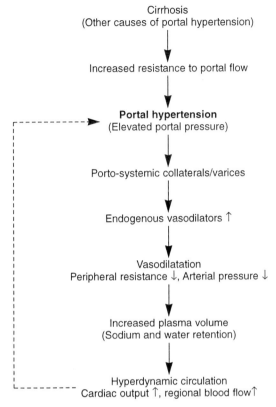

Figure 2. Hyperdynamic circulatory state in portal hypertension. Modified from Genecin and Groszmann (1994, The biology of portal hypertension. In Arias IM et al (eds) *The Liver: Biology and Pathobiology*, 3rd edn, pp 1327–1341. Philadelphia: Lippincott-Raven).

ameliorated by preventing an increase in splanchnic blood flow without any decrease in portal pressure. Thus, increased portal pressure does not appear to be an absolutely necessary component of collateral development in portal hypertensive states. Therefore, propranolol and clonidine may prevent collateral formation, in part at least, by decreasing flow, not by their effect on portal pressure. On the other hand, Sikuler et al (1985) studied PVL rats on post-operative day 3 and found no relationship between porto-systemic shunting and portal venous inflow. Therefore, the development of portosystemic shunting does not appear to be exclusively dependent upon either portal pressure or portal venous inflow. Evidence from studies conducted in PVL rats suggest that increased NO may be responsible for the initial collateralization of the portal system. Increased NO could result from progressive increases in splanchnic flow, a potent stimulus known to be present in portal hypertensive states. In addition, development of a new portocollateral bed renders available a new endothelial surface capable of producing NO (Lee et al, 1993a).

Mosca et al (1992) determined the vascular responsiveness of collateral vessels to various vasoconstrictors and vasodilators using an *in situ* perfused animal model. By administering norepinephrine, 5-hydroxy-tryptamine, isoproterenol and acetylcholine in the presence and absence of their respective blockers, phentolamine, propranolol, and L-NNA, they determined that collateral vessels have functional α-adrenoreceptors, 5-hydroxytryptamine receptors, and β-adrenoreceptors. In addition, collateral veins appear to be as sensitive to NO as arteries.

Regardless of the specific initiating stimulus, at least at the beginning, the mechanism of collateral formation appears to be recruitment of preformed channels, as opposed to *de novo* formation of new vessels. Portosystemic shunting can be detected almost immediately after the induction of portal hypertension, a pattern of timing that is consistent with the rapid dilatation of preformed vessels (Mosca et al, 1992). Whether these preformed vessels expand as the result of active dilatation mediated by increased flow or as a passive response to increased portal pressure is unclear. Neoformation of vessels cannot be excluded.

In humans, the portosystemic shunting of blood occurs between the short gastric, coronary veins, and the oesophageal azygos and the intercostal veins; superior and the middle and inferior haemorrhoidal veins; the paraumbilicus venous plexus and the venous system of abdominal organs juxtaposed with the retroperitoneum and abdominal wall; the left renal vein and the splanchnic, adrenal and spermatic veins. As discussed earlier, the dilatation of the pre-existing embryonic channels is thought to be the main mechanism of evolution of these collaterals. With progression of portal hypertension, the number and diameter of these collaterals increases.

The development of gastro-oesophageal varices constitute a major complication of portal hypertension. A threshold portal pressure gradient (HPVG) of 11 to 12 mmHg has been shown to exist in humans with oesophageal varices, below which varices are not encountered (Garcia-Tsao et al, 1985). Elevation above this pressure, however, does not always result in varices, since many patients with HPVG in excess of 12 mmHg do not have varices.

PATHOPHYSIOLOGY OF VARICEAL HAEMORRHAGE

The earlier concept of *erosion theory*, which suggested that the oesophageal varices bleed due to external trauma to thin-walled varices, has been abandoned because of lack of supporting objective evidence. Factors involved in the variceal haemorrhage appear to be multiple. A certain increase in the portal venous pressure is required for the initiation of oesophageal collateral formation. The volume of blood traversing the collateral vein has a role in the enlarging collateral as does the perivascular tissue, which gives support to the vessel. Tissue support is particularly important in the oesophageal and rectal varices since the surrounding tissue provides very little support to the variceal wall. With continuing increase in intravariceal pressure, the varices expand in size and the variceal wall thickness decreases. Bleeding probably occurs when the expanding force can no longer be counter-balanced by the variceal wall tension; at this point the varices ruptures and bleed (Polio and Groszmann, 1986). The factors regulating the tension exerted by the wall of varices to contain the expanding force can be described according to the Laplace's law (Figure 3):

$$T = TP \times r/w$$

in which T is the wall tension, TP the transmural pressure, r the radius and w the wall thickness of the varices. The transmural pressure is the difference between intravariceal pressure and the pressure in the oesophageal lumen. The entire varix is in equilibrium between the outwardly directed force $(TP \times r/w)$ and the inwardly directed force of wall tension. The inwardly directed force is augmented by the surrounding tissue structures, which provide reinforcement for the vessel wall.

The larger variceal size multiplies the deleterious effect of high intravariceal pressure by increasing the expanding force. When varix distension increases, the radius increases and wall thickness decreases (Figure 3). The wall tension increases in an attempt to contain the expanding force. Since venous structures have little musculature, this limits their capacity to develop wall tension. Eventually, the expanding force in a enlarging varix exceeds the limit of wall tension and variceal rupture occurs.

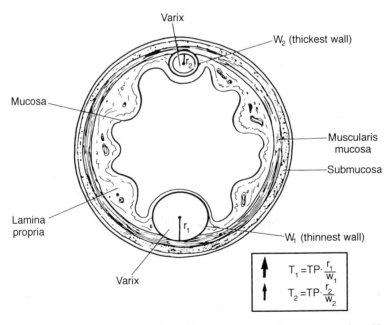

Figure 3. Relative position and size of varices with respect to the oesophagus and oesophageal lumen. At equal transmural pressure (TP), the tension (T) developed will be greater in T_1 than in T_2 due to increased radius (r) and smaller wall thickness (w). Reproduced from Jensen and Groszmann (1992, Complications of liver disease: pathophysiology and management. In Kaplowitz N. ed. *Liver and Biliary Diseases*, p 502. Baltimore: Williams & Wilkins).

The sequence of events leading to portal variceal bleeding are initiated by increased portal pressure, which results in the opening of collaterals. With progression of portal hypertension, the variceal blood flow and intravariceal pressure increases. The variceal size increases and the wall becomes thinner. Further increase in portal pressure, or a defect in the variceal wall leads to variceal haemorrhage. Portal pressure and blood flow are not static and vary markedly with various physiological stimuli. Portal flow increases transiently after meals because of postprandial hyperaemia. Similarly, fluctuations in portal pressure has been observed during circadian rhythm: portal pressure being higher at night and lower during afternoon and evening (Garcia-Pagan et al, 1994b). These variations in portal pressure may influence the onset of bleeding in patients with already elevated baseline portal pressure.

RATIONAL BASIS OF PHARMACOTHERAPY OF PORTAL HYPERTENSION

Drug therapy of portal hypertension is primarily the treatment and prevention of the complications of portal hypertension, mainly variceal haemorrhage. The aim of therapy is to reduce oesophageal varix wall tension, which is accomplished pharmacologically by decreasing transmural variceal pressure by a reduction in portal and intravariceal venous pressure. Since the portal pressure is elevated due to an increase in both resistance and portal venous inflow, the reduction in portal pressure can be achieved pharmacologically by decreasing portal venous and/or portocollateral blood flow or by reducing intrahepatic or portocollateral resistance. As discussed in earlier sections, part of the increased intrahepatic resistance is because of an increased vascular tone, which can be modulated. Vasodilators can reduce intrahepatic and/or portocollateral resistance.

The pharmacological agents currently available for the treatment of portal hypertension primarily act by modulation of the hyperdynamic splanchnic circulation. Vasoconstrictors decrease portal pressure by reducing splanchnic arterial flow. Since increased plasma volume is an important component of hyperdynamic circulation, drugs that modulate plasma volume like diuretics may help in reducing splanchnic blood flow. The last 5 years have clearly seen a general acceptance of drug therapy for portal hypertension. This is not a fad that will wane away with time, but is an important advance in medical treatment of a syndrome that has a mortality as high as an acute myocardial infarction.

REFERENCES

Albillos A, Colombato LA & Groszmann RJ (1992) Vasodilatation and sodium retention in prehepatic portal hypertension. *Gastroenterology* **102:** 931–935.
Albillos A, Colombato LA, Lee FY et al (1993) Octreotide ameliorates vasodilatation and sodium retention in portal hypertensive rats. *Gastroenterology* **104:** 575–579.

Baldus WP & Hoffbauer FW (1963) Vascular changes in the cirrhotic liver as studied by injection technique. *American Journal of Digestive Disease* **8:** 689–692.

Beker S & Valencia-Parparcen J (1968) Portal hypertension syndrome. A comparative analysis of bilharzial fibrosis and hepatic cirrhosis. *American Journal of Digestive Disease* **13:** 1047–1054.

Bhathal PS & Grossman HJ (1985) Reduction of the increased portal vascular resistance of the isolated perfused cirrhotic rat liver by vasodilators. *Journal of Hepatology* **1:** 325–337.

Benoit JN, Barrowman JA, Harper SL et al (1984) Role of humoral factors in the intestinal hyperemia associated with chronic portal hypertension. *American Journal of Physiology* **247:** G486–G493.

Brion E, Brenard R, Pariente EA et al (1991) Sinusoidal portal hypertension in hepatic amyloidosis. *Gut* **32:** 227–230.

*Casadevall M, Panes J, Pique JM et al (1993) Involvement of nitric oxide and prostaglandins in gastric mucosal hyperemia of portal-hypertensive anesthetized rats. *Hepatology* **18:** 628–634.

Claria J, Jimenez W, Ros J et al (1993) Pathogenesis of arterial hypotension in cirrhotic rats with ascites: role of endogenous nitric oxide. *Hepatology* **15:** 343–349.

*Colombato LA, Albillos A & Groszmann RJ (1992) Temporal relationship of peripheral vaso-dilatation, plasma volume expansion and the hyperdynamic circulatory state in portal-hyper-tensive rats. *Hepatology* **15:** 323–328.

Doni MG, Whittle BJ, Palmer RM et al (1988) Action of nitric oxide on the release of prosta-cyclin from bovine endothelial cells in culture. *European Journal of Pharmacology* **151:** 19–25.

Garcia-Pagan JC, Fernandez M, Bernadich C et al (1994a) Effect of continued NO inhibition on portal hypertensive syndrome after portal vein stenosis in rat. *American Journal of Physiology* **267:** G984–G990.

Garcia-Pagan JC, Feu F, Castells A et al (1994b) Circadian variations of portal pressure and variceal hemorrhage in patients with cirrhosis. *Hepatology* **19:** 595–601.

*Garcia-Tsao G, Groszmann RJ, Fisher RL et al (1985) Portal pressure, presence of gastroesophageal varices and variceal bleeding. *Hepatology* **5:** 419–424.

*Genecin P & Groszmann RJ (1993) Portal hypertension. In Schiff E & Schiff L (eds) *Diseases of the Liver*, pp 935–973. Philadelphia: JB Lippincott Company.

Genecin P, & Groszmann RJ (1994) The biology of portal hypertension. In Arias IM et al (eds) *The Liver: Biology and Pathobiology*, 3rd edn, pp 1327–1341. Philadelphia: Lippincott-Raven.

Genecin P, Polio J & Groszmann RJ (1990a) Sodium restriction blunts expansion of plasma volume and ameliorates hyperdynamic circulation in portal hypertension. *American Journal of Physiology* **259:** G498–G503.

Genecin P, Polio J, Ferraioli G et al (1990b) Bile acids do not mediate the hyperdynamic circulation in portal hypertensive rats. *American Journal of Physiology* **259:** G21–G25.

Gomis R, Fernandez-Alvarez J, Pizcueta P et al (1994) Impaired function of pancreatic islets from rats with portal hypertension resulting from cirrhosis and partial portal vein ligation. *Hepatology* **19:** 1257–1261.

Greenway CV & Stark RD (1971) Hepatic vascular bed. *Physiological Review* **51:** 23–65.

Groszmann RJ & Atterbury CE (1982) The pathophysiology of portal hypertension. A basis for classification. *Seminars in Liver Disease* **2:** 177–186.

Gupta TK & Groszmann RJ (1994) Administration of L-arginine, the physiological precursor of nitric oxide, reduces portal perfusion pressure and ameliorates hepatic vascular hyperreactivity in experimental cirrhosis. *Hepatology* **20(4):** 200A.

Gupta TK, Chung M, Sessa WC et al (1995) Impaired endothelial function in the intrahepatic circulation in cirrhosis. *Hepatology* **22(4):** 156A.

Halvorsen JF & Myking AO (1974) The portosystemic collateral pattern in the rat. *European Surgical Research* **6:** 183–195.

Jensen JE and Groszmann RJ (1992) Complications of liver disease: pathophysiology and manage-ment. In Kaplowitz N (ed.) *Liver and Biliary Diseases*, pp 494–504. Baltimore: Williams & Wilkins.

Johnson SJ, Hines JE & Burt AD (1992) Phenotypic modulation of perisinusoidal cells following acute liver injury—a quantitative analysis. *International Journal of Experimental Pathology* **73:** 765–772.

Karatapanis S, McCormick PA, Kakad S et al (1994) Alteration in vascular reactivity in isolated aortic rings from portal vein-constricted rats. *Hepatology* **20:** 1516–1521.

Lee F-Y, Colombato LA, Albillos A et al (1993a) Administration of *N*-omega-nitro-L-arginine ameliorates portal-systemic shunting in portal-hypertensive rats. *Gastroenterology* **105:** 1464–1470.

*Lee F-Y, Colombato LA, Albillos A et al (1993b) N^w-nitro-L-arginine administration corrects vasodilatation and systemic capillary hypotension, and ameliorates plasma volume expansion and sodium retention in portal hypertensive rats. *Hepatology* **17:** 84–90.

van Leeuwen DJ, Howe SC, Scheuer PJ, et al (1991) Portal hypertension in chronic hepatitis: relationship to morphological changes. *Gut* **31:** 339–343.

Lieber CS, Zimmon DS, Kessler RE et al (1976) Portal hypertension in experimental alcoholic liver injury. *Clinical Research* **24:** 478(a).

Liebermann FL & Reynolds TB (1967) Plasma volume in cirrhosis of the liver. *Journal of Clinical Investigation* **46:** 1279–1308.

*Lopez-Talavera JC, Merrill WW & Groszmann RJ (1995) Tumor necrosis factor α: a major contributor to the hyperdynamic circulation in prehepatic portal-hypertensive rats. *Gastroenterology* **108:** 761–767.

Lopez-Talavera JC, Cadelina GW, Olchowski J et al (1996) Thalidomide inhibits tumor necrosis factor-α, decreases nitric oxide synthesis and ameliorates the hyperdynamic circulatory syndrome in portal hypertensive rats. *Hepatology* **23(6):** 1616–1621.

Mittal MK, Gupta TK, Lee FY et al (1994) Nitric oxide modulates vascular tone in normal rat liver. *American Journal of Physiology* **267:** G416–G422.

Mosca P, Lee F-Y, Kaumann AJ et al (1992) Pharmacology of portal-systemic collaterals in portal hypertensive rats: role of endothelium. *American Journal of Physiology* **263:** G544–G550.

Pinzani M, Failli P, Ruocco C et al (1992) Fat-storing cells as liver-specific pericytes—spatial dynamics of agonist-stimulated intracellular calcium transients. *Journal of Clinical Investigation* **90:** 642–646.

Pizcueta P, Garcia-Pagan JC, Fernandez M et al (1991) Glucagon hinders the effects of somatostatin on portal hypertension. *Gastroenterology* **101:** 1710–1715.

Pizcueta MP, Casamitjana R, Bosch J et al (1995) Decreased systemic vascular sensitivity to norepineprine in portal hypertensive rats: role of hyperglucagonemia. *American Journal of Physiology* **258:** G191–G195.

*Polio J & Groszmann RJ (1986) Hemodynamic factors involved in the development and rupture of esophageal varices: a pathophysiologic approach to treatment. *Seminars of Liver Disease* **6:** 318–331.

Popper H & Zak FG (1958) Pathological aspects of cirrhosis. *American Journal of Medicine* **24:** 593–625.

Reynolds TB, Hidmura R, Mitchell H et al (1969) Portal hypertension without cirrhosis in alcoholic liver disease. *Annals of Internal Medicine* **70:** 497–506.

Rockey DC & Weisiger RA (1996) Endothelin induced contractility of stellate cell from normal and cirrhotic rat liver: implication for regulation of portal pressure and resistance. *Hepatology* **24(1):** 233–240.

Rodriguez-Perez F, Isales CM & Groszmann RJ (1993) Platelet cytosolic calcium, peripheral hemodynamics, and vasodilatory peptides in liver cirrhosis. *Gastroenterology* **105:** 863–867.

Rubanyi GM (1990) Endothelium-derived relaxing and contracting factors. *Journal of Cellular Biochemistry* **46:** 27–36.

Rudolph R, McClure WJ & Woodward M (1979) Contractile fibroblasts in chronic alcoholic cirrhosis. *Gastroenterology* **76:** 704–709.

Schaffner F & Popper H (1963) Capillarization of the hepatic sinusoids in man. *Gastroenterology* **44:** 239–251.

*Sieber CC & Groszmann RJ (1992a) Nitric oxide mediates hyporeactivity to vasopressors in mesenteric vessels of portal hypertensive rats. *Gastroenterology* **103:** 235–239.

Sieber CC & Groszmann RJ (1992b) *In vitro* hyporeactivity to methoxamine in portal hypertensive rats: reversal by nitric oxide blockade. *American Journal of Physiology* **262:** G996–G1001.

Sikuler E & Groszmann RJ (1986) Hemodynamic studies in long- and short-term portal hypertensive rats: the relation of systemic glucagon levels. *Hepatology* **6(3):** 414–418.

Sikuler E, Kravetz D & Groszmann RJ (1985) Evolution of portal hypertension and mechanisms involved in its maintenance in a rat model. *American Journal of Physiology* **248:** G618–G625.

Sitzmann JV, Campbell KA, Wu Y et al (1993) Effect of portosystemic shunting on PGI$_2$ and glucagon levels in humans. *Annals of Surgery* **217:** 248–252.

*Vallance P & Moncada S (1991) Hyperdynamic circulation in cirrhosis: a role for nitric oxide? *Lancet* **337:** 776–778.

Vane JR, Anggard EE & Botting RM (1990) Regulatory functions of vascular endothelium. *New England Journal of Medicine* **323:** 27–36.

Wu Y, Burns C & Sitzmann JV (1993) Effects of nitric oxide and cyclooxygenase inhition on splanchnic hemodynamics in portal hypertension. *Hepatology* **18:** 1416–1421.

2

Evaluation of patients with portal hypertension

DIDIER LEBREC MD, FRCP

Director of Research
Splanchnic Haemodynamic and Vascular Biology Laboratory, INSERM U-24, and Department of Hepatology, Hôpital Beaujon, 100 Blvd du General Lecler, 92118 Clichy, France

PHILIPPE SOGNI MD

Practicien Hospitalier Universitaire
Department of Hepatology and Gastroenterology, Hôpital Cochin, 75674 Paris, France

VALERIE VILGRAIN MD

Professor of Radiology
Department of Radiology, Hôpital Beaujon, 100 Blvd du General Lecler, 92118 Clichy, France

Patients with suspected portal hypertension must first be evaluated by physical examination, upper digestive endoscopy and ultrasonography with Doppler. Moreover, the evaluation of patients with portal hypertension depends on the cause of portal hypertension, the presence of complications and the specific treatment considered. Haemodynamic assessment with measurement of the hepatic venous pressure gradient is useful in confirming the origin of portal hypertension. This technique is the 'gold-standard' for evaluating haemodynamic treatments. Splanchnic and systemic circulation must also be measured. Quantitative evaluation of the splanchnic territory by Doppler sonography and other non-invasive investigations, may be performed. Further clinical studies are, however, needed to determine their interest in portal hypertension.

Key words: portal pressure; variceal pressure; hepatic venous pressure gradient; collateral circulation; haemodynamics; ultrasonography; Doppler; endoscopy

The presence of portal hypertension must be evaluated in all patients with cirrhosis or non-cirrhotic diseases that may cause portal hypertension (Table 1). At present, many methods have been developed to evaluate patients with portal hypertension. The increasing use of non-invasive techniques, such as echo-Doppler combined with endoscopic evaluation have reduced the necessity of angiographic techniques. In the same way, haemodynamic assessments have been developed and the hepatic venous pressure gradient measurement is the reference value to confirm the presence and location of portal hypertension (Bolondi et al, 1996).

Baillière's Clinical Gastroenterology —
Vol. 11, No. 2, June 1997
ISBN 0–7020–2339–6
0950–3528/97/020221 + 21 $12.00/00

Moreover, the measurement of the pressure gradient is strongly recommended in patients who are treated for the prevention of bleeding (Groszmann et al, 1996). Other techniques are being evaluated to confirm their use in this indication. This chapter reviews the main physical and endoscopic invasive and non-invasive investigative techniques used for the management of portal hypertension.

Table 1. Methods to evaluate portal hypertension.

Evaluation	Methods
Non-invasive evaluation	• physical signs • oesophagogastro-endoscopy • ultrasonography with duplex Doppler
Haemodynamic evaluation	• hepatic venous pressure gradient • systemic and pulmonary haemodynamics
Pharmacological haemodynamic studies	• variceal pressure • azygos blood flow • hepatic blood flow • renal blood flow • endoscopic sonography • other imaging techniques

PHYSICAL SIGNS

Splenomegaly

Splenomegaly is frequent but not always present in portal hypertension. There is no clear relationship between portal pressure or presence of the oesophageal varices and splenic size (Simpson and Finlayson, 1995). The only consequence of splenomegaly is hypersplenism, which corresponds to a reduction of some blood elements (most frequently a low platelet count) with a normal bone-marrow function. In fact, hypersplenism is not only associated with portal hypertension but can be present in any condition associated with splenomegaly and peripheral cytopenia. In portal hypertension and splenomegaly, other causes of cytopenia should be considered, such as folate deficiency, gastrointestinal bleeding, haemolysis or drug toxicity. The presence of splenomegaly and portal hypertension can also be related to common disorders involving both the liver and spleen such as infiltrative or infectious diseases. On the other hand, the association of splenomegaly and pancytopenia may result in the false diagnosis of malignant blood disease. Splenomegaly and pancytopenia can persist after surgical shunts for portal hypertension. Spontaneous rupture and infarction are rare. Splenomegaly can be more accurately diagnosed with ultrasound examination.

Abdominal collateral circulation

The abdominal collateral circulation can be visualized if the obstacle is distal from or at the level of the left branch of the portal vein corresponding to a recanalization of the umbilical or paraumbilical veins. In Cruveilhier–Baumgarten syndrome, an association with umbilical varicosities (*caput medusae*) and a collateral ascending circulation between the umbilicus and the xyphoid process may be observed. The collateral circulation in portal hypertension must be distinguished from cavo–caval circulation, which is not ascending and is located in the flanks. When it is associated with the *caput medusae*, a venous hum is detectable in rare cases (Salmi et al, 1990).

ENDOSCOPIC EVALUATION

Oesophagogastro-endoscopy

Endoscopic investigation is essential for evaluating portal hypertension. This procedure may detect the three main lesions responsible for gastro-oesophageal bleeding in portal hypertension: gastro-oesophageal varices, hypertensive gastropathy and antral vascular ectasia. The presence of oesophageal varices is considered to be pathognomonic of portal hypertension. However, hanging oesophageal varices can be observed in patients with superior vena cava obstruction, mediastinal tumours or fibrosis, or after thyroid resection (Fleig et al, 1982). Bleeding events from these downhill varices are rare. The presence of oesophagogastric varices at endoscopy is a major risk factor for bleeding and survival (see Chapter 3). The best classification of oesophageal varices should associate a good predictive value for the risk of haemorrhage and easy clinical use with low interobserver variability. Variceal size and wall abnormalities seem to be the most accurate predictive factors for the risk of bleeding.

Endoscopic sonography

The portal venous system is studied by exploring the oesophagus and stomach (Caletti et al, 1992). Oesophageal and gastric varices are seen at endoscopic sonography as anechoic structures beneath the mucosal and submucosal layers. Detection of oesophageal or gastric varices depends on the grade of the varices. In patients with oesophageal varices, the sensitivity of endoscopic sonography is inferior to endoscopy in patients with small varices (Caletti et al, 1992; Burtin et al, 1996). In patients with gastric varices, endoscopic sonography is more sensitive than endoscopy, especially for fundal varices (Caletti et al, 1992; Burtin et al, 1996). Peri-oesophageal and perigastric veins are seen as anechoic structures outside the oesophageal or gastric walls. These vessels are more often seen in patients with endoscopic grade 2 and 3 varices than in patients with grade 1 oesophageal varices (Caletti et al, 1992; Burtin et al, 1996). Perforating veins are mostly visualized in patients with large varices at endoscopy (Caletti et al, 1992). The azygos vein is observed in all subjects and in patients with portal hypertension. The diameter of the azygos vein is significantly larger in patients with portal hypertension.

Abnormalities such as anechoic structures are observed at endoscopic sonography in the submucosa of the stomach in patients with endoscopic signs of portal hypertension and gastropathy.

HAEMODYNAMIC EVALUATION

Portal and hepatic venous pressures

The measurement of elevated portal pressure gradient (the difference from portal venous pressure and inferior vena cava pressure) is used to define the presence of portal hypertension. In normal fasted subjects at rest and in the supine position, portal pressure ranges from 7 to 12 mmHg and the portal pressure gradient is below 5 mmHg. Many methods have been described to measure portal pressure. Direct methods of inserting a needle or a catheter in the portal vein or in the umbilical vein have been used, but these are invasive and must be performed under general anaesthesia, which modifies haemodynamic values. Indirect methods by direct puncture of the splenic pulp or the liver are also invasive and unreliable (Feyves et al, 1988).

At present, the procedure of choice is the measurement of the hepatic venous pressure gradient by inserting a catheter in the internal jugular, femoral or humeral vein, under local anaesthesia. The catheter is guided under fluoroscopic control into a hepatic vein. Wedged hepatic venous pressure, which is similar to the occluded pressure obtained with balloon catheters, is recorded when the tip of the catheter is wedged in a small hepatic venule. Free hepatic venous pressure is measured with the tip of the catheter placed in the hepatic vein close to the inferior vena cava junction (Valla et al, 1984). The difference between wedged and free hepatic pressures corresponds to the hepatic venous pressure gradient. Normal values of hepatic venous pressure gradient range from 1 to 4 mmHg. The hepatic venous pressure gradient is normal in patients with extrahepatic portal hypertension (Table 2). In patients with pre-sinusoidal intrahepatic portal hypertension, the hepatic venous pressure gradient is normal or moderately elevated. In patients with cirrhosis, the hepatic venous pressure gradient is elevated but differs greatly from one patient to another, usually ranging from 8 to 30 mmHg. In patients with alcoholic or hepatitis B-related cirrhosis, the wedged hepatic venous pressure is identical to the portal pressure (Boyer et al, 1977; Lin et al, 1989). In patients with cirrhosis and hepatocellular carcinoma, a heterogeneous hepatic venous pressure gradient can be observed (Lee et al, 1990). In patients with cirrhosis, the hepatic venous pressure gradient has been shown to increase after a meal (McCormick et al, 1990) or physical exercise (García-Pagán et al, 1996) and circadian variations of the hepatic venous pressure gradient have also been described (García-Pagán et al, 1994). Thus, for comparisons in pharmacological investigations, the hepatic venous pressure gradient should be measured in fasted patients at rest and at the same time of day.

Several studies had focused on determining the lowest hepatic venous pressure gradient necessary to reduce the risk of bleeding. A value of

Table 2. Causes of portal hypertension and hepatic venous pressure gradient (adapted from Lebrec and Benhamou, 1986).

Diseases	Hepatic venous pressure gradient
Cirrhosis	elevated
Non-cirrhotic portal hypertension	
Extrahepatic	
Portal vein thrombosis, compression or invasion	normal
Intrahepatic	
Chronic liver lesions commonly associated with portal hypertension	
Schistosomiasis	normal or moderately elevated
Chronic veno-occlusive disease	elevated
Primary or secondary biliary cirrhosis	elevated
Alcoholic fibrosis	moderately elevated
Chronic active hepatitis	moderately elevated
Hepatoportal sclerosis or idiopathic portal hypertension	normal or moderately elevated
Congenital hepatic fibrosis	normal or moderately elevated
Nodular regenerative hyperplasia	normal or moderately elevated
Partial nodular transformation	normal
Peliosis hepatis	elevated
Chronic liver diseases, portal hypertension unfrequent	
Sarcoidosis, tuberculosis, amyloidosis, mastocytosis	normal or moderately elevated
Rendu–Osler disease	elevated
Myeloma, Waldenström disease	normal or moderately elevated
Lymphoma, myeloproliferative diseases	normal or moderately elevated
Polycystic disease	normal or moderately elevated
Metastatic carcinoma	normal or moderately elevated
Acute liver lesions associated with portal hypertension	
Acute veno-occlusive disease	elevated
Acute alcoholic hepatitis	normal or moderately elevated
Acute or fulminant hepatitis	moderately elevated
Acute fatty liver of pregnancy	moderately elevated
Suprahepatic	
Right heart insufficiency	normal
Vena cava obstruction	normal
Budd–Chiari syndrome	normal

12 mmHg was retrospectively determined (Lebrec et al, 1980; Garcia Tsao et al, 1985). However some studies were not in agreement with these results (Triger et al, 1991) and one measurement of the hepatic venous pressure gradient at the beginning of follow-up is probably insufficient (see Chapter 3). Recent studies have emphasized the prognostic usefulness of the measurement of hepatic venous pressure gradient in cirrhotic patients. Retrospective (Merkel et al, 1992) and prospective (Vorobioff et al, 1996) studies have demonstrated that the hepatic venous pressure gradient measurement was an independent risk factor for bleeding and mortality in cirrhosis.

Variceal pressure

The risk of variceal rupture depends in part on wall tension. The Laplace law states that wall tension (T) depends on transmural pressure (p), the radius of the varix (r) and is inversely dependent on the wall thickness (t) and may be expressed as: $T = p \times r/t$. Except for preliminary results from new endoscopic ultrasonography techniques (Schiano et al, 1996), the variceal pressure corresponding to the transmural pressure is the only value that can be measured in humans. Direct puncture of the variceal wall has been first proposed, but this technique is invasive and should be performed immediately before sclerotherapy, since bleeding occurs in 10% of cases (Gertsch et al, 1993).

Non-invasive measurement by endoscopic gauge has been shown to be well correlated with results obtained by direct variceal puncture (Bosch et al, 1986). Non-invasive measurement seems to have a low interobsever variability (Gertsch et al, 1993) and a good reproducibility in the same patient under placebo conditions at 6 weeks, 3 months and 1 year (Nevens et al, 1996). Variceal pressure could provide additional information for standard haemodynamic measurements. Variceal pressure was approximately 15% lower than portal pressure measured by the hepatic venous pressure gradient (Bosch et al, 1986), and there was no correlation between the hepatic venous pressure gradient and variceal pressure in patients with cirrhosis (Bosch et al, 1986). On the other hand, variceal pressure may provide a useful reflection of collateral circulation, since a good correlation has been found between variceal pressure and azygos blood flow (Bosch et al, 1986). Haemodynamic changes induced by pharmacological treatment are not strictly correlated with variceal pressure modifications (Feu et al, 1993). Among the endoscopic signs of portal hypertension, red spots on oesophageal varices is the sign that is most highly correlated with high variceal pressure (Kleber et al, 1989).

Systemic and pulmonary haemodynamics

At present, cardiac output and pulmonary pressures are measured with a Swan–Ganz catheter inserted into the pulmonary artery. Both systemic and pulmonary vascular resistances are then calculated. In patients with cirrhosis, as in animal models of portal hypertension, a decrease in systemic (and pulmonary) vascular resistance and an increase in cardiac output has been observed. These changes are more marked in patients with severe liver disease (Braillon et al, 1986), but no correlation between cardiac index and the size of oesophageal varices or the presence of previous episodes of gastrointestinal bleeding has been found (Calès et al, 1984).

Pulmonary arterial hypertension, which is a well-known complication of portal hypertension, is defined by an elevated pulmonary artery pressure (> 25 mmHg) in the presence of a normal wedged pulmonary pressure (see Chapter 11). It is important to diagnose this syndrome because the prognosis is poor and specific vasoactive treatment may be beneficial before pulmonary arterial resistance becomes chronic (Hadengue et al, 1991).

Azygos blood flow

The measurement of azygos venous blood flow provides the best haemodynamic estimation of superior portosystemic collateral circulation. Measurements of azygos blood flow are used in the assessment of the effects of pharmacological therapy. A catheter is inserted into the azygos vein under fluoroscopic control and the continuous thermodilution method is used (Bosch and Groszmann, 1984; Calès et al, 1984; Bosch et al, 1986). In patients without portal hypertension the azygos blood flow has been found to be between 0.08 and 0.19 litre/minute (Calès et al, 1984). In patients with cirrhosis, the azygos blood flow is higher than in normal subjects, it is dependent on the severity of cirrhosis and is correlated with the hepatic venous pressure gradient. In these patients, azygos blood flow averages from 0.48 ± 0.24 to 1.06 ± 0.48 litre/minute in patients in good and poor condition, respectively (Braillon et al, 1986). In patients with cirrhosis and portal hypertension, azygos blood flow is not correlated with the presence of oesophageal varices or with previous episodes of gastro-intestinal bleeding (Calès et al, 1984). Azygos blood flow is an index of blood flow through gastro-oesophageal collaterals and varices draining into the azygos vein, but cannot distinguish between variceal and non-variceal collateral flow.

Hepatic blood flow

Hepatic blood flow can be measured directly during surgery or indirectly by analysis of the dilution curve obtained in the hepatic vein after injection of a non-metabolized radioactive marker in the portal vein. At present, during haemodynamic procedures, the method of choice for hepatic blood flow measurement is based on the clearance technique. In the case of low hepatic extraction ($< 10\%$), calculation errors are too large and thus the hepatic blood flow cannot be calculated. The normal hepatic blood flow in humans is 1 to 2 litre/minute. In cirrhosis, the hepatic blood flow can be increased or decreased (Gadano et al, 1997). No relationship between portal hypertension and hepatic blood flow has been demonstrated. The measurement of hepatic blood flow is mainly of interest in pharmacological studies.

Renal haemodynamics

Renal haemodynamics may also be studied during the haemodynamic evaluation of portal hypertension. The renal clearance of inulin and p-aminohippuric acid is the method of choice to measure the glomerular filtration rate and 'effective' renal plasma flow. In patients with cirrhosis and with ascites, a lower renal blood flow has been reported (Moreau et al, 1993). However, no relationship between the severity of liver disease and renal hypoperfusion has been found.

Haemodynamic evaluation in post-transplant patients

Haemodynamic disturbances in the post-transplantation period are because of the transplantation procedure per se and to its complications such as sepsis, anaemia, graft rejection or dysfunction. In patients with cirrhosis undergoing liver transplantation, cardiac index, azygos blood flow and hepatic blood flow are elevated in the first 6 months and progressively normalized (Gadano et al, 1995). Certain complications can result in haemodynamic changes. It has been demonstrated that acute graft rejection produces an increase in the hepatic venous pressure gradient. Sepsis is responsible for haemodynamic changes including an increase in heart rate and cardiac index with a decrease in systemic vascular resistance (Gadano et al, 1995).

DOPPLER SONOGRAPHY

Diagnosis of portal hypertension

Portal vein

Enlargement of the portal vein is a sign of portal hypertension, but studies have shown that a diameter greater than 13 mm or 15 mm only has a sensitivity of 40% and 12%, respectively (Bolondi et al, 1982; Vilgrain et al, 1990). These findings confirm an angiographic study that also demonstrated that the diameter of the portal vein did not increase with the hepatic venous pressure gradient (Lafortune et al, 1984).

In normal subjects, portal blood flow goes towards the liver and has a continuous spectrum, with mild waves. In most patients with portal hypertension, there is a continuous flow towards the liver. In some cases, alterations of portal blood flow appear as an absence of end-diastolic, arterialized flow or bi-directional (back and forth) flow (Lafortune et al, 1990). Reversed flow is rarely observed in the portal vein (1.1%) and is associated with a significant reduction in the portal vein diameter (Gaiani et al, 1991).

Compared with angiography in patients with portal hypertension, Doppler sonography has been shown to be accurate in determining the direction of portal flow (Nelson et al, 1987). The sensitivity and specificity of duplex Doppler for main portal vein disorders are 83% and 93%, respectively (Alpern et al, 1987).

Splanchnic veins

One study has demonstrated that the diameters of the superior mesenteric and splenic veins were different in control subjects and patients with cirrhosis (Zoli et al, 1985). The best discriminant findings were expiration measurements (Zoli et al, 1985).

A lack of variation in calibre of the superior mesenteric vein during breathing was first considered highly sensitive and specific for diagnosis (Bolondi et al, 1982). Reversed flow may be detected in the superior mesenteric or splenic vein at Doppler sonography (Gaiani et al, 1991). Reversed flow is not related to the cause of cirrhosis, but is more frequently observed in patients with severe cirrhosis.

In control subjects, the diameter of the coronary vein measured up to 6 mm. In patients with portal hypertension, dilatation of the coronary vein was seen in 26% of the cases (Figure 1), while hepatofugal flow in the coronary vein was seen in 78% of patients (Wachsberg and Simmons, 1994).

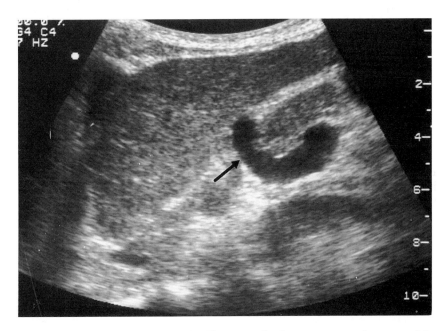

Figure 1. Dilatation of the coronary vein. Ultrasonography demonstrates an enlargement of the coronary vein (arrow).

Collaterals

Detection of collaterals is a sensitive and specific sign for the diagnosis of portal hypertension at sonography (Subramanyam et al, 1983; Vilgrain et al, 1990). The three most frequent collaterals detected are the gastro-oesophageal veins, the paraumbilical vein and the splenorenal or gastro-renal veins (Figure 2). A correlation was observed between the degree of portal hypertension and the number of portosystemic pathways (Vilgrain et al, 1990). Other collateral pathways are rarely observed, such as the pancreaticoduodenal veins, the retroperitoneal veins and the omental veins. Usually, conventional sonography cannot detect rectal and pararectal varices. The use of transvaginal sonography to detect pararectal varices can be performed and should be used especially in patients with lower gastro-intestinal bleeding (Malde et al, 1993). Gallbladder varices, which may be observed in portal hypertension, are defined as serpentine areas in the wall of the gallbladder, and are portosystemic shunts between the cystic vein and the systemic anterior abdominal wall veins or patent portal vein branches within the liver (Figure 3). They are most often observed in association

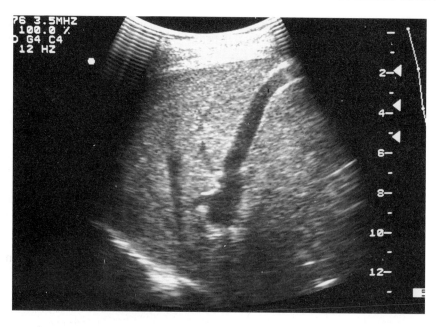

Figure 2. Paraumbilical vein. Ultrasonography reveals a dilatation of the paraumbilical vein.

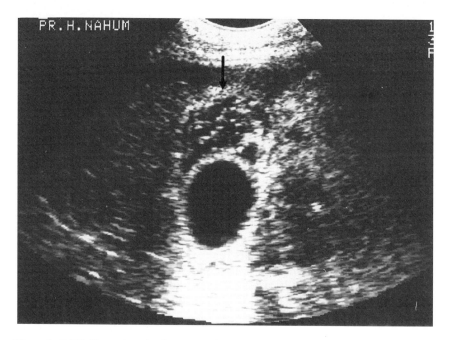

Figure 3. Gallbladder varices. At ultrasonography, vessels are identified within the gallbladder wall (arrow). The patient had portal vein obstruction.

with portal vein thrombosis (Chawla et al, 1994). Duplex Doppler and colour Doppler are very useful in the detection of collaterals because they increase the reliability of the diagnosis by demonstrating continuous flow similar to that of the portal vein.

Quantitative evaluation of the portal vein at Doppler sonography

Mean portal velocity. Portal velocity is measured in supine, fasting patients and multiple measurements are performed to avoid flow fluctuations. Comparison of mean portal velocities in healthy subjects and in patients with cirrhosis shows that the velocity is reduced to a greater or a lesser extent in patients with cirrhosis (Bolondi et al, 1990) (Table 3). In patients with portal hypertension, the mean portal vein velocity may differ depending on the presence and the location of spontaneous shunts. In patients with cirrhosis, no correlation was found with the Child–Pugh's score whereas a negative correlation was found with the hepatic venous pressure gradient (Figure 4). Thus, an increased hepatic venous pressure gradient reflects an

Table 3. Mean portal velocity and blood flow in controls and patients with cirrhosis.

	Mean portal velocity (cm/s)		Mean portal blood flow (ml/minute)	
	Controls	Cirrhosis	Controls	Cirrhosis
Gaiaini et al, 1989	19.0±2.1	11.4±3.7	919±285	1197±625
Moriyasu et al, 1986	15.3±4.0	9.7±2.6	899±284	870±289
Ohnishi et al, 1985	17.0±3.9	12.1±3.2	648±186	690±258
Okazaki et al, 1986	21.2±5.2	10.2±3.5	966±344	579±262
Zoli et al, 1986	16.0±0.5	10.5±0.6	694±23	736±46

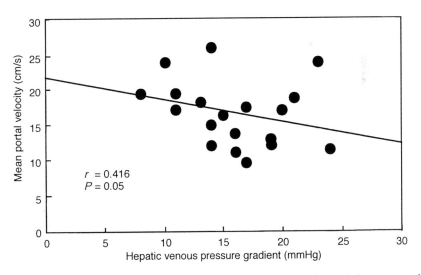

Figure 4. Negative relationship between the hepatic venous pressure gradient and the mean portal velocity measured at Doppler flowmetry.

elevated intrahepatic resistance and is associated with decreased mean portal velocity (Vilgrain et al, 1993).

Portal blood flow. Portal blood flow is calculated from the mean portal velocity multiplied by the cross-sectional area of the vessel. As in portal velocity, portal blood flow is different between healthy subjects and patients with cirrhosis. However, these results are more variable than those of velocities (Bolondi et al, 1990). Of greater interest is the difference in portal blood flow in normal subjects and in patients with portal hypertension after a meal. It has been demonstrated that a significant increase in mean calibre, mean velocity and flow volume occurs in the portal vein of healthy subjects and not in patients with portal hypertension (Gaiani et al, 1989).

Congestion index. The congestion index was defined by Moriyasu et al (1986) as the ratio of the cross-sectional area to portal flow velocity. The authors have found a significant increase in this index in patients with cirrhosis compared with normal subjects.

Limitations. Although measurements by Doppler sonography have been extensively used for many years, the limitations should be mentioned. There are numerous errors in measurement caused by this technique, including the measurement of the beam-vessel angle, the measurement of the cross-sectional area of the vessel and the calculations of mean velocity. Another limitation of the usefulness of quantitative data is the low inter-observer agreement (Sabbà et al, 1990; de Vries et al, 1991). For these reasons Doppler sonography cannot be used in clinical practice to establish a diagnosis. However, under certain conditions (examinations performed by the same observers with the same equipment) Doppler sonography may be suitable for monitoring changes induced by a meal or medical treatment.

Consequences on the other vessels

Hepatic arteries. In normal subjects, the hepatic artery has a positive diastolic component because of a low resistance peripheral bed. The hepatic arterial resistance index increases in cirrhosis (Joynt et al, 1995; Sacerdoti et al, 1995). However, the results when cirrhosis is complicated by portal vein thrombosis are still controversial because some authors have found an increase in hepatic arterial resistance, whereas others have shown a reduction.

Splanchnic arteries. In patients with cirrhosis, an increase in splanchnic artery blood flow and a decrease in arterial resistance has been observed (Sato et al, 1987; Darnault et al, 1989). At Doppler sonography, both the resistive and pulsatility index decrease (Darnault et al, 1989). After a meal, the splanchnic artery index is reduced in all patients, however, this reduction is less marked in patients with cirrhosis (Sabbà et al, 1991).

Hepatic veins. In healthy subjects, the flow in the hepatic veins is mainly antegrade but multiphasic, reflecting the variations during the cardiac cycle. A small retrograde wave is observed and corresponds to atrial systole. In patients with cirrhosis, the waveform of hepatic veins may have lower oscillations without a reversed phase or may be completely flat (Bolondi et al, 1991). These abnormalities in the Doppler waveform of the hepatic veins are correlated with the amount of fibrosis and steatosis analysed after liver biopsy (Colli et al, 1994).

Causes of portal hypertension

Extrahepatic portal hypertension

Doppler sonography is helpful in identifying portal vein obstruction. At sonography the portal vein is usually enlarged and contains intraluminal material (Figure 5). The absence of flow signals at duplex Doppler and at colour Doppler confirm the diagnosis. When portal obstruction is complete, a cavernous transformation is observed as multiple, small tortuous tubular structures, which replace the portal vein in the porta hepatis. With Doppler these vessels have a continuous and hepatopetal flow (Parvey et al, 1994).

Intrahepatic portal hypertension

Doppler sonography shows features suggestive of chronic liver disease. These findings include morphological changes in the liver such as the association of atrophy–hypertrophy. The most frequent combination is atrophy of the right liver and segment 4, and hypertrophy of the left lobe and segment 1. Furthermore, changes in liver structure at sonography (irregular contours, coarse pattern) suggest chronic liver disease. Doppler is also helpful in demonstrating localized inversion of the intrahepatic portal branches, the paraumbilical vein and the absence of suprahepatic obstruction.

Suprahepatic portal hypertension

Diagnosis of this condition is usually made by Doppler sonography. The specific features are echogenic material in the lumen of the main hepatic veins or the vena cava, stenosis of the inferior vena cava and/or main hepatic veins with upstream dilatation, hyperechogenic cord replacing one of the main hepatic veins, and intrahepatic venous collaterals (Valla and Benhamou, 1996) (Figure 6). Comparisons between ultrasonography findings and venography or necropsy have shown that sonography is a very useful imaging technique. Duplex Doppler and colour Doppler improve the diagnostic accuracy of sonography by demonstrating absence of flow, flow reversal and continuous flow in collaterals (Ralls et al, 1992). The usefulness of Doppler sonography has been also emphasized for the detection of membranous obstruction of the hepatic veins or the inferior vena cava (Vilgrain et al, 1995).

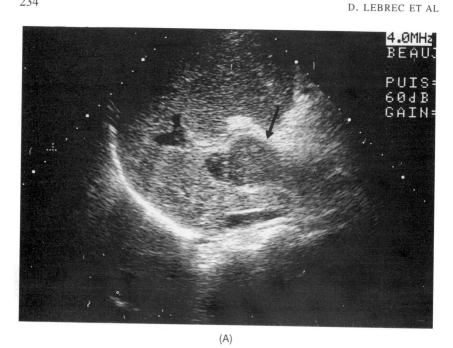

(A)

(B)

Figure 5. Portal vein thrombosis. (A) Ultrasonography: longitudinal view of the portal vein, which is enlarged and hyperechoic (arrow). (B) Post-contrast computed tomography in enlargement of the partially obstructed portal vein (arrow).

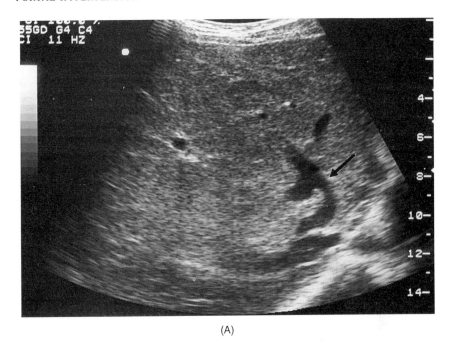

(A)

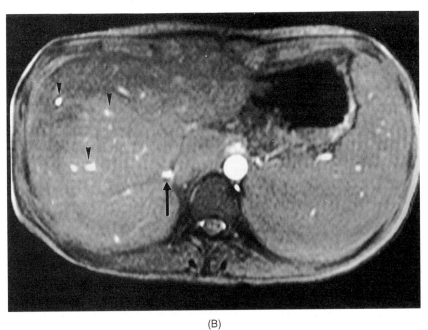

(B)

Figure 6. Hepatic venous obstruction. (A) Ultrasonography shows an irregular left hepatic vein (arrow). (B) Magnetic resonance imaging demonstrates multiple intrahepatic collaterals (arrowheads). The inferior vena cava is patent but compressed by the liver (arrow).

Complications of portal hypertension

Gastrointestinal bleeding

Although there is no direct correlation between Doppler signs and risk of bleeding, some authors have demonstrated features that may increase or decrease the risk of bleeding. For example, spontaneous hepatofugal portal flow was rarely observed in patients with variceal bleeding (Gaiani et al, 1991). Dilatation of the coronary vein was also a poor indicator of the risk of bleeding. Conversely, preservation of hepatopetal flow in the coronary vein was associated with a higher risk of variceal haemorrhage (Wachsberg and Simons, 1994). A splenic venous flow exceeding the portal venous flow at Doppler sonography may be observed in patients with an increased prevalence of varices, which tend to be larger and more likely to bleed (Nelson et al, 1993). Finally, other authors have established scores based on Doppler sonography alone, or in association with physical, biochemical, and endoscopic parameters to evaluate the risk of bleeding or rebleeding. For the timing of the first variceal haemorrhage, the only Doppler variable that improved the classification of patients was the congestive index (Siringo et al, 1994). For the prediction of recurrent bleeding, a Doppler sonoscore calculated after the first occurrence of variceal haemorrhage provides useful prognostic information (Schmassmann et al, 1993).

COMPUTED TOMOGRAPHY (CT)

Improvement in the CT technique, including the helical mode, allows an excellent identification of portal venous structures. Especially in patients with suspicion of portal venous obstruction with doubtful Doppler results, CT is a useful tool to determine the presence of an obstruction and to provide signs suggesting recent obstruction (Figure 5). Also, helical CT allows the acquisition of consistent volumetric data of the upper abdomen during the peak of vascular enhancement. From these volumetric results, detailed 3D images can be created, representing the portal venous system and the collaterals in patients with portal hypertension. However, the main limitation of CT is its incapacity to determine the direction of the flow.

MAGNETIC RESONANCE IMAGING (MR)

For qualitative data, MR imaging is indicated when Doppler studies are inconclusive. MR imaging is especially useful for the detection of porto-systemic collaterals (Rafal et al, 1990), for the diagnosis of portal vein thrombosis (Levy and Newhouse, 1988; Zirinsky et al, 1988), and for the diagnosis and evaluation of hepatic vein obstruction (Figures 6 and 7). In the later condition, MR imaging is complementary to Doppler sonography

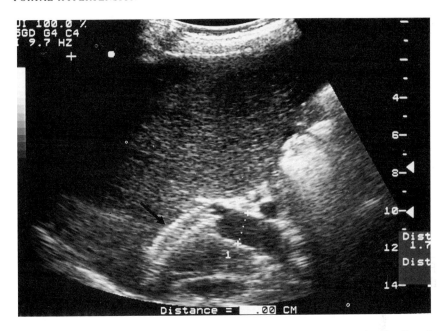

Figure 7. Splenorenal collaterals. Magnetic resonance imaging demonstrates large collaterals between the spleen and the left kidney (arrow).

and is particularly helpful in identifying the morphological changes of the liver parenchyma and for assessment of patency of the portal vein and inferior vena cava (Kane and Eustace, 1995). MR angiography of hepatic veins can be used when the diagnosis is not clear after sonographic examination. MR imaging is also an effective non-invasive method of visualization of surgical portosystemic shunts when Doppler sonography is effective. Moreover, MR imaging has also been used to measure blood flow in the portal vein. Two different methods have been evaluated: the time-of-flight bolus tracking technique and the quantitative phase-contrast technique (Applegate et al, 1993; Burkart et al, 1993). Both are rapid techniques to assess portal venous patency, and flow direction. Correlation studies have shown that the mean portal velocities on MR were well correlated with Doppler sonography values (Burkart et al, 1993). Calculations of the portal vein flow by phase-contrast MR imaging were significantly lower in patients with portal hypertension with hepatopetal flow. However, this technique has several limitations: it requires good quality MR angiography sequences, it is costly and time consuming. Furthermore the inter- and intraobserver variability is not high enough to use MR angiography as a first choice imaging technique in patients with portal hypertension. Several authors have also shown that azygos blood flow rate and velocity are increased in patients compared with control subjects (Lomas et al, 1995; Debatin et al, 1996; Wu et al, 1996). However these measurements have not been compared with invasive methods.

REFERENCES

Alpern MB, Rubin JM, Williams DM & Capek P (1987) Porta hepatis: duplex Doppler US with angiographic correlation. *Radiology* **162**: 53–56.

Applegate GR, Thaete FL, Meyers SP et al (1993) Blood flow in the portal vein: velocity quantitation with phase-contrast MR angiography. *Radiology* **187**: 253–256.

Bolondi L, Li Bassi S, Gaiani S & Barbara L (1990) Doppler portal flowmetry in portal hypertension. *Journal of Gastroenterology and Hepatology* **5**: 459–467.

Bolondi L, Gandolfi L, Arienti V et al (1982) Ultrasonography in the diagnosis of portal hypertension: diminished response of portal vessels to respiration. *Radiology* **142**: 167–172.

Bolondi L, Li Bassi S, Gaiani S et al (1991) Liver cirrhosis: changes of Doppler waveform of hepatic veins. *Radiology* **178**: 513–516.

*Bolondi L, Gatta A, Groszmann R et al (1996) Baveno II consensus statements: imaging techniques and haemodynamic measurements in portal hypertension. In de Franchis R (ed.) *Portal Hypertension II. Proceedings of the Second Baveno International Consensus Workshop on Definitions, Methodology and Therapeutic Strategies*, p 67. Oxford: Blackwell Science

Bosch J & Groszmann RJ (1984) Measurement of azygos venous blood flow by a continuous thermal dilution technique: an index of blood flow through gastroesophageal collaterals in cirrhosis. *Hepatology* **4**: 84–89.

*Bosch J, Bordas JM, Rigau J et al (1986) Noninvasive measurement of the pressure of esophageal varices using an endoscopic gauge: comparison with measurements by variceal puncture in patients undergoing endoscopic sclerotherapy. *Hepatology* **6**: 667–672.

Boyer TD, Triger DR, Horisawa M et al (1977) Direct transhepatic measurement of portal vein pressure using a thin needle. Comparison with wedged hepatic vein pressure. *Gastroenterology* **72**: 584–589.

Braillon A, Calès P, Valla D et al (1986) Influence of the degree of liver failure on systemic and splanchnic haemodynamics and on response to propranolol in patients with cirrhosis. *Gut* **27**: 1204–1209.

*Burkart DJ, Johnson CD, Morton MJ et al (1993) Volumetric flow rates in the portal venous system: measurement with cine phase-contrast MR imaging. *American Journal of Roentgenology* **160**: 1113–1118.

Burtin P, Calès P, Oberti F et al (1996) Endoscopic ultrasonographic signs of portal hypertension in cirrhosis. *Gastrointestinal Endoscopy* **44**: 257–261.

Calès P, Braillon A, Jiron MI & Lebrec D (1984) Superior portosystemic collateral circulation estimated by azygos blood flow in patients with cirrhosis. Lack of correlation with oesophageal varices and gastrointestinal bleeding. Effect of propranolol. *Journal of Hepatology* **1**: 34–46.

Caletti GC, Brocchi E, Ferrari A et al (1992) Value of endoscopic ultrasonography in the management of portal hypertension. *Endoscopy* **24**: 342–346.

Chawla Y, Dilawari JB & Katariya S (1994) Gallbladder varices in portal vein thrombosis. *American Journal of Roentgenology* **162**: 643–645.

Colli A, Cocciolo M, Riva C et al (1994) Abnormalities of Doppler waveform of the hepatic veins in patients with chronic liver disease: correlation with histologic findings. *American Journal of Roentgenology* **162**: 833–837.

Darnault P, Bretagne JF, Fournier V & Raoul J (1989) Splenic haemodynamic assessment in patients with liver cirrhosis and hypersplenism. *Gastroenterology* **96**: A589 (Abstract).

Debatin JF, Zahner B, Meyenberger C et al (1996) Azygos blood flow: phase contrast quantitation in volunteers and patients with portal hypertension pre- and postintrahepatic shunt placement. *Hepatology* **24**: 1109–1115.

Feu F, Bordas JM, Luca A et al (1993) Reduction of variceal pressure by propranolol: comparison of the effects on portal pressure and azygos blood flow in patients with cirrhosis. *Hepatology* **18**: 1082–1089.

Feyves D, Pomier-Laymargues G, Willems B & Cote J (1988) Intrahepatic pressure measurement: not an accurate reflection of portal vein pressure. *Hepatology* **8**: 211–216.

Fleig WE, Stange EF & Ditschuneit H (1982) Upper gastrointestinal hemorrhage from downhill esophageal varices. *Digestive Diseases and Sciences* **27**: 23–27.

*Gadano A, Hadengue A, Widmann JJ et al (1995) Hemodynamics after orthotopic liver transplantation: study of associated factors and long-term effects. *Hepatology* **22**: 458–465.

Gadano A, Hadengue A, Vachiery F et al (1997) Relationship between hepatic blood flow, liver tests, haemodynamic values and clinical characteristics in patients with chronic liver disease. *Journal of Gastroenterology and Hepatology* **12:** 167–171.

Gaiani S, Bolondi L, Li Bassi S et al (1989) Effect of a meal on portal haemodynamics in healthy humans and in patients with chronic liver disease. *Hepatology* **9:** 815–819

Gaiani S, Bolondi L, Li Bassi S et al (1991) Prevalence of spontaneous hepatofugal portal flow in liver cirrhosis. Clinical and endoscopic correlation in 228 patients. *Gastroenterology* **100:** 160–167.

García-Pagán JC, Feu F, Castells A et al (1994) Circadian variations of portal pressure and variceal hemorrhage in patients with cirrhosis. *Hepatology* **19:** 595–601.

García-Pagán JC, Santos C, Barbera JA et al (1996) Physical exercise increases portal pressure in patients with cirrhosis and portal hypertension. *Gastroenterology* **111:** 1300–1306.

Garcia-Tsao G, Groszmann RJ, Fisher RL et al (1985) Portal pressure, presence of gastroesophageal varices and variceal bleeding. *Hepatology* **5:** 419–424.

*Gertsch P, Fischer G, Kleber G et al (1993) Manometry of esophageal varices: comparison of an endoscopic balloon technique with needle puncture. *Gastroenterology* **105:** 1159–1166.

*Groszmann R, Bendtsen F, Bosch J et al (1996) Baveno II consensus statements: drug therapy for portal hypertension. In de Franchis R (ed.) *Portal Hypertension II. Proceedings of the Second Baveno* International Consensus Workshop on Definitions, Methodology and Therapeutic Strategies, pp 98–99. Oxford: Blackwell Science

Hadengue A, Benhayoun MK, Lebrec D & Benhamou JP (1991) Pulmonary hypertension complicating portal hypertension: prevalence and relation to splanchnic hemodynamics. *Gastroenterology* **100:** 520–528.

Joynt LK, Platt JF, Rubin JM et al (1995) Hepatic artery resistance before and after standard meal in subjects with diseased and healthy livers. *Radiology* **196:** 489–492.

Kane R & Eustace S (1995) Diagnosis of Budd–Chiari syndrome: comparison between sonography and MR angiography. *Radiology* **195:** 117–121.

Kleber G, Sauerbruch T, Fischer G & Paumgartner G (1989) Pressure of intraoesophageal varices assessed by fine needle puncture: its relation to endoscopic signs and severity of liver disease in patients with cirrhosis. *Gut* **30:** 228–232.

*Lafortune M, Marleau D, Breton G et al (1984) Portal venous system measurements in portal hypertension. *Radiology* **151:** 27–30.

Lafortune M, Patriquin H & Burns P (1990) Doppler ultrasound in the evaluation of portal and splanchnic blood flow. In Ferrucci JT & Mathieu DG (eds) *Advances in Hepatobiliary Radiology*, pp 29–73. St Louis: CV Mosby.

Lebrec D & Benhamou JP (1986) Non cirrhotic intrahepatic portal hypertension. *Seminars in Liver Disease* **6:** 332–340.

*Lebrec D, de Fleury P, Rueff B et al (1980) Portal hypertension, size of esophageal varices, and risk of gastrointestinal bleeding in alcoholic cirrhosis. *Gastroenterology* **79:** 1139–1144.

Lee SS, Koshy A, Hadengue A & Lebrec D (1990) Heterogeneous hepatic venous pressures in patients with liver cancer. *Journal of Clinical Gastroenterology* **12:** 53–56.

Levy HM & Newhouse JH (1988) MR imaging of portal vein thrombosis. *American Journal of Roentgenology* **151:** 283–286.

Lin HC, Tsai YT, Lee FY et al (1989) Comparison between portal vein pressure and wedged hepatic vein pressure in hepatitis B-related cirrhosis. *Journal of Hepatology* **9:** 326–330.

Lomas DJ, Hayball MP, Jones DP et al (1995) Non-invasive measurement of azygos venous blood flow using magnetic resonance. *Journal of Hepatology* **22:** 399–403.

McCormick PA, Dick R, Graffeo M et al (1990) The effect of non-protein liquid meals on the hepatic venous pressure gradient in patients with cirrhosis. *Journal of Hepatology* **11:** 221–225.

Malde H, Nagral A, Shah P et al (1993) Detection of rectal and pararectal varices in patients with portal hypertension: efficacy of transvaginal sonography. *American Journal of Roentgenology* **161:** 335–337.

Merkel C, Bolognesi M, Bellon S et al (1992) Prognostic usefulness of hepatic vein catheterization in patients with cirrhosis and esophageal varices. *Gastroenterology* **102:** 973–979.

Moreau R, Gaudin C, Hadengue A et al (1993) Renal hemodynamics in patients with cirrhosis: relationship with ascites and liver failure. *Nephron* **65:** 359–363

Moriyasu F, Ban N, Nishida O et al (1985) Clinical application of an ultrasonic duplex system in the quantitative measurement of portal blood flow. *Journal of Clinical Ultrasound* **14:** 579–588.

Moriyasu F, Nishida O, Ban N et al (1986) 'Congestion index' of the portal vein. *American Journal of Roentgenology* **146:** 735–739.

Nelson RC, Sherbourne GM, Spencer HB & Chezmar JL (1993) Splenic venous flow exceeding portal venous flow at Doppler sonography: relationship to portosystemic varices. *American Journal of Roentgenology* **161**: 563–567.

Nelson RC, Lovett KE, Chezmar JL et al (1987) Comparison of pulsed Doppler sonography and angiography in patients with portal hypertension. *American Journal of Roentgenology* **149**: 77–81.

Nevens F, Spengers D, Feu F, Bosch J & Fevery J (1996) Measurement of variceal pressure with an endoscopic pressure sensitive gauge: validation and effect of propranolol therapy in chronic conditions. *Journal of Hepatology* **24**: 66–73.

Ohnishi K, Saito M, Nakayama T et al (1985) Portal venous haemodynamics in chronic liver disease: effects of posture change and exercise. *Radiology* **155**: 757–761.

Okazaki K, Miyazaki M, Onishi S & Ito K (1986) Effects of food intake and various extrinsic hormones on portal blood flow in patients with liver cirrhosis demonstrated by pulsed Doppler with the Octoson. *Scandinavian Journal of Gastroenterology* **21**: 1029–1038.

Parvey HR, Raval B & Sandler CM (1994) Portal vein thrombosis: imaging findings. *American Journal of Roentgenology* **162**: 77–81.

Rafal RB, Kosovsky PA, Jennis R & Markisz JA (1990) Magnetic resonance imaging evaluation of spontaneous portosystemic collaterals. *Cardiovascular and Interventional Radiology* **13**: 40–43.

Ralls PW, Johson MB, Radin DR et al (1992) Budd–Chiari Syndrome: detection with color Doppler sonography. *American Journal of Roentgenology* **159**: 113–116.

*Sabbà C, Weltin GG, Cicchetti DV et al (1990) Observer variability in echo-Doppler measurements of portal flow in cirrhotic patients and normal volunteers. *Gastroenterology* **98**: 1603–1611.

Sabbà C, Ferraioli G, Genecin P et al (1991) Evaluation of postprandial hyperemia in superior mesenteric artery and portal vein in healthy and cirrhotic humans: an operator-blind echo-Doppler study. *Hepatology* **13**: 714–718.

Sacerdoti D, Merkel C, Bolognesi M et al (1995) Hepatic arterial resistance in cirrhosis with and without portal vein thrombosis: relationships with portal hemodynamics. *Gastroenterology* **108**: 1152–1158.

Salmi A, De Cotis R & Rusconi C (1990) On the rarity of Cruveilhier–Baumgarten's venous hum. *Journal of Hepatology* **11**: 279–280.

Sato S, Ohnishi K, Sugita S & Okuda K (1987) Splenic artery and superior mesenteric artery blood flow: non surgical Doppler US measurement in healthy subjects and patients with chronic liver disease. *Radiology* **164**: 347–352.

Schiano TD, Adrain AL, Cassidy MJ et al (1996) Use of high-resolution endoluminal sonography to measure the radius and the wall thickness of esophageal varices. *Gastrointestinal Endoscopy* **44**: 425–428.

Schmassmann A, Zuber M, Livers M et al (1993) Recurrent bleeding after variceal hemorrhage: predictive value of portal venous duplex sonography. *American Journal of Roentgenology* **160**: 41–47.

Simpson KJ & Finlayson NDC (1995) Clinical evaluation of liver disease. *Clinics in Gastroenterology* **9**: 639–659.

Siringo S, Bolondi L, Gaiani S et al (1994) Timing of the first variceal hemorrhage in cirrhotic patients: prospective evaluation of Doppler flowmetry, endoscopy and clinical parameters. *Hepatology* **20**: 66–73.

Subramanyam BR, Balthazar EJ, Madamba MR et al (1983) Sonography of portosystemic venous collaterals in portal hypertension. *Radiology* **146**: 161–166.

Triger DR, Smart HL, Hosking SW & Johnson AG (1991) Prophylactic sclerotherapy for esophageal varices: long-term results of a single-center trial. *Hepatology* **13**: 117–123

Valla D & Benhamou JP (1996) Obstruction of the hepatic veins or suprahepatic inferior vena cava. *Digestive Diseases and Sciences* **14**: 99–118

Valla D, Bercoff E, Menu Y et al (1984) Discrepancy between wedged hepatic venous pressure and portal venous pressure after acute propranolol administration in patients with alcoholic cirrhosis. *Gastroenterology* **86**: 1400–1403.

Vilgrain V, Lebrec D, Menu Y et al (1990) Comparison between ultrasonographic signs and the degree of portal hypertension in patients with cirrhosis. *Gastrointestinal Radiology* **15**: 218–222.

Vilgrain V, Hadengue A, Zins M et al (1993) Estimation of total hepatic blood flow (HBF) by Doppler sonography: comparison with the clearance method in patients with cirrhosis. *Journal of Hepatology* **18**: S38 (Abstract).

Vilgrain V, Laure S, Henri L et al (1995) Doppler sonography: a non invasive method for diagnosis of membranous obstruction of IVC or hepatic vein. *European Journal of Radiology* **20:** 205–207.

Vorobioff J, Groszmann RJ, Picabea E et al (1996) Prognostic value of hepatic venous pressure gradient measurements in alcoholic cirrhosis: a 10-year prospective study. *Gastroenterology* **111:** 701–709.

de Vries PJ, van Hattum J, Hoekstra JBL & de Hooge P (1991) Duplex Doppler measurements of portal venous flow in normal subjects. Inter- and intra-observer variability. *Journal of Hepatology* **13:** 358–363.

Wachsberg RH & Simmons MZ (1994) Coronary vein diameter and flow direction in patients with portal hypertension: evaluation with duplex sonography and correlation with variceal bleeding. *American Journal of Roentgenology* **162:** 637–641.

Wu MT, Pan HB, Chan C et al (1996) Azygos blood flow in cirrhosis: measurement with MR imaging and correlation with variceal hemorrhage. *Radiology* **198:** 457–462.

Zirinsky K, Markisz JA, Rubenstein WA et al (1988) MR imaging of portal venous thrombosis: correlation with CT and sonography. *American Journal of Roentgenology* **150:** 283–288.

Zoli M, Dondi C, Marchesini G et al (1985) Splanchnic vein measurements in patients with liver cirrhosis: a case-control study. *Journal of Ultrasound in Medicine* **4:** 641–646.

Zoli M, Marchesini G, Cordiani MR et al (1986) Echo-doppler measurement of splanchnic blood flow in control and in cirrhotic subjects. *Journal of Clinical Ultrasound* **14:** 429–435.

3

Natural history. Clinical–haemodynamic correlations. Prediction of the risk of bleeding

GENNARO D'AMICO MD
Professor on Tenure of Gastroenterology

ANGELO LUCA MD
Research Fellow in Clinical Radiology

Divisione di Medicina, Ospedale V Cervello, Via Trabucco 180, 90146 Palermo, Italy

Promoting the development of oesophageal varices and ascites, portal hypertension dominates the clinical course of cirrhosis. Varices appear in patients with portal pressure gradient above 10 mmHg and enlarge in 10–20% within 1–2 years of their detection. Bleeding occurs in patients with portal pressure gradient above 12 mmHg when the wall tension causes the rupture of varices, with an incidence of about 10% per year. Indicators of bleeding risk are portal pressure gradient, variceal pressure, large varices and liver dysfunction. Mortality per bleeding episode is 30–50%. Among survivors 60% will rebleed and 30% will die in the following year. The risk of rebleeding decreases in patients with spontaneous or treatment induced reduction of portal pressure gradinent or variceal pressure. Ascites develops in almost all patients along the course of the disease. Median survival after its appearance is less than 2 years. Less than 5% of cirrhotic patients die without ascites or without a previous bleeding. Thus portal hypertension is a major determinant of survival in cirrhosis.

Key words: portal hypertension; natural history of cirrhosis; oesophageal varices; variceal bleeding risk indicators.

Portal hypertension in cirrhosis is determined by an increase of intrahepatic vascular resistance resulting from the architectural distortion of the liver and from increased sinusoidal tone. The consequent hyperdynamic circulation and increased plasma volume, result in increased portal blood inflow, which further enhances portal hypertension. Collateral circulation then develops in response to the increased portal pressure by opening and dilating pre-existing vessels and possibly by active angiogenesis. Oesophago-gastric varices are the most important clinical expression of collateral circulation in portal hypertension: they increase in size with increasing severity of portal hypertension and rupture when the tension of their wall exceeds a critical point.

Baillière's Clinical Gastroenterology—
Vol. 11, No. 2, June 1997
ISBN 0–7020–2339–6
0950–3528/97/020243 + 14 $12.00/00

Bleeding from oesophageal varices, ascites and complications of ascites mark the clinical course of portal hypertension. Here we report a synthetic review of the most important clinical aspects of the natural history of portal hypertension in cirrhosis.

THE SIZE OF THE PROBLEM

Cirrhosis accounts for almost 90% of the causes of portal hypertension in Europe and in North America. Other causes such as hepato-splenic schistosomiasis, non-cirrhotic portal fibrosis and extrahepatic portal vein thrombosis are more common in Asia and South America.

The median mortality for cirrhosis in 38 selected countries of the Americas, Europe, Africa and Asia was 10/100 000 inhabitants (range from 3 to 40) between 1985 and 1990 (La Vecchia et al, 1994). Considering a median survival of 6 years after diagnosis (Pagliaro et al, 1994) and that about 40% of cirrhotic patiens die before the disease is recognized (Dufour et al, 1993) the median expected prevalence of the disease is 100/100 000 inhabitants with a range from 25 to 400 all around the world. In Italy, 18 000 people died from cirrhosis in 1988 (Capocaccia and Farchi, 1988) suggesting a prevalence of about 110 000. A recent survey estimated that in the USA there were approximately 900 000 people with cirrhosis in 1980 (Dufour et al, 1993).

About one-third of deaths from cirrhosis are related to portal hypertension, mainly because of upper digestive bleeding. The hospital admission rate for upper digestive bleeding ranges between 48 and 150/100 000 inhabitants per year in Europe and USA (Cutler and Mendeloff, 1981; Gilbert, 1990; Longstreth, 1995): portal hypertension related bleeding (70% from varices) accounts for 6% to 20% of all the causes. Mortality per episode of variceal bleeding is about 30% as compared with about 8% for bleeding not related to portal hypertension (Silverstein et al, 1981; Morgan and Clamp, 1988).

DEVELOPMENT OF VARICES

When cirrhosis is diagnosed, varices are present in about 60% of decompensated and 30% of compensated patients.

There is little information on the incidence of oesophageal varices. Two large studies report a similar incidence of about 8% per year (Christensen et al, 1981; Pagliaro et al, 1994) (Figure 1A). Once varices develop, they tend to increase in size before they eventually rupture and bleed. Increase in the size of varices occurs in 10% to 20% after 1 to 2 years of their first observation (Calès et al, 1990; Pagliaro et al, 1994; Calès et al, 1995, Zoli et al, 1996). Further prospective studies are needed to validate these observations and to identify subgroups of patients at higher risk of developing or enlarging varices, in order to obtain a more complete approach to prophylaxis of bleeding and possibly for prevention of varices.

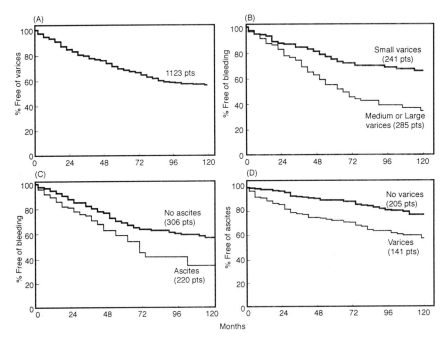

Figure 1. Incidence of varices, bleeding and ascites in liver cirrhosis. Data from two studies of the natural history of cirrhosis including a total of 1649 patients (D'Amico et al, 1986; Pagliaro et al, 1994). (A) Proportion free of oesophageal varices among 1123 patients without varices at the diagnosis. (B) The proportion who were free of bleeding, among 241 patients with small and 285 with medium or large oesophageal varices at diagnosis ($P = 0.0000077$; log-rank test). (C) The proportion who were free of bleeding among patients with oesophageal varices of which 306 were without and 220 with ascites at diagnosis ($P = 0.005$; log-rank test). (D) The proportion who were free of ascites among 205 patients without and 141 with varices at the diagnosis ($P = 0.000012$; log-rank test).

The presence and size of oesophageal varices is associated with the severity of liver disease and alcohol abuse. Abstinence from alcohol and improvement in liver function may result in decreasing or even disappearance of varices (Vorobioff et al, 1996). Whatever the degree of liver dysfunction and the alcohol drinking status, oesophageal varices have been observed only in patients with a portal pressure gradient (HVPG (hepatic venous pressure gradient): the difference between portal pressure and the inferior vena cava pressure) of above 10 mmHg (Viallet, 1975; Lebrec, 1980; Garcia-Tsao, 1985); however, not all patients with HVPG above this level have oesophageal varices (Garcia-Tsao, 1985). Variations in portal pressure gradient are accompanied by parallel variations in the size of oesophageal varices, which may disappear when HVPG decreases to less than 12 mmHg or when it decreases to $\geq 15\%$ of the baseline value (Groszmann et al, 1990; Vorobioff et al, 1996). Thus HVPG has a key role in the development and severity of oesophageal varices and it will probably become a main target in monitoring prophylactic treatment for variceal bleeding.

INCIDENCE AND RISK INDICATORS OF FIRST VARICEAL BLEEDING

Clinical and endoscopic indicators

The incidence of variceal bleeding in unselected patients who have never bled at the time of diagnosis is low. In two prospective studies of natural history of cirrhosis, including a total of 1649 patients at our unit (D'Amico et al, 1986; Pagliaro et al, 1994), the incidence of upper digestive bleeding was 4.4/100 patients/year in the first 5 years after diagnosis. This figure was 5/100 among patients with small oesophageal varices and 9/100 among those with medium or large sized varices (Figure 1B). Among patients with oesophageal varices the bleeding incidence was significantly lower in the Child–Pugh class A (Pugh et al, 1973) (4/100 patients/year) than in class B or C (8/100 patients/year) as well as in patients without ascites compared with those with ascites (Figure 1C), independently of variceal size.

Several other studies (NIEC, 1988; Kleber et al, 1991) confirmed the relationship between variceal size, severity of liver dysfunction and the risk of variceal bleeding. The incidence of bleeding is also significantly greater when newly formed vessels (cherry red spots and red weal marks) may be seen on the variceal wall (NIEC, 1988; Kleber et al, 1991). Platelet count may be a far more easily found indicator of the bleeding risk: patients with primary biliary cirrhosis and platelet count less than 150×10^9 have a 5-year incidence of bleeding more than twice that of patients with platelet counts above this level (Plevris et al, 1995). This figure is confirmed by our ongoing study of natural history of cirrhosis (Pagliaro et al, 1994).

Haemodynamic indicators

Variceal bleeding depends on portal pressure. No bleeding has been reported in patients with hepatic venous pressure gradient (HVPG) below the threshold value of 12 mmHg in cross-sectional studies (Viallet et al, 1975; Lebrec et al, 1980; Garcia-Tsao et al, 1985) and in three prospective studies (Groszmann et al, 1990; Villanueva et al, 1996; Vorobioff et al, 1996). The incidence of variceal bleeding is significantly greater in patients with higher baseline HVPG (Merkel et al, 1992) and in patients in whom HVPG either increases or does not change with time, whereas it is lower in patients whose HVPG decreases (Groszmann et al, 1990; Villanueva et al, 1996; Vorobioff et al, 1996). Similarly, two prospective studies of β-blockers alone (Feu et al, 1995) or associated with nitrates (Villanueva et al, 1996) for prevention of rebleeding, showed a significant reduction of the relative risk of rebleeding in patients with a decrease of HVPG ≥20% after 3 months of treatment. Finally, in several studies, multivariable Cox regression analysis showed that HVPG is an independent and significant risk indicator of variceal bleeding (Groszmann et al, 1990; Merkel et al, 1992; Feu et al, 1995; Villanueva et al, 1996) and death (Groszmann et al, 1990; Merkel et al, 1992; Villanueva et al, 1996).

However, in patients with HVPG greater than 12 mmHg, a linear relationship between HVPG and the risk of bleeding has not been identified. Moreover variceal bleeding has been found to be associated with increased variceal pressure more than with increased HVPG in a cross-sectional study (Rigau et al, 1989). This might depend on the resistance of the collaterals feeding the varices: the higher this resistance is, the higher the difference between HVPG and variceal pressure is and the lower the risk of bleeding. Variceal pressure is significantly related with variceal size, red signs, and severity of liver dysfunction; moreover a recent prospective study showed variceal pressure to be significantly associated with the risk of bleeding and death (Nevens et al, 1996),

The relationship between variceal pressure and the risk of bleeding probably reflects the increase in variceal wall tension with the increase of variceal pressure and size (Polio and Groszmann, 1986). Wall tension is directly related to the radius of the varix and to the transmural pressure and is inversely related to the thickness of the wall. According to this concept, variceal pressure and wall tension (empirically measured on an arbitrary scale) are higher in patients who had bled than in those who had not (Rigau et al, 1989). Actual variceal wall tension cannot be measured because the endoscopic measure of the variceal diameter is only approximate and it is not possible to measure the variceal wall thickness. However, high resolution endoluminal sonography allows a more precise and reliable measure of variceal diameter than endoscopy (Miller et al, 1996). If these results can be confirmed in further studies, this method will allow a quantitative even though approximate measure of variceal wall tension. Moreover it is conceivable that high resolution endoluminal sonography will allow measurement of variceal wall thickness: if so, a precise measure of variceal wall tension will be definitely possible, and will be able to contribute to further improvement in the assessment of the risk of variceal bleeding.

In clinical practice the assessment of bleeding risk is presently based mainly on the NIEC index (NIEC, 1988), a score combining variceal size, red weal marks and Child–Pugh classification. However, in the NIEC study, less than 20% of patients were in the two highest risk classes making the prediction of bleeding of limited clinical value. Other simple variables such as the platelet count could be incorporated in the NIEC index in further prospective studies to assess if its efficiency may be improved.

Haemodynamic parameters, alone or combined with clinical and endoscopic criteria, are expected to improve the accuracy of the bleeding risk assessment: clearly, further large enough prospective studies using multi-variable analysis are needed to confirm that they are bleeding risk indicators independent of those currently used, before they are introduced in clinical practice. Furthermore non-invasive assessment of portal haemodynamics could be of help to identify patients at high risk of bleeding. There is very little information in this area. It has been reported that Doppler sonographic assessment of portal blood flow may be predictive of bleeding (Gaiani et al, 1991) and survival (Zoli et al, 1993) in cirrhosis and that echo-Doppler femoral blood flow variations are related to the variations of HVPG in cirrhotic patients treated with β-blockers (Luca et al, 1996). However, several variables affect echo-Doppler haemodynamic assessment and although its reliability may be much improved (Sabbà et al, 1995), at present it cannot be recommended for prognostic assessment or for monitoring response to β-blockers in clinical practice. Further evaluation of non-invasive techniques for the haemodynamic assessment of portal circulation is needed.

THE ACUTE VARICEAL BLEEDING

Even with emergency endoscopy, active variceal bleeding (blood spurting from the ruptured varix) is seen in about 20–30% of patients with a final diagnosis of variceal bleeding. This finding and the clinical evidence of repeated haematemesis or fresh blood in the gastric aspirate lasting for many hours, have led to the concept that variceal bleeding is a stop and start event. Thus it is difficult to define the active bleeding duration and when a new haematemesis or melena should be considered a rebleeding episode. For these reasons three large consensus conferences stated several definitions for events and timing of events related to the variceal bleeding episode, in order to design and report clinical studies (Burroughs, 1987; De Franchis et al, 1992; De Franchis, 1996).

Data on the *duration of the active bleeding* is scanty. In about half of untreated control groups of RCTs of emergency treatments bleeding stopped spontaneously within 24–48 hours (D'Amico et al, 1995). In a trial comparing glypressin with vasopressin plus transdermal nitrate we considered the bleeding as having been controlled when naso-gastric aspirate was clear for 6 consecutive hours. With this definition the mean bleeding control rate in that trial was about six patients/hour with 24/165 patients still bleeding after 24 hours; the median duration of the bleeding was 10 hours (D'Amico et al, 1994).

Data on *immediate mortality* from uncontrolled bleeding is insufficient for a reliable estimate. In eight recent studies that included a total of 1488 patients, the median mortality for uncontrolled variceal bleeding was 8% and occurred within 1 to 2 days from admission (Graham and Smith, 1981; D'Amico et al, 1986; Melchior et al, 1987; Burroughs et al, 1989; D'Amico et al, 1994; Gatta et al, 1994; Thomsen et al, 1994; Feu et al, 1996). Prognostic indicators of this very early mortality could allow immediate invasive salvage treatment, but there is presently no information about them.

Early rebleeding is significantly associated with the risk of death within 6 weeks (Graham and Smith, 1981; D'Amico et al, 1986; Burroughs et al, 1989) suggesting that its prevention should be a primary objective in the therapeutic approach to variceal bleeding. The incidence of early rebleeding ranges between 30% and 40% in the first 6 weeks. The risk peaks in the first 5 days with 40% of all rebleeding episodes occurring in this very early period, remains high during the first 2 weeks and then declines slowly in the next 4 weeks. After 6 weeks the risk of rebleeding becomes virtually equal to that of before bleeding (Graham and Smith, 1981).

Low albuminaemia, gastric varices (Heresbach et al, 1991), high blood urea nitrogen (BUN) (D'Amico et al, 1986) and HVPG > 16 mmHg measured the first or second day after hospital admission (Ready et al, 1991), have been reported as prognostic indicators of early rebleeding risk. Active bleeding at emergency endoscopy has been found to be a significant indicator of the risk of early rebleeding (Siringo et al, 1991; Ben-Ari et al, 1996), but this finding has not been confirmed (Graham and Smith, 1981; Balanzò, 1991; Gatta et al, 1994). A white nipple on a varix is diagnostic of variceal bleeding but has no prognostic value (Siringo et al, 1991).

Six-week mortality after variceal bleeding ranges between 30 and 50%. About 60% of deaths are caused by uncontrolled bleeding, either the initial episode or early rebleeding. Like rebleeding, mortality peaks in the first days after bleeding (Graham and Smith, 1981), slowly declines thereafter and after 6 weeks becomes constant and virtually equal to that of before bleeding (Sorenson et al, 1987).

Accurate indicators of early death risk could allow selection of patients for emergency shunt or TIPS before their conditions deteriorate hindering further therapy. Unfortunately the risk indicators so far identified are mainly indicators of poor liver and/or renal function, which are also associated with high operative risk and consequently are of limited clinical value.

On hospital admission, the most consistently reported death risk indicators are Child–Pugh classification or its components, BUN or creatininaemia, age and active alcohol abuse (Poynard et al, 1980; Graham and Smith, 1981; Garden et al, 1985; D'Amico et al, 1986; Melchior et al, 1987; Pagliaro et al, 1987; Ohmann et al, 1990; Heresbach et al, 1991; Gatta et al, 1994). The prognostic role of active bleeding on endoscopy is still unsettled probably because of different time-intervals between the start of bleeding and endoscopy across the reported studies.

Early rebleeding is the most important and the most consistently reported among *late* prognostic indicators of the 6-week death risk (Graham and Smith, 1981; D'Amico et al, 1986; Pagliaro et al, 1987; Cardin et al, 1990; Heresbach et al, 1991; Ben-Ari et al, 1996). HVPG measured within 48 hours of admission is significantly higher in patients with higher 2-week mortality (Vinel et al, 1986).

However, although many studies have investigated the prognostic indicators of early rebleeding and death after variceal bleeding, a clinically sound prediction rule is not yet available: this suggests that further studies possibly investigating new candidate indicators together with those so far identified, are needed.

INCIDENCE AND RISK INDICATORS OF LONG-TERM RECURRENT VARICEAL BLEEDING

Patients surviving a first episode of variceal bleeding have a very high risk of rebleeding and death. Median rebleeding incidence within 1 to 2 years in untreated controls of 20 RCTs of non-surgical treatment for prevention of recurrent bleeding, reported after 1981, is 63% (D'Amico et al, 1995). The corresponding mortality figure is 33%.

Therefore, in clinical practice the risk indicators of long-term rebleeding are of less clinical value than those for first bleeding, because all patients must be treated for prevention of rebleeding. RCTs for prevention of rebleeding suggest that the risk is higher in patients in Child–Pugh Class C than in those in A or B class. Continued alcohol abuse and hepatocellular carcinoma are also associated with higher incidence of rebleeding (Poynard et al, 1987).

It has been reported that patients with large varices have higher incidence of rebleeding than patients with small varices (Lebrec et al, 1980; Rector and Reynolds, 1985). However, data on variceal size as risk indicator of recurrent bleeding is insufficient. Although a higher risk in patients with larger varices would be coherent with the present knowledge on the risk of first bleeding it is also conceivable that the high portal and variceal pressure causing the first variceal rupture may cause a second rupture irrespective of the variceal size.

According to this concept, in a prospective study of 63 patients given propranolol after a variceal bleeding, HVPG change was the only independent predictor of rebleeding identified by a multivariable analysis including sex, active drinking, Child–Pugh score, ascites, variceal size, HVPG and cardiac output (Feu et al, 1995). This finding suggests that recurrent variceal bleeding depends almost entirely on portal pressure and that other clinical risk indicators are possibly related to it. This hypothesis is strengthened by the recent finding that HVPG changes are paralleled by changes in Child–Pugh class and variceal size (Vorobioff et al, 1996) and that variceal pressure is significantly related to both these variables (Nevens et al, 1996). Also abstinence from alcohol, which is significantly related with a reduction in rebleeding risk (Poynard et al, 1987), is accompanied by a significant reduction in HVPG (Vorobioff et al, 1996).

Thus, present knowledge suggests that the risk of rebleeding is higher in Child–Pugh C patients, in those who continue to drink and in those with large varices and also that the risk is dependent on portal and variceal pressure. Consequently, it seems that the target of therapy for prevention of rebleeding will be, in the near future, the reduction of HVPG and of variceal pressure: of course, this concept should be confirmed in further prospective and large enough studies before it is applied in clinical practice.

PORTAL HYPERTENSIVE GASTROPATHY (PHG)

When cirrhosis is first diagnosed the prevalence of PHG is about 30% and its incidence is about 12% per year (D'Amico et al, 1990); these figures may be as high as 80% and 30% respectively, in patients with previously known cirrhosis (Primignani et al, 1996). Patients with severe liver dysfunction, large oesophageal varices or undergoing endoscopic therapy for oesophageal varices are at higher risk of developing PHG (Sarin, 1996).

The clinical course of PHG is characterized by overt or chronic gastric mucosal bleeding, which is less frequent and severe in patients with a mosaic like mucosal pattern than in those with red signs (similar to cherry red spots on varices). For this reason the mosaic pattern has been termed *mild* and the red sign pattern *severe* PHG. Prevalence and incidence figures indicate that overall, during the course of cirrhosis, mild PHG may be observed in 50–60% of patients and severe PHG in 10–20% (D'Amico et al, 1990).

The incidence of overt bleeding from any source in patients with mild HPG is about 5% per year as compared with 15% in those with severe PHG. The source of bleeding is the gastric mucosa in about 40% episodes in patients with mild, and 80% in those with severe PHG; variceal rupture is the source in almost all the remaining episodes. Overt bleeding from PHG has a far better prognosis than variceal bleeding with less than 5% mortality per episode.

The incidence of minor mucosal blood loss without overt bleeding is about 8% per year in patients with mild and 25% in those with severe PHG in whom it may result in severe chronic iron deficiency anaemia which requires frequent hospital admissions and blood transfusions. These figures were drawn from a study of the natural history of PHG performed at our unit about 10 years ago (D'Amico et al, 1990) and confirmed in a clinical trial (Perez-Ayuso et al, 1991). It is now our impression that both chronic and overt bleeding from PHG is far less frequent, probably because of the wide use of β-blockers in cirrhotic patients. In fact it has been proven that β-blockers significantly reduce the rebleeding risk in patients who bled from PHG (Perez-Ayuso et al, 1991). Mortality is higher in patients with severe PHG, but this has been found to be dependent on the severity of liver dysfunction (D'Amico et al, 1990).

ASCITES

The median prevalence of patients with ascites is 50% and ranges between 10% and 89% in 36 studies of natural history of cirrhosis reported after 1980 (Pagliaro et al, 1994). The incidence of ascites ranges from 3% to 10% per year (D'Amico et al, 1986; Gines et al, 1987; Pagliaro et al, 1994). Since it is difficult to define a homogeneous start point to describe the natural course of compensated cirrhosis (frequently casually discovered), reliable indicators of the risk of developing ascites have not been identified. In our ongoing study including 399 patients without ascites at diagnosis and showing ascites incidence of 3% per year, the risk is significantly greater in patients with oesophageal varices (Figure 1D).

Once developed, ascites marks the ending phase of the disease. In fact the median survival time after appearance of ascites is consistently reported to be between 1 and 2 years (Saunders et al, 1981; Gines et al, 1987; Pagliaro et al, 1994) whereas the mortality while free of ascites is 2% per year in our ongoing study after more than 10 years of follow-up (Pagliaro et al, 1994). Accordingly, ascites has been found to be the first or the second more important independent death risk indicator in all the 10 studies using multivariable regression analysis reported after 1980 in which it has been assessed.

This high mortality of patients with ascites is largely accounted for by the high risk of further complications of the disease. The incidence of variceal bleeding is significantly higher in patients with ascites (Figure 1C).

Spontaneous bacterial peritonitis (SBP) is mostly caused by Gram-negative enteric bacteria (65%) or by streptococci (25%) spreading by haematogenous or lymphatic route. Its prevalence ranges from 4 to 20% in prospective studies. The incidence of the first episode of SBP is 20% in the first year following the appearance of ascites with higher risk for patients surviving a bleeding episode, or with protein concentration in the ascitic fluid of < 1.5 g/dl (Pinzello et al, 1993). The mortality rate per episode of SBP was very high (80–97%) in studies reported in the 1970s whereas the median mortality in 10 studies published between 1982 and 1991, and including a total of 507 patients, is 50% (Pinzello et al, 1993). This lower mortality in recent studies probably reflects earlier detection of the infection and a more appropriate treatment. Independent risk indicators of death risk are the first episode of SBP, the Child–Pugh score and creatininaemia (Llovet et al, 1993; Pinzello et al, 1993). Patients surviving a first episode have a 70% incidence of recurrent SBP (Tito et al, 1988; Gines et al, 1990), which is reduced by prophylactic norfloxacin (Gines et al, 1990).

Hepatorenal syndrome (HRS) is the extreme expression of the haemodynamic impairment and sodium retention in patients with ascites and marks the impending conclusion of the disease. It results from intense renal vasoconstriction with selective cortical hypoperfusion induced by the sympathetic response to peripheral vasodilatation and vascular underfilling. A progressive renal failure develops with oliguria or anuria, urinary sodium concentration < 10 mml/l, urine osmolality greater than serum osmolality and urine to plasma creatinine ratio > 30:1. The incidence of HRS is about 8% ascitic patients per year (Gines et al, 1993). Severe bacterial infection and gastro-intestinal bleeding may act as precipitating factors but the syndrome is unrelated to any event in half of patients. Serum sodium ≤ 133 mEq/l and plasma renin activity > 3.5 ng/ml are independent risk indicators of the syndrome. The prognosis of patients developing HRS is very poor with a median survival of 2 weeks and 95% of patients dying within 10 weeks (Gines et al, 1993).

THE OUTCOME OF PATIENTS WITH PORTAL HYPERTENSION

The markers of clinically relevant portal hypertension are oesophageal varices, bleeding from portal hypertension related sources and ascites. The incidence of these events (Figure 1) has been discussed above, together with the corresponding risk indicators. Mortality of patients presenting each of these signs at the time of the diagnosis is reported in Figure 2.

Either incidence or survival figures reported in Figures 1 and 2 are drawn from two prospective studies performed at our unit (D'Amico et al, 1986; Pagliaro et al, 1994) and including a total of 1649 patients. Median survival times for patients with small varices at the time of diagnosis, or with bleeding, ascites or both ascites and bleeding are, respectively, 84, 24, 18 and 20 months as compared with a 10-year survival of 60% for patients without varices (Figure 2). Thus there is a clear worsening of the prognosis from the absence of varices, to their appearance, to the first manifestation of overt decompensation of the disease, either bleeding or ascites or both. This suggests that these conditions (absence of varices, varices, bleeding and ascites) mark definite stages of the ongoing disease, corresponding to the progression of portal hypertension, and that the prognosis of the disease is more reliably assessed within each stage rather than when disease was first diagnosed. This concept is supported by the observation that only 90 of the 1649 (5%) patients included in the two studies performed at our unit died while free of bleeding or ascites after more than 10 years of follow-up. Similarly the mortality of patients who remain in Child–Pugh class A is

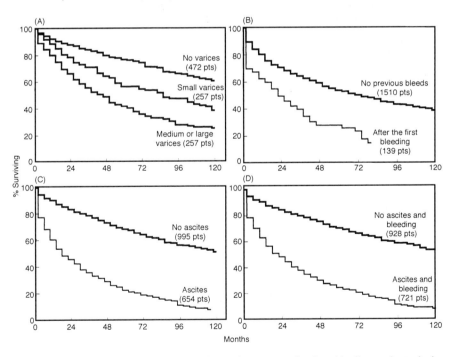

Figure 2. Survival of cirrhotic patients according to the presence of varices, bleeding, ascites or both ascites and bleeding at the time of the diagnosis. Data from two studies of the natural history of cirrhosis included a total of 1649 patients (D'Amico et al, 1986; Pagliaro et al, 1994). (A) The proportion surviving among 472 patients without varices, 257 with small and 352 with medium or large varices ($P < 10^{-7}$). (B) The proportion surviving among 1510 patients without and 139 with previous bleeding at diagnosis ($P < 10^{-7}$). (C) The proportion surviving among 995 patients without and 654 with ascites at diagnosis ($P < 10^{-7}$). (D) The proportion surviving among 928 patients without and 721 with ascites or bleeding at diagnosis ($P < 10^{-7}$).

only 9% after 6 years (Pagliaro, 1994). Thus liver function and markers of portal hypertension should be probably combined for a more accurate assessment of prognostic indicators of death in cirrhosis in future studies.

REFERENCES

D'Amico G, Pagliaro L & Bosch J (1995) The treatment of portal hypertension. A metanalytic review. *Hepatology* **22**: 332–354.

D'Amico G, Morabito A, Pagliaro L & Marubini E (1986) Survival and prognostic indicators in compensated and decompensated cirrhosis. *Digestive Diseases and Sciences* **31**: 468–475.

D'Amico G, Morabito A, Pagliaro L et al (1986) Six-week prognostic indicators in upper gastro-intestinal hemorrhage in cirrhosis. In Dianzani MU & Genntilini P (eds) *Frontiers in Gastrointestinal Research: Chronic Liver Disease*, pp 247–257. Basel: Karger.

D'Amico G, Montalbano L, Traina M et al (1990) Natural history of congestive gastropathy in cirrhosis. *Gastroenterology* **99**: 1558–1564.

D'Amico G, Traina M, Vizzini G et al (1994) Terlipressin or vasopressin plus transdermal nitro-glycerin in a treatment strategy for digestive bleeding in cirrhosis. A randomized clinical trial. *Journal of Hepatology* **20**: 206–212.

Balanzò J, Villanueva C, Espinòs JC et al (1991) Predictive value of the endoscopic signs in variceal bleeding. [Abstract]. *Journal of Hepatology* **13 (supplement 2)**: S93.

Ben-Ari Z, Cardin F, Wannamethee G et al (1996) Prognostic significance of endoscopic bleeding and early rebleeding from oesophageal varices. [Abstract] *Journal of Hepatology* **(supplement)**: S92.

Burroughs AK (ed.) (1987) *Methodology and Review of Clinical Trials in Portal Hypertension*. Excerpta Medica, Amsterdam, 1987.

Burroughs AK, Mezzanotte G, Phillips A et al (1989) Cirrhotics with variceal hemorrhage: the import-ance of the time interval between admission and the start of analysis for survival and rebleeding rates. *Hepatology* **9**: 801–807.

Calès P, Desmorat H, Vinel JP et al (1990) Incidence of large esophageal varices in patients with cirrhosis: application to prophylaxis of first bleeding. *Gut* **31**: 1298–1302.

Calès P. Groupe francais de la prevention pré-primaire (1995) Propranolol does not decrease the development of large esophageal varices in patients with cirrhosis. A controlled study. [Abstract] *Hepatology* **22 (supplement)**: 155A.

Capocaccia R & Farchi G (1988) Mortality from liver cirrhosis in Italy: proportion associated with consumption of alcohol. *Journal of Clinical Epidemiology* **41**: 347–357.

Cardin F, Gori G, McCormick PA & Burroughs AK (1990) A predictive model for very early rebleed-ing from varices. [Abstract] *Gut* **31**: A1204.

Christensen E, Faverholdt L, Schlichting P et al (1981) Aspects of natural history of gastrointestinal bleeding in cirrhosis and the effect of prednisolone. *Gastroenterology* **81**: 944–952.

Cutler JA & Mendeloff AI (1981) Upper gastrointestinal bleeding. Nature and magnitude of the problem in the US. *Digestive Diseases and Sciences* **26 (supplement)**: S90–S96.

Dufour MC, Stinson F & Fe Caces M (1993) Trends in cirrhosis morbidity and mortality: United States, 1979–1988. *Seminars in Liver Disease* **13**: 109–125.

Feu F, Garcia-Pagan JC, Bosch J et al (1995) Relation between portal pressure response to pharmaco-therapy and risk of recurrent variceal haemorrhage in patients with cirrhosis *Lancet* **346**: 1056–1059.

Feu F, Ruiz del Arbol L, Banares R et al (1996) Double-blind randomized controlled trial comparing terlipressin and somatostatin for acute variceal hemorrhage. *Gastroenterology* **111**: 1291–1299.

*De Franchis R (ed.) (1996) *Portal Hypertension II. Proceedings of the Second Baveno International Consensus Workshop on Definitions, Methodology, and Therapeutic Strategies*. Oxford: Blackwell Science.

De Franchis R, Pascal JP, Ancona E et al (1992) Definitions, methodology and therapeutic strategies in portal hypertension. A consensus development workshop, Baveno, Lake Maggiore, Italy, April 5 and 6, 1990. *Journal of Hepatology* **15**: 256–261.

Gaiani S, Bolondi L, Li Bassi S et al (1991) Prevalence of spontaneous hepatofugal portal flow in liver cirrhosis. Clinical and endoscopic correlations in 228 patients. *Gastroenterology* **100**: 160–167.

*Garcia-Tsao G, Groszmann RJ, Fisher RL et al (1985) Portal pressure, presence of gastroesophageal varices and variceal bleeding. *Hepatology* 5: 419–424.

Garden OJ, Motyl H, Gilmour WH et al (1985) Prediction of outcome following acute variceal haemorrhage. *British Journal of Surgery* 72: 91–95.

Gatta A, Merkel C, Amodio P et al (1994) Development and validation of a prognostic index predicting death after upper gastrointestinal bleeding in patients with liver cirrhosis: a multicenter study. *American Journal of Gastroenterology* 89: 1528–1536.

Gilbert DA (1990) Epidemiology of upper gastrointestinal bleeding. *Gastrointestinal Endoscopy* 36 (supplement): S8–S13.

Gines P, Quintero E, Arroyo V et al (1987) Compensated cirrhosis: natural history and prognostic factors. *Hepatology* 7: 122–128.

Gines P, Rimola A, Planas R et al (1990) Norfloxacin prevents spontaneous bacterial peritonitis recurrence in cirrhosis: results of a double blind, placebo-controlled trial. *Hepatology* 12: 716–724.

Gines A, Escorsell A, Gines P et al (1993) Incidence, predictive factors, and prognosis of the hepatorenal syndrome in cirrhosis with ascites. *Gastroenterology* 105: 229–236.

*Graham DY & Smith JL (1981) The course of patients after variceal hemorrhage. *Gastroenterology* 80: 800–809.

*Groszmann RJ, Bosch J, Grace ND et al (1990) Hemodynamic events in a prospective randomized trial of propranolol versus placebo in the prevention of a first variceal hemorrhage. *Gastroenterology* 99: 1401–1407.

Heresbach D, Bretagne JF, Raoul JL et al (1991) Pronostic et facteurs pronostiques de l'hémorragie par rupture de varice chez le cirrhotique à l'ère de la sclérose endoscopique. *Gastroenterologie Clinique et Biologique* 15: 838–844.

Kleber G, Sauerbruch T, Ansari H & Paumgartner G (1991) Prediction of variceal hemorrhage in cirrhosis: a prospective follow-up study. *Gastroenterology* 100: 1332–1337.

La Vecchia C, Levi F, Lucchini F et al (1994) Worldwide patterns and trends in mortality from liver cirrhosis, 1955 to 1990. *Annals of Epidemiology* 4: 480–486.

*Lebrec D, Fleury P, Rueff B et al (1980) Portal hypertension, size of esophageal varices, and risk of gastrointestinal bleeding in alcoholic cirrhosis. *Gastroenterology* 79: 1139–1144.

Llovet JM, Planas R, Morillas R et al (1993) Short term prognosis of cirrhotics with spontaneous bacterial peritonitis: multivariate study. *American Journal of Gastroenterology* 88: 388–392.

Longstreth FG (1995) Epidemiology of hospitalization for acute upper gastrointestinal hemorrhage: a population based study. *American Journal of Gastroenterology* 90: 206–210.

Luca A, Garcia-Pagan JC, Feu F et al (1995) Noninvasive measurement of femoral blood flow and portal pressure response to propranolol in patients with cirrhosis. *Hepatology* 21: 83–88.

Melchior JC, Poupon RE, Verrier J et al (1987) Analyse des facteurs liés à la mortalité précoce au cours des hémorragies dues à l'hypertension portale. *Gastroenterologie Clinic Biologic* 11: 402–408.

Merkel C, Bolognesi M, Bellon S et al (1992) Prognostic usefulness of hepatic vein catheterization in patients with cirrhosis and esophageal varices. *Gastroenterology* 102: 973–979.

Miller LS, Schiano TD, Adrian A et al (1996) Comparison of high-resolution endoluminal sonography to videoendoscopy in the detection and evaluation of esophageal varices *Hepatology* 24: 552–555.

Morgan AG & Clamp SE (1988) OMGE International upper gastrointestinal bleeding survey, 1978–1986. *Scandinavian Journal of Gastroenterology* 23 (supplement 144): S51–S58.

Nevens F, Sprengers D, Feu F et al (1996) Measurement of variceal pressure with an endoscopic pressure sensitive gauge: validation and effect of propranolol therapy in chronic conditions. *Journal of Hepatology* 24: 66–73.

*NIEC (North Italian Endoscopic Club for the Study and Treatment of Esophageal Varices) (1988) Prediction of the first variceal hemorrhage in patients with cirrhosis of the liver and esophageal varices. *New England Journal of Medicine* 319: 983–989.

Ohmann C, Stoltzing H & Wins L (1990) Prognostic scores in oesophageal or gastric variceal bleeding. *Scandinavian Journal of Gastroenterology* 25: 501–512.

Pagliaro L, D'Amico G, Malizia G et al (1987) *Methodology and Reviews of Clinical Trials in Portal Hypertension*, Burroughs AK (ed.) pp 53–62. Amsterdam: Excerpta Medica.

Pagliaro L, D'Amico G, Pasta L et al (1994) Portal hypertension in cirrhosis: natural history. In Bosch J & Groszmann R (eds) *Portal Hypertension: Pathophysiology and Treatment*, pp 72–92. Cambridge, MA: Blackwell Scientific.

Perez-Ayuso RM, Piqué JM, Bosch J et al (1991) Propranolol in prevention of recurrent bleeding from severe portal hypertensive gastropathy in cirrhosis. *Lancet* 337: 1431–1434.

Pinzello G, Simonetti R, Camma C et al (1993) Spontaneous bacterial peritonitis: an update. *Gastroenterology International* **6:** 54–60.

Plevris JN, Dhariwal A, Elton RA et al (1995) The platelet count as a predictor of variceal hemorrhage in primary biliary cirrhosis. *American Journal of Gastroenterology* **90:** 959–961.

Polio J & Groszmann RJ (1986) Hemodynamic factors in the development and rupture of esophageal varices: a pathophysiologic approach to treatment. *Seminars in Liver Disease* **6:** 318–326.

Poynard T, Chaput JC, Mary JY et al (1980) Analyse critique des facteurs lié au trentième jour dans les hemorrhagies digestives hautes du cirrhotique. *Gastoenterologie Clinic Biologic* **4:** 655–665.

Poynard T, Lebrec D, Hillon P et al (1987) Propranolol in prevention of recurrent gastrointestinal bleeding in patients with cirrhosis: a prospective study of factors associated with rebleeding. *Hepatology* **7:** 447–451.

Primignani M, Carpinelli L, Preatoni P et al (1996) Portal hypertensive gastropathy in liver cirrhosis: natural history. A multicenter study of the New Italian Endoscopic Club. *Journal of Hepatology* **24 (supplement):** S71.

Pugh RNH, Murray-Lyon IM, Dawson JL et al (1973) Transection of the oesophagus for bleeding oesophageal varices. *British Journal of Surgery* **60:** 646–649.

Ready JB, Robertson DA, Goff SJ & Rector WG (1991) Assessment of the risk of bleeding from varices by continuous monitoring of portal pressure. *Gastroenterology* **100:** 1403–1410.

Rector WG & Reynolds TB (1985) Risk factors for hemorrhage from esophageal varices and acute gastric erosions. *Clinics in Gastroenterology* **14:** 139.

Rigau J, Bosch J, Bordas JM et al (1989) Endoscopic measurement of variceal pressure in cirrhosis: correlation with portal pressure and variceal hemorrhage. *Gastroenterology* **96:** 873–880.

Sabbà C, Merkel C, Zoli M et al (1995) Interobserver and interequipment variability of echo-doppler examination of the portal vein: effect of a cooperative training program. *Hepatology* **21:** 428–433.

Sarin KS (1996) Diagnostic issues: portal hypertensive gastropathy and gastric varices. In De Franchis R (ed.) *Portal Hypertension II. Proceedings of the Second Baveno International Consensus Workshop on Definitions, Methodology, and Therapeutic Strategies,* pp 30–54. Oxford: Blackwell Science.

Saunders JB, Walters JRF, Davies P & Paton A (1981) A 20-year prospective study of cirrhosis. *British Journal of Medicine* **282:** 263–266.

Silverstein FE, Gilbert DA, Tedesco FJ et al (1981) The National ASGE survey on upper gastro-intestinal bleeding. I. Study design and baseline data. II. Clinical prognostic factors. *Gastrointestinal Endoscopy* **27:** 73–93.

Siringo S, McCormick PA, Mistry P et al (1991) Prognostic significance of the white nipple sign in variceal bleeding. *Gastrointestinal Endoscopy* **37:** 51–55.

Sorensen TIA (1987) Definition of death in relation to variceal bleeding. In Burroughs AK (ed.) *Methodology and Reviews of Clinical Trials in Portal Hypertension,* pp 31–35. Amsterdam: Excerpta Medica.

Thomsen LB, Moller S, Sorensen TIA et al (1994) Optimized analysis of recurrent bleeding and death in patients with cirrhosis and esophageal varices. *Journal of Hepatology* **21:** 367–375.

Tito L, Rimola A & Gines P (1988) Spontaneous bacterial peritonitis in cirrhosis: frequency and predictive factors. *Hepatology* **8:** 27–31.

Viallet A, Marleau D, Huet M et al (1975) Hemodynamic evaluation of patients with intrahepatic portal hypertension: relationship between bleeding varices and the portohepatic gradient. *Gastroenterology* **69:** 1297–1300.

Villanueva C, Balanzò J, Novella M et al (1996) Nadolol plus isosorbide mononitrate compared with sclerotherapy for the prevention of variceal bleeding. *New England Journal of Medicine* **334:** 1624–1629.

Vinel JP, Cassigneul J, Levade M et al (1986) Assessment of short-term prognosis after variceal bleed-ing in patients with alcoholic cirrhosis by early measurement of portohepatic gradient. *Hepatology* **6:** 116–117.

*Vorobioff J, Groszmann RJ, Picabea E et al (1996) Prognostic value of hepatic venous pressure gradient measurements in alcoholic cirrhosis: a 10-year prospective sudy. *Gastroenterology* **111:** 701–709.

Zoli M, Iervese T, Merkel C et al (1993) Prognostic significance of portal hemodynamics in patients with compensated cirrhosis. *Journal of Hepatology* **17:** 56–61.

Zoli M, Merkel C, Magliotti D et al (1996) Small esophageal varices in patients with liver cirrhosis: bleeding risk and natural history. [Abstract] *Italian Journal of Gastroenterology* **28 (supplement 1):** S242.

4

Portal hypertensive gastropathy

JOSEP M. PIQUÉ MD

Chief
Gastroenterology Department, Hospital Clínic i Provincial, University of Barcelona, Villarroel 170, 08036 Barcelona, Spain

The term portal hypertensive gastropathy (PHG) defines a wide spectrum of diffuse macroscopic lesions that appear in the gastric mucosa of patients with portal hypertension. Histologically, these lesions correspond to dilated vessels in the mucosa and submucosa in the absence of erosions or inflammation. Endoscopically, the lesions are classified as mild when mosaic pattern or superficial reddening are present, and severe when gastric mucosa appear with diffuse cherry red spots. Mild lesions are highly prevalent (65–90%), whereas severe lesions are present in only 10–25% of cirrhotic patients.

The pathogenesis of PHG is not well known, but both venous congestion related with raised portal pressure and increased gastric blood flow seem to be crucial factors for its development. Variceal sclerosis may contribute to the development or aggravation of the lesions.

Bleeding is the unique clinical manifestation of PHG, and occurs only in those patients with severe lesions. During a 5-year follow-up, the risk of overt bleeding or chronic bleeding, which induces anaemia, is 60% and 90%, respectively, for patients with severe PHG.

Propranolol is the only pharmacological treatment that has been proven useful in preventing bleeding from PHG. Porto-systemic shunts and liver transplantation are also effective.

Key words: portal hypertensive gastropathy; portal hypertension; mosaic pattern; gastric red spots; upper GI-bleeding; propranolol.

Under the term of portal hypertensive gastropathy (PHG), the occurrence of several diffuse macroscopic lesions that appear in the gastric mucosa of patients with portal hypertension, can be included. This term has been proposed within the last 10 years to group the previously named 'haemorrhagic gastritis' or 'diffuse gastric lesions' in patients with cirrhosis. This was the result of several studies demonstrating that dilated vessels in the mucosa, and not erosions or inflammation, is the histological hallmark of endoscopic diffuse gastric lesions in patients with portal hypertension (McCormack et al, 1985; Quintero et al, 1987). For that reason the term 'gastritis' was considered inappropriate for describing this mucosal gastric alteration. In addition, the term 'congestive gastropathy', which has also been used alternatively to PHG, is not fully accurate since venous congestion seems not to be the only pathogenic mechanism involved in the development of such gastric lesions.

ENDOSCOPIC AND PATHOLOGICAL DIAGNOSIS

Endoscopically, PHG includes several mucosal lesions which have been classified as mild or severe (Table 1) (McCormack et al, 1985; Spina and Archidiacomo, 1994; Hashizume and Sugimachi, 1995). Despite the subjectivity of the description and classification of these lesions, an acceptable inter-observer agreement has been found in its assessment, especially when severe lesions are present (Calès et al, 1990).

Table 1. Classification of portal hypertension gastropathy.

Mild	Severe
Mosaic pink in centre	Red spots
Fine red speckling	Brown spots
Scarlatina type rash	Diffuse haemorrhagic lesions
Snake skin pattern	

The mosaic pattern is defined by a white reticular network separating areas of raised red or pink mucosa resembling a snake skin. This is the most common gastric mucosal alteration in patients with portal hypertension and is predominantly found in the corpus and in the fundus. A mosaic pattern is not a specific lesion for portal hypertension unless pink or red oedematous mucosa is present in the centre of the white reticula. When only mosaic with this feature is considered, it has been reported in up to 90% of patients with portal hypertension and only in 0.3% of patients without portal hypertension (Papazian et al, 1986). Other mucosal lesions included in mild PHG are superficial reddening on the surface of the rugae and a fine pink speckling or 'scarlatina' type rash.

The severe endoscopic lesion of PHG is characterized by discrete cherry-red spots, which may progress to confluent areas of diffuse bleeding. These red spots may appear in any part of the gastric mucosa, including fundus, corpus and antrum. When the red spots are located in the antrum of cirrhotic patients, some authors have proposed different terminology such as gastric antral vascular ectasia (GAVE). This is based on some differential histological features, which may imply distinct pathogenesis according to the author's suggestion (Payen et al, 1995a). However, it is likely that the same gastric vascular alteration related to portal hypertension may appear slightly different macroscopically and histologically according to the anatomical peculiarities of each gastric region.

Another different endoscopic finding also reflecting an underlying vasculopathy is that of red strips in the gastric antrum converging on the pyloric area. This macroscopic lesion, which has been named 'watermelon stomach', can be seen in cirrhotic patients but also in other diseases, mainly autoimmune or connective tissue disorders such as scleroderma, sclerodactylyl, hypothyroidism, pernicious anaemia, or primary biliary cirrhosis (Gosutout et al, 1992).

Although the mucosal vascular lesions are more common in the stomach of patients with portal hypertension, similar lesions can also be found in other parts of the digestive tract such as the small intestine or colon (Kozarek et al, 1991; Naveau et al, 1991; Nagral et al, 1993).

Concerning the histological findings, two early studies came to similar conclusion that the unique feature of PHG is a marked dilation of the capillaries and collecting venules in the gastric mucosa (McCormack et al, 1985; Quintero et al, 1987). In addition, submucosal veins appear ectatic, irregular and with areas of intimal thickening. These vascular alterations are present in the absence of any significant inflammatory cell infiltrate or erosion in the gastric mucosa, making incorrect the previous classification of these lesions as gastritis. When the red spots are located in the antrum, fibromuscular hyperplasia, fibrohyalinosis and thrombi are usually encountered in the histological examination. Whether these features represent different pathogenic factors from those involved in the lesions observed in the corpus and fundus or merely reflect the influence of distinct anatomic or motility patterns in the antral area, remains unclear.

The diagnosis of PHG is usually endoscopic, although it may be difficult some times to endoscopically distinguish such lesions from other gastric disorders not related with portal hypertension (Corbishley et al, 1988). Routine endoscopic biopsies obtained by conventional forceps are often unhelpful to diagnose PHG, since from specimens obtained by such device it is difficult to ascertain the presence or absence of vessel dilation because of the patchy nature of the alteration. In contrast, large snare biopsies can easily ascertain the presence or absence of dilated vessels, but this procedure is not recommended for routine use (Saperas et al, 1989). In addition, endoscopic ultrasonography may detect a characteristic thickening of the gastric wall reflecting the oedema usually present in the gastric mucosa and submucosa of patients with PHG.

PREVALENCE AND NATURAL HISTORY

The reported prevalence of PHG largely depends on the classification used to define mild lesions. If any type of mosaic pattern is included, a prevalence ranging from 63% to 90% has been described in cirrhotic patients (Papazian et al, 1986; Iwao et al, 1992; NIEC, 1992). However, if only mosaic pattern with red and prominent centre is included, the prevalence reported is that of 27% (D'Amico et al, 1990). In addition, if any type of mosaic pattern is excluded and only red spots or reddening is considered, then the prevalence reported is around 11% (Sarin et al, 1992).

Little is known about the natural history of the disease, but it is a common observation that the endoscopic appearance of the lesions may vary with time. Triger and Hosking (1989) reported minor progression of the lesions in a small group of cirrhotic patients with PHG during 2 years follow-up. However, D'Amico et al (1990) reported that 72 patients (46%)

developed PHG during 5 years follow-up (65 developed mild gastropathy and seven severe gastropathy) among a series of 154 cirrhotic patients without gastric mucosal lesions at baseline.

Several authors have provided evidence suggesting that esclerotherapy may increase the risk of bleeding from PHG (McCormack et al, 1985; D'Amico et al, 1990; Kotzampasi et al, 1990; Triger and Hosking, 1989; Tanoue et al, 1992). However, the mechanism by which variceal obliteration may lead to the development of PHG is unknown. Sclerosis might cause a rise in pressure within the gastric veins and subsequent increase in gastropathy. Alternatively, an increased blood flow velocity might occur in the gastric vessels after oesophageal vein obliteration. It has been shown that hepatofugal flow velocity is increased in the left gastric vein in direct relationship with enlarged size of oesophageal varices (Matsutani et al, 1993), and that gastric mucosal blood flow is higher in cirrhotic patients whose extrahepatic collaterals are predominantly via oesophageal varices (Yamamoto et al, 1992). According to these observations, it is possible that obliteration of oesophageal collateral vein network may lead to a higher flow velocity in the gastric vascular bed.

Although some authors have suggested that PHG is more common in patients with advanced liver disease (D'Amico et al, 1990; Iwao et al, 1992), many investigators have failed to demonstrate any significant correlation between PHG and the degree of liver damage (McCormack et al, 1985; Quintero et al, 1987; Vigneri et al, 1991). It is likely that portal hypertension, rather than liver damage, would be the key factor for developing gastric vasculopathy. This is in keeping with the observation that PHG may also appear in patients with portal hypertension and without liver disease (Sarin et al, 1988).

PATHOGENESIS

The mechanisms by which gastric vasodilation and mucosal red spots appear in patients with portal hypertension remain unknown. Acid secretion does not play a major role. In fact, it has been demonstrated that cirrhotic patients with PHG have not only enhanced acid output but also reduced gastric acid secretion (Pérez et al, 1989). This functional hyposecretion is more commonly observed in patients with antral PHG, it is not related to corpus or fundus gastric atrophy, and it is commonly associated with hypergastrinaemia (Quintero et al, 1987; Pérez et al, 1989).

PHG seems not to be related to the presence of *Helicobacter pylori* in the gastric mucosa. The prevalence of this micro-organism in cirrhotic patients is similar to that in the general population, the chronic gastritis induced by the infection is not affected by cirrhosis, and no correlation has been found between *H. pylori* colonization and the presence of PHG (McCormick et al, 1991).

Portal hypertension is a prerequisite for the development of PHG, since only patients with this alteration, with or without hepatic cirrhosis, develop such a complication. Therefore, impairment of gastric venous drainage towards the portal system may be, at least initially, an important component of the dilated vessels in the gastric mucosa and submucosa. However, raised portal pressure and splanchnic venous congestion seem not to be the only pathogenic mechanisms inducing gastric vessel dilation, since no direct correlation is usually found between severity of portal hypertension assessed by portal venous gradient or oesophageal variceal size and the degree of gastric vasodilation or prevalence of gastric red spots (Quintero et al, 1987; Vigneri et al, 1991).

It is well known that chronically raised portal pressure is followed by the development of extensive collateralization of the portal venous system. This phenomenon, which tends to decompress the portal system, does not effectively reduce portal pressure because it is accompanied by a general splanchnic vasodilation that increases portal venous inflow and contributes to an enhanced portal pressure. This hyperdynamic splanchnic circulation has been demonstrated in patients with cirrhosis and in several experimental models of portal hypertension (Kotelanski et al, 1972; Vorobioff et al, 1983; Benoit et al, 1986a).

According to this generalized arteriolar splanchnic vasodilation, it is probable that an enhanced blood flow may also be present in the stomach. This issue was extensively investigated in different experimental models of portal hypertension and highly uniform results were obtained, confirming an enhanced total gastric blood flow (Benoit and Granger, 1986; Benoit et al, 1986; Geraghty et al, 1989; Pizcueta et al, 1992). This has been demonstrated by using radiolabelled microspheres in cirrhotic rats and in rats with partial portal vein occlusion (Benoit and Granger, 1986; Benoit et al, 1986; Pizcueta et al, 1992), and by [^{14}C]iodo-antipyrine autoradiographic technique in partial portal vein ligated rats (Geraghty et al, 1989). It would be possible that despite an enhanced total gastric blood flow, wall redistribution may lead to a hyperperfused serosal and muscularis layer with mucosal hypoperfusion. This assumption is based on the description of few arteriovenous shunts in the submucosa of cirrhotic patients (Hashizume et al, 1983). However, this seems not to be the case, since several investigations have provided evidence ruling out such possibility. Benoit et al (1986) have demonstrated by means of a radioactive microspheres technique that the increase in flow in the stomach wall of portal hypertensive rats is mainly observed in the mucosal layer, and that the proportional distribution of flow between different layers is not altered in portal hypertensive rats in comparison with sham operated animals. In addition, different investigators using different techniques have shown an increased blood flow in the mucosal layer of portal hypertensive animals (Kitano et al, 1982; Benoit et al, 1986; Piqué et al, 1988, 1990).

It has been described that portal hypertensive animals have an impaired hyperaemic response when the gastric mucosa is challenged by different noxious agents (Ferraz et al, 1995; Nishizaki et al, 1996). Whether this impairment reflects true defective vascular reactivity or merely the lack of response because of the presence of increased basal gastric blood flow remains unknown.

Few studies have investigated the gastric mucosal perfusion in humans with cirrhosis. In contrast with the highly reproducible results obtained in experimental models of portal hypertension, human studies using laser-Doppler flowmetry and reflectance spectrophotometry through the endoscope, have come to some contradictory results. Some investigators have found increased gastric blood perfusion (Chung et al, 1988; Panés et al, 1992a), while others reported decreased perfusion (Nishiwaki et al, 1990; Iwao et al, 1993) or a combination of both congestion and hyperaemia (Otha et al, 1994). These heterogeneous findings probably reflect the lack of good reproducibility of the techniques estimating gastric blood flow in humans or the presence of confounding factors in the interpretation of the results obtained with those techniques. In that regard, it has described the potential influence of red blood cell content in the gastric mucosa in the assessment of blood flow by either laser-Doppler or reflectance spectrophotometry (Casadevall et al, 1992).

The pathophysiology of the splanchnic hyperdynamic circulation, including the stomach, is not well known and it probably has a multifactorial component. It was proposed that increased circulating levels of vasodilators such as glucagon (Benoit et al, 1984) or a reduced sensitivity to endogenous vasoconstrictors (Kiel et al, 1985; Pizcueta et al, 1990) may play a significant role. This hypothesis is supported by the fact that several vasodilators including glucagon, norepinephrine, VIP, gastrin or secretin have been found increased in the plasma of cirrhotic patients or in animals with portal hypertension (Chey et al, 1971; Henriksen et al, 1980; Quintero et al, 1987; Pizcueta et al, 1990). However, the finding of similar plasma levels of such vasodilators in cirrhotic patients with and without PHG (Saperas et al, 1990), does not support a major role for those peptides in the pathophysiology of gastric vasculopathy.

More recently, it has been suggested that several endothelial factors, including prostaglandins and nitric oxide, may be involved. It has been shown that the administration of specific inhibitors of both prostaglandin and nitric oxide may significantly attenuate the gastric hyperaemia of portal hypertensive rats (Piqué et al, 1988; Pizcueta et al, 1992a; Casadevall et al, 1993; Fernandez et al, 1996). Moreover, gastric microcirculation of cirrhotic rats appears to be more sensitive to PGE_1 administration and to endogenous prostaglandin inhibition (Beck et al, 1993). Both vasoactive factors, prostaglandins and nitric oxide seem to interact to some extent modulating the gastric hyperaemia of portal hypertension (Casadevall et al, 1993; Ferraz and Wallace, 1996) and both factors are also involved in the hyperdynamic circulation of splanchnic organs other than the stomach (Sitzmann et al, 1988; Pizcueta et al, 1992b; Sieber et al, 1993; Cahill et al, 1994).

How these two endothelial factors interact modulating splanchnic vasodilation, what stimuli are responsible for their enhanced release or increased microcirculatory sensitivity in portal hypertension, and how these factors may interact with other possible vasodilatory substances, remains to be elucidated. In addition, it is not completely known if the origin of the enhanced release of nitric oxide in portal hypertension comes from the constitutive or the inducible enzyme. Although some evidence suggests that the constitutive enzyme may be the main factor responsible for the enhanced release (Fernández et al, 1995; Martinez-Cuesta et al, 1996), it cannot be ruled out that additional nitric oxide formation from the inducible enzyme occurs in advanced stages of liver disease (Guarner et al, 1993).

It has been suggested that portal hypertension renders the gastric mucosa more susceptible to damage (Sarfeh et al, 1983, 1988; Beck et al, 1992; Nishizaki et al, 1994). This hypothesis, which has not definitively been proven in humans, arises from several studies performed in experimental models of portal hypertension. An increased gastric mucosal damage has been reported in rats with total portal vein occlusion, common bile duct ligation or cirrhosis induced by carbon tetrachloride (Sarfeh et al, 1983, 1988; Beck et al, 1992; Nishizaki et al, 1994). The mechanisms by which gastric mucosa becomes more susceptible in these animal models is unclear. Several factors have been proposed, including decreased trans-mucosal potential difference, impaired reactive hyperaemia, impaired gastric mucosal oxygenation, thinner gastric mucous gel layer and decreased surface cell intracellular pH (Sarfeh et al, 1989; Beck et al, 1992; Nishizaki et al, 1994; Ferraz et al, 1995).

In humans with cirrhosis, some contradictory results have been published regarding this issue. While decreased gastric potential difference (Payen et al, 1995b) and decreased gastric ATP and energy charge level have been reported (Kawano et al, 1996), other investigators have not found any significant change in the gastric intramucosal pH of cirrhotic patients with PHG in comparison with controls (Lamarque et al, 1994).

From the clinical point of view, several reports have pointed out the increased incidence of peptic ulcer or gastric erosions in patients with cirrhosis (Rabinovitz et al, 1990; Siringo et al, 1995; Chen et al, 1996). However, it is not clear whether this phenomenon is related to portal hypertension or may be influenced by co-factors such as chronic endotoxaemia or renal impairment commonly present in patients with advanced liver disease.

CLINICAL MANIFESTATIONS

The presence of PHG does not promote dyspeptic symptoms. The single clinical manifestation of this gastric vascular alteration is overt or chronic upper-GI bleeding. This complication usually occurs in cirrhotic patients with severe PHG, whereas this is uncommon in patients with mild vascular lesions. Chronic gastric mucosal bleeding and recurrent iron-deficiency anaemia, some times requiring blood transfusion, are the most character-istic clinical features of patients with PHG. Overt bleeding is less frequent, and it is usually presented by repeated episodes of self-limited haemorrhage. However, in a few patients bleeding can be persistent or recurrent and life-threatening.

In the series of patients reported by D'Amico et al (1990), overt bleed-ing occurred in 60% of patients with severe PHG during a 5-year follow-up. A cumulative risk of bleeding of 75% was calculated in these patients during the follow-up period. A higher risk (90%) of minor and/or chronic bleeding was documented for patients with severe PHG. Once the first episode of bleeding from PHG has occurred, the risk of rebleeding from the same source is as high as 62% at 12 months after the index haemorrhage, and up to 75% in 2 years of follow-up (Pérez et al, 1991).

Sustained chronic anaemia, which is usually present in cirrhotic patients with severe PHG, may be a deleterious factor worsening the hyperdynamic circulation of such patients. In that regard, it has been demonstrated that chronic anaemia enhances gastric mucosal blood flow in cirrhotic patients with PHG (Cirera et al, 1995), and there is preliminary evidence showing that anaemia may worsen the systemic vasodilation of cirrhotic patients (Elizalde et al, 1996). This effect could be produced by the increment of nitric oxide availability in the blood stream as a consequence of the reduced blood haemoglobin, one of the most important natural scavengers of nitric oxide in the vessel lumen (Panés et al, 1992b).

Bleeding from PHG is an unusual direct cause of death and it has been shown in multivariate regression analysis that it is not an independent risk factor that affects survival in patients with cirrhosis (D'Amico et al, 1990). However, repeated bleeding episodes or maintained chronic anaemia that requires blood transfusions may probably contribute to the deterioration of liver function.

THERAPEUTIC OPTIONS

The therapeutic approach to bleeding gastric mucosal lesions in cirrhotic patients has significantly improved within the last 10–15 years (Table 2).

When bleeding gastric mucosal lesions in cirrhosis were considered a characteristic form of gastritis, antisecretory drugs or antacids were used. This kind of treatment has proven unsuccessful (Rector and Reynolds, 1965; McCormack et al, 1985), and we now know that there is no rationale basis for its use, because there is a lack of evidence supporting a role for acid secretion in the pathogenesis of this alteration. At that time, the only reported effective treatment for gastric mucosal bleeding in patients with

Table 2. Therapeutic approaches to bleeding gastric mucosal lesions in cirrhotic patients in the last 10–15 years.

Treatment	Years	Efficacy	Risk
Antisecretory drugs	Prior to 1986	Ineffective	None
Portocaval shunt	Prior to 1986	Effective	High risk in advanced liver disease
Propranolol	From 1987	Effective in 50% of the patients	Some contraindications
Endoscopic haemostasis is confined to a restricted area	From 1987	Effective if bleeding	Minor
Somatostatin/glypressin	From 1993	Unknown	Minor
TIPSS	From 1994	Uncertain	Moderate
Transplantation	From 1986	Effective	High risk

cirrhosis was decompressive shunt surgery. Reynolds et al (1981), and Sarfeh et al (1982) reported no rebleeding episodes from gastric lesions after a portocaval shunt. More recently, Orloff et al (1995) have reported the results of 12 cirrhotic patients with bleeding PHG who were submitted to portocaval shunt. In all patients definitive haemostasis was obtained with the surgical procedure, the mucosal lesions disappeared in further endoscopic controls, and no recurrent bleeding was observed during follow-up. Although the shunt surgery seems to be an effective treatment for bleeding PHG, this procedure has not been considered up to now as the first option for treating such complications. This is because of the universal decline in the use of surgery to prevent rebleeding in cirrhotic patients, and the introduction of effective pharmacological options for the control of upper-GI bleeding in cirrhosis.

Two open studies performed 10 years ago in a limited number of cirrhotic patients had reported beneficial effects of propranolol in the control of bleeding PHG (Quintero et al, 1985; Hosking et al, 1987). The rationale for the use of β-adrenergic blockers in this pathological condition is based on both experimental and clinical investigations demonstrating that this drug reduces portal pressure and induces significant vasoconstriction in the overall splanchnic vascular bed. It has been shown in rats with partial portal vein ligation that propranolol, at a dose that consistently reduces portal pressure, induces a slight but significant reduction in gastric mucosal blood flow (Piqué et al, 1990). Similar results were obtained in patients with cirrhosis and PHG where a significant fall in gastric mucosal blood flow assessed by laser-Doppler and reflectance spectrophotometry was observed after acute double-blind infusion of propranolol in comparison with placebo (Panés et al, 1993).

Up to now, only one prospective controlled study is available that demonstrates the efficacy of propranolol to prevent rebleeding from PHG in cirrhosis (Pérez et al, 1991). In that study, the actuarial proportion of patients free of rebleeding during follow-up was significantly higher in patients treated with propranolol than in those included in the control group. The multivariate analysis showed that propranolol therapy was the only predictive variable for rebleeding. In addition, patients under propranolol treatment presented a lower number of bleeding episodes and required fewer blood transfusions than controls. However, despite the proven efficacy of this drug for preventing rebleeding from PHG, 50% of cirrhotic patients under such therapy still presented with rebleeding episodes within 2 years of follow-up.

Spontaneous haemostasis usually occurs in cirrhotic patients with overt bleeding from PHG, but in some cases repeated bleeding episodes that require blood transfusion may lead to a critical situation in these patients. In such cases, propranolol is often not helpful and may introduce some inconvenience in assessing the usual haemodynamic response to hypovolaemic shock. If the bleeding lesions are confined to a restricted area in the gastric mucosa, endoscopic photocoagulation or electrocoagulation may be effective to arrest active bleeding. Several reports have suggested that haemostasis of gastric vascular lesions can be achieved by repeated sessions of different modalities of endoscopic therapy (Rutgeerts et al, 1985, Gosutout et al, 1989).

When bleeding is diffuse or comes from different regions of the stomach, the endoscopic treatment is not useful. In this situation, drugs acutely reducing gastric perfusion might be effective, but no clinical trials are available to assess its effectiveness in arresting bleeding from gastric mucosal lesions in cirrhosis. Preliminary studies have demonstrated that i.v. infusion of vasopressin, glypressin or somatostatin is effective in reducing gastric blood perfusion in cirrhotic patients with PHG (Panés et al, 1994a,b). Somatostatin and glypressin would be preferable since both drugs reduce gastric blood flow without impairing gastric mucosal oxygenation, a deleterious effect that can be usually seen by using vasopressin (Panés et al, 1994a).

Other therapeutic alternatives to stop bleeding or to prevent rebleeding from PHG may be the transjugular intrahepatic portosystemic shunt (TIPSS) or the orthotopic liver transplantation. Single clinical observations have provided evidence that liver transplantation may prevent bleeding from PHG. With regard to TIPSS, a few reports that included a small number of patients have suggested that this procedure can be useful in preventing bleeding from PHG (Simpson et al, 1993; Nolte et al, 1995). However, no specific study has been published that directly addresses the effectiveness of that procedure for preventing bleeding from PHG, and some caution needs to be used since there is evidence that this procedure may worsen the hyperdynamic circulatory state of the cirrhotic patient (Azoulay et al, 1994).

Finally, since patients with severe PHG have an increased risk of bleeding, prospective controlled trials are needed to address whether or not drugs such as propranolol or other β-blockers may be useful in preventing the first bleeding episode from gastric mucosal vascular lesions.

REFERENCES

*D'Amico G, Montalabano L, Traina M et al (1990) Natural history of congestive gastropathy. *Gastroenterology* 99: 1558–1564.

Azoulay D, Castaing D, Dennison A et al (1994) Transjugular intrahepatic portosystemic shunt worsens the hyperdynamic circulation state of the cirrhotic patient: preliminary report of a prospective study. *Hepatology* 19: 129–132.

Beck PL, Lee SS, McKnight W & Wallace JL (1992) Characterization of spontaneous and ethanol-induced gastric damage in cirrhotic rats. *Gastroenterology* 103: 1048–1055.

Beck PL, McKnight W, Lee SS & Wallace JL (1993) Prostaglandin modulation of the gastric vasculatures and musosal integrity in cirrhotic rats. *American Journal of Physiology* 265: G453–G458.

Benoit JN & Granger DN (1986) Splanchnic hemodynamics in chronic portal hypertension. *Seminars in Liver Disease* 6: 287–298.

Benoit J, Barrowman JA, Harper SL et al (1984) Role of humoral factors in the intestinal hyperemia associated with chronic portal hypertension. *American Journal of Physiology* 247: G486–G493.

Benoit J, Womack RA, Korthius RJ et al (1986) Chronic portal hypertension: effects of gastro-intestinal flow distribution. *American Journal of Physiology* 1250: G535–G539.

Cahill PA, Wu Y & Sitzmann JV (1994) Altered adenylcyclase activities and G-protein abnormalities in portal hypertensive rabbits. *Journal of Clinical Investigation* 93: 2691–2700.

Calès P, Zabotto B, Meskens C et al (1990) Gastroesophageal endoscopic features in cirrhosis. Obesrver variability, interassociations, and relationship to hepatic dysfunction. *Gastroenterology* **98**: 156–162.

Casadevall M, Panés J, Piqué JM et al (1992) Limitations of laser-Doppler and reflectance spectro-photometry in estimating gastric blood flow. *American Journal of Physiology* **263**: G810–G815.

*Casadevall M, Panés J, Piqué JM et al (1993) Involvement of nitric oxide and prostaglandins in gastric mucosal hyperemia of portal hypertensive anesthetized rats. *Hepatology* **18**: 628–634.

Casadevall M, Piqué JM, Cirera I et al (1996) Increased blood hemoglobin attenuates splanchnic vasodilation in portal-hypertensive rats by nitric oxide inhibition. *Gastroenterology* **110**: 1156–1165.

Chen L–S, Lin H–C, Hwang S–J et al (1996) Prevalence of gastric ulcer in cirrhotic patients and its relation to portal hypertension. *Journal of Gastroenterology and Hepatology* **11**: 59–64.

Chey WY, Hendricks J & Lorber SH (1971) Inactivation of secretin by the liver. *Clinical Research* **19**: 389–405.

Chung RS, Bruch D & Dearlove J (1988) Endoscopic measurement of gastric mucosal blood flow by laser-Doppler velocimetry: effect of chronic esophageal variceal sclerosis. *American Surgeon* **54**: 116–120.

Cirera I, Panés J, Bordas JM et al (1995) Anemia increases gastric blood flow in noncirrhotic and cirrhotic patients. *Gastrointestinal Endoscopy* **42**: 403–407.

Corbishley CM, Saverymuttu SH & Maxwell JD (1988) Use of endoscopic biopsy for diagnosing congestive gastropathy *Journal of Clinical Pathology* **41**: 1187–1190.

Elizalde JI, García-Pagán JC, Bandi JC et al (1996) Effects of increasing hemoglobin concentration on the hyperdynamic circulation of patients with liver cirrhosis and anemia. [abstract] *Gastroenterology* **110**: A1186.

Fernández M, García-Pagán JC, Casadevall M et al (1995) Evidence against a role for inducible nitric oxide synthase in the hyperdynamic circulation of portal hypertensive rats. *Gastroenterology* **108**: 1487–1495.

Fernandéz M, García-Pagán JC, Casadevall M et al (1996) Acute and chronic cyclooxygenase blockade in portal-hypertensive rats: influence on nitric oxide biosynthesis. *Gastroenterology* **110**: 1529–1535.

Ferraz JP & Wallace JL (1996) Prostaglandins modulate the responsiveness of the gastric micro-circulation to sodium nitroprusside in cirrhotic rats. *Hepatology* **23**: 123–129.

Ferraz JGP, McKnight W, Sharkey KA & Wallace JL (1995) Impaired vasodilatory responses in the gastric microcirculation of anesthetized rats with secondary biliary cirrhosis. *Gastroenterology* **108**: 1183–1191.

Geraghty JG, Angerson WJ & Carter DC (1989) Autoradiographic study of the regional distribution of gastric blood flow in portal hypertensive rats. *Gastroenterology* **97**: 1108–1114.

Gosutout CJ, Ahlquist DA, Radford CM et al (1989) Endoscopic laser therapy for watermelon stomach. *Gastroenterology* **96**: 1462–1465.

Gosutout CVJ, Viggiano TR, Ahlquist DA et al (1992) The clinical and endoscopic spectrum of the watermelon stomach. *Journal of Clinical Gastroenterology* **15**: 256–263.

Guarner C, Soriano G, Tomás A et al (1993) Increased serum nitrite and nitrate levels in patients with cirrhosis: relationship to endotoxemia. *Hepatology* **18**: 1139–1143.

Hashizume M & Sugimachi K (1995) Classification of gastric lesions associated with portal hyper-tension. *Journal of Gastroenterology and Hepatology* **10**: 339–343.

Hashizume M, Tanaka K & Inokuchi K (1983) Morphology of gastric micro-circulation in cirrhosis. *Hepatology* **3**: 1008–1012.

Henriksen JH, Staun-Olsen P & Fahrenkrug T (1980) Vasoactive intestinal polypeptide (VIP) in cirrhosis: arteriovenous extraction in different vascular beds *Scandinavian Journal of Gastroenterology* **15**: 787–792.

Hosking SW, Kennedy HJ, Seddon Y & Triger DR (1987) The role of propranolol in congestive gastropathy of portal hypertension. *Hepatology* **7**: 437–441.

Iwao T, Toyonaga A, Sumino M et al (1992) Portal hypertensive gastropathy in patients with cirrhosis. *Gastroenterology* **102**: 2060–2065.

Iwao T, Toyonaga A, Ikegami M et al (1993) Reduced gastric mucosal blood flow in patients with portal-hypertensive gastropathy. *Hepatology* **18**: 36–40.

Kawano S, Tanimura H, Tsuji S et al (1996) Gastric mucosal metabolism and intracellular mucin content changes in patients with liver cirrhosis. *Journal of Gastroenterology and Hepatology* **11**: 380–384.

Kiel JW, Pitts V, Benoit J et al (1985) Reduced vascular sensitivity to norepinephrine in portal hypertensive rats. *American Journal of Physiology* **248**: G192–G195.

Kitano S, Koyanagi M, Sugimuchi K et al (1982) Mucosal blood flow and modified vascular responses to norepinephrine in the stomach of rats with liver cirrhosis. *European Journal of Surgical Research* **14**: 221–230.

Kotelanski B, Groszmann RJ & Cohn JN (1972) Circulation times in the splanchnic and hepatic beds in alcoholic liver disease. *Gastroenterology* **63**: 102–111.

Kotzampasi K, Eleftheriadis E & Aletras H (1990) The 'mosaic-like' pattern of portal hypertensive gastric mucosa after variceal eradication of sclerotherapy. *Journal of Gastroenterology and Hepatology* **5**: 659–663.

Kozarek RA, Botoman VA, Bredfeldt JE et al (1991) Portal colopathy: prospective study of colopathy in patients with portal hypertension. *Gastroenterology* **101**: 1192–1197.

Lamarque D, Levoir D, Duvoux C et al (1994) Measurement of gastric intramucosal pH in patients with cirrhosis and portal hypertensive gastropathy. *Gastroenterology and Clinical Biology* **18**: 969–974.

*McCormack TT, Sims J, Eyre-Brook Y et al (1985) Gastric lesions in portal hypertension: inflammatory gastritis or congestive gastropathy? *Gut* **26**: 1226–1232.

McCormick PA, Sankey EA, Cardin F et al (1991) Congestive gastropathy and *Helicobacter pylori*: an endoscopic and morphometric study. *Gut* **32**: 351–354.

Martínez-Cuesta MA, Moreno L, Piqué JM et al (1996) Nitric oxide mediated β_2-adrenorecpetor relaxation is impaired in mesenteric veins from portal hypertensive rats. *Gastroenterology* **111**: 727–735.

Matsutani S, Furuse J, Ishii H et al (1993) Hemodynamics of the left gastric vein in portal hypertension. *Gastroenterology* **105**: 513–518.

Nagral AS, Joshi AS, Bhatia SJ et al (1993) Congestive jejunopathy in portal hypertension. *Gut* **34**: 694–697.

Naveau S, Bedossa P, Poynard T et al (1991) Portal hypertensive colopathy: a new entity. *Digestive Diseases in Science* **36**: 1774–1781.

NIEC Proceedings of III National Congress. Milano, 1992.

Nishiwaki H, Asai T, Sowa M & Umeyama K (1990) Endoscopic measurement of gastric mucosal blood flow with special reference to the effect of sclerotherapy in patients with liver cirrhosis. *American Journal of Gastroenterology* **85**: 34–37.

Nishizaki Y, Kaunitz JD, Oda M & Guth PH (1994) Impairment of gastric mucosal defense measured *in vivo* in cirrhotic rats. *Hepatology* **20**: 445–452.

Nishizaki Y, Guth PH, Sternini C & Kaunitz JD (1996) Impairment of the gastric hyperemic response to luminal acid in cirrhotic rats. *American Journal of Physiology* **270**: G71–G78.

Nolte W, Wiltfang JG, Kunert HJ et al (1995) Initial experiences with TIPS (transjugular intrahepatic portasystemic stent-shunt). *Leber Magen Damm* **25**: 264–266.

*Orloff MJ, Orloff MS, Orloff S & Haynes KS (1995) Treatment of bleeding from portal hypertensive gastropathy by portocaval shunt. *Hepatology* **21**: 1011–1017.

Otha M, Hashizume M, Higashi H et al (1996) Portal and gastric mucosal hemodynamics in cirrhotic patients with portal-hypertensive gastropathy. *Hepatology* **20**: 1432–1436.

*Panés J, Bordas JM, Piqué JM et al (1992a) Increased gastric mucosal perfusion in cirrhotic patients with portal hypertensive gastropathy. *Gastroenterology* **103**: 1875–1882.

Panés J, Casadevall M, Piqué JM et al (1992b) Effects of acute normovolemic anemia on gastric mucosal blood flow in rats: role of nitric oxide. *Gastroenterology* **103**: 407–413.

Panés J, Bordas JM, Piqué JM et al (1993) Effects of propranolol on gastric mucosal perfusion in cirrhotic patients with portal hypertensive gastropathy. *Hepatology* **17**: 213–218.

Panés J, Piqué JM, Bordas JM et al (1994a) Reduction of gastric hyperemia by glypressin and vasopressin administration in cirrhotic patients with portal hypertensive gastropathy. *Hepatology* **19**: 55–60.

Panés J, Piqué JM, Bordas JM et al (1994b) Effect of bolus injection and continuous infusion of somatostatin on gastric perfusion in cirrhotic patients with portal-hypertensive gastropathy. *Hepatology* **20**: 336–341.

*Papazian A, Braillon A, Duppas JL et al (1986) Portal hypertensive gastric mucosa: and endoscopic study. *Gut* **27**: 1199–1203.

Payen JL, Calès P, Voigt JJ et al (1995a) Severe portal hypertensive gastropathy and antral vascular ectasia are distinct entities in patients with cirrhosis. *Gastroenterology* **108**: 138–144.

Payen JL, Calès P, Pienkowski P, Sozzani P et al (1995b) Weakness of mucosal barrier in portal hypertensive gastropathy of alcoholic cirrhosis. Effect of propranolol and enprostil. *Journal of Hepatology* **23:** 689–696.

Pérez RM, Piqué JM, Saperas E et al (1989) Gastric vascular ectasia in cirrhosis: association with hypoacidity not related with gastric atrophy. *Scandinavion Journal of Gastroenterology* **24:** 1073–1078.

*Pérez Ayuso RM, Piqué JM, Bosch J et al (1991) Propranolol in the prevention of rebleeding from portal hypertensive gastropathy. *Lancet* **337:** 1431–1434.

*Piqué JM, Leung FW, Kitahora T et al (1988) Gastric mucosal blood flow and acid secretion in portal hypertensive rats. *Gastroenterology* **95:** 727–733.

Piqué JM, Pizcueta P, Pérez RM et al (1990) Effects of propranolol on gastric mucosal blood flow and acid secretion. *Hepatology* **12:** 476–480.

Pizcueta P, Casamitjana R, Bosch J & Rodés J (1990) Decreased systemic vascular sensitivity to norepinephrine in portal hypertensive rats. Role of hyperglucagonism. *American Journal of Physiology* **258:** G191–G195.

*Pizcueta P, Piqué JM, Fernández M et al (1992a) Modulation of the hyperdynamic circulation of cirrhotic rats by nitric oxide inhibition. *Gastroenterology* **103:** 1909–1915.

Pizcueta P, Piqué J, Bosch J et al (1992b) Effects of inhibiting nitric oxide biosynthesis on the systemic and splanchnic circulation of rats with portal hypertension. *British Journal of Pharmacology* **105:** 184–190.

Quintero E, Piqué JM, Bombí JA et al (1985) Antral mucosal hyperemia: characterization of a portal hypertension related syndrome causing bleeding in patients with cirrhosis. *Journal of Hepatology* **1 (supplement 2):** S315.

*Quintero E, Piqué JM, Bombí JA et al (1987) Gastric vascular ectasia causing bleeding in patients with cirrhosis: a distinct entity associated with hypergastrinemia and low serum levels of pepsinogen Y. *Gastroenterology* **93:** 1054–1061.

Rabinovitz M, Yoo YK, Schade RR et al (1990) Prevalence of endoscopic findings in 510 consecutive individuals with cirrhosis evaluated prospectively. *Digestive Diseases of Science* **35:** 705–710.

Rector WG & Reynolds TB (1965) Risk factors for hemorrhage from esophageal varices and acute gastric lesions. *Clinical Gastroenterology* **15:** 139–153.

Reynolds TB, Donovan AJ, Mikkelsen WP et al (1981) Results of a 12-year randomized trial of porto-caval shunt in patients with liver disease and bleeding varices. *Gastroenterology* **80:** 1005–1011.

Rutgeerts P, Van Gompel F, Geboes K et al (1985) Long term results of treatment of vascular malformations of the gastrointestinal tract by neodymium Yag laser photocoagulation. *Gut* **26:** 586–593.

Saperas E, Piqué JM, Pérez RM et al (1989) Comparison between jumbo and large forceps biopsies in the histologic diagnosis of gastric vascular ectasia in cirrhosis. *Endoscopy* **21:** 165–167.

Saperas E, Pérez RM, Poca E et al (1990) Increased gastric PGE2 biosynthesis in cirrhotic patients with gastric vascular ectasia. *American Journal of Gastroenterology* **85:** 138–140.

Sarfeh IJ, Juler GL, Stemmer EA & Mason GR (1982) Results of surgical management of hemorrhagic gastritis in patients with gastroesophageal varices. *Surgical and Gynecological Obstetrics* **155:** 167–170.

Sarfeh IJ, Tarnawski A, Malki A et al (1983) Portal hypertension and gastric mucosal injury in rats. Effects of alcohol. *Gastroenterology* **84:** 987–993.

Sarfeh IJ, Tarnawski A, Hajduczeck A et al (1988) The portal hypertensive gastric mucosa: histological, ultrastructural, and functional analysis after aspirin-induced damage. *Surgery* **104:** 79–85.

Sarfeh IJ, Soliman H, Waxman K et al (1989) Impaired oxygenation of gastric mucosa in portal hypertension. The basis for increased susceptibility to injury. *Digestive Diseases and Science* **2:** 225–228.

Sarin SK, Misra SP, Singal A et al (1988) Evaluation of the incidence and significance of the mosaic pattern in patients with cirrhosis, noncirrhotic portal fibrosis and extrahepatic obstruction. *American Journal of Gastroenterology* **83:** 1235–1239.

Sarin SK, Sreenivas DV, Lahoti D & Saraya A (1992) Factors influencing development of portal hypertensive gastropathy in patients with portal hypertension. *Gastroenterology* **102:** 994–999.

Sieber C, López-Talavera JC & Groszmann RJ (1993) Role of nitric oxide in the *in vitro* splanchnic vascular hyporeactivity in ascitic cirrhotic rats. *Gastroenterology* **104:** 1750–1754.

Simpson KJ, Chalmers N, Redhead DN et al (1993) Transjugular intrahepatic portasystemic shunting for control of acute and recurrent upper gastrointestinal haemorrhage related to portal hypertension. *Gut* **34:** 968–973.

Siringo S, Burroughs AK, Bolondi L et al (1995) Peptic ulcer and its course in cirrhosis: an endo-scopic and clinical prospective study. *Journal of Hepatology* **22**: 633–641.

Sitzmann JV, Bulkley GB, Mitchell M & Campbell K (1988) Role of prostacyclin in the splanchnic hyperemia contributing to portal hypertension. *Annals of Surgery* **209**: 322–327.

Spina GP, Arcidiacono R, Bosch J et al (1994) Gastric endoscopic features in portal hypertension: final report of a consensus conference, Milan, Italy, September 19, 1992. *Journal of Hepatology* **21**: 461–467.

Tanoue K, Hashizume M, Wada H et al (1992) Effect of endoscopic injection sclerotherapy on portal hypertensive gastropathy: a prospective study. *Gastrointestinal Endoscopy* **38**: 582–585.

Triger Dr & Hosking SW (1989) The gastric mucosa in portal hypertension. *Journal of Hepatology* **8**: 267–272.

Vigneri S, Termini R, Piraino A et al (1991) The stomach in liver cirrhosis. Endoscopic, morpho-logical, and clinical correlations. *Gastroenterology* **101**: 472–478.

Vorobioff J, Bredfeldt JE & Groszmann RJ (1983) Hyperdynamic circulation in portal-hypertensive rat model: a primary factor for maintenance of chronic portal hypertension. *American Journal of Physiology* **244**: G52–G57.

Yamamoto Y, Sezai S, Sakurabayashi S et al (1992) Effect of hepatic collateral hemodynamics on gastric mucosal blood flow in patients with liver cirrhosis. *Digestive Diseases and Sciences* **37**: 1319–1323.

5

Pharmacological prevention of variceal bleeding. New developments

JOAN CARLES GARCÍA-PAGÁN* MD

Staff Member

JAUME BOSCH MD

Professor of Medicine

Hepatic Haemodynamic Laboratory, Liver Unit, Department of Medicine, Hospital Clínic i Provincial, University of Barcelona, Villarroel 170, 08036 Barcelona, Spain

The introduction of pharmacological therapy has been one of the major advances in the treatment of the complications of portal hypertension. Many drugs have been shown to reduce portal hypertension in patients with cirrhosis. However, the most widely used drugs and the only ones for which there is sufficient evidence, are the beta-blockers. These drugs have been, up to now, the only accepted prophylactic therapy for oesophageal variceal bleeding and are also an alternative treatment to sclerotherapy or surgery to prevent variceal rebleeding. A reduction in portal pressure gradient by beta-blockers below 12 mmHg or by more than 20% of baseline values is associated with almost a total protection from oesophageal bleeding. Such a marked response in portal pressure is only achieved in some patients receiving propranolol. New pharmacological approaches with a greater portal pressure reducing effect may improve the beneficial effect of drugs in preventing variceal bleeding. The more promising approach is the combined administration of beta-blockers and isosorbide-5-mononitrate, which has been shown to potentiate the reduction in portal pressure and to be highly effective in initial randomized clinical trials.

Key words: portal hypertension; cirrhosis; pharmacological therapy; beta-blockers; nitrates.

Portal hypertension is a major complication of chronic liver disease. Its main clinical consequence, bleeding from ruptured oesophagogastric varices, represents a dramatic medical emergency with a mortality rate ranging from 30 to 50% (García-Pagán et al, 1989).

* Address for correspondence

Baillière's Clinical Gastroenterology—
Vol. 11, No. 2, June 1997
ISBN 0–7020–2339–6
0950–3528/97/020271 + 17 $12.00/00

271

Many efforts have been made over the past three decades in the treatment and prevention of variceal bleeding. During the last decade, marked improvement in the knowledge of the pathophysiology of portal hypertension has opened the scene to pharmacological treatments, resulting in a dramatic change in the therapeutic approach to portal hypertension. This field has experienced substantial advances after the introduction of the concept that portal hypertension, in analogy with arterial hypertension, can be treated effectively by continuous drug administration (Bosch et al, 1993).

RATIONAL BASIS FOR PHARMACOLOGICAL THERAPY

The pharmacological treatment of portal hypertension is based on the assumption that a sustained reduction in portal pressure shall reduce the incidence of the complications of portal hypertension.

As it has been previously discussed that portal pressure is determined by the product of the blood flow circulating through the portal venous system and the vascular resistance that opposes that flow. Increased resistance to portal blood flow is the primary factor in the pathophysiology of portal hypertension. There is now a great body of evidence indicating that there is an active component in the increased hepatic resistance of cirrhosis, which can be influenced by several stimuli, including pharmacological agents (Bathal and Grossman, 1985; Ballet et al, 1988). Recent studies suggest that increased hepatic resistance in cirrhosis may be in part because of an insufficient release of nitric oxide at the hepatic microcirculation (Pizcueta et al, 1992; Mittal et al, 1994). These observations provide the rational basis for the use of vasodilators (and especially of nitrovasodilators) in the treatment of portal hypertension (see below). Another factor contributing to the maintenance and aggravation of the portal pressure elevation is an increased inflow of blood into the portal venous system, as a result of splanchnic arteriolar vasodilatation (Vorobioff et al, 1983). Up to now, most attempts at the pharmacological treatment of portal hypertension have been aimed at correcting this increased portal blood inflow by the use of splanchnic vasocontrictors.

Splanchnic vasodilatation is characteristically associated with peripheral vasodilatation and hyperkinetic circulation, with reduced arterial pressure and peripheral resistance, and increased cardiac output (Bosch et al, 1992). Peripheral vasodilatation plays a major role in the activation of neurohumoral systems leading to sodium retention and expansion of plasma volume. Expansion of the plasma volume is thought also to play a role in the maintenance of portal hypertension (Zimmon and Kessler, 1974; García-Pagán et al, 1994b), which provides the rationale for using diuretic agents in the treatment of portal hypertension. Therefore, the pharmacological treatment of portal hypertension is based on the use of drugs that reduce the porto-hepatic vascular resistance, the portal blood flow, the blood volume or any combination of these parameters.

EFFECTS OF PHARMACOLOGICAL AGENTS ON PORTAL HYPERTENSION

Many drugs have been shown to reduce portal pressure in man (Table 1). For practical purposes, only orally administered drugs are suitable for continuous administration (i.e. for the prevention of oesophageal variceal bleeding). These are listed in Table 1, and include beta-adrenergic blockers, nitrovasodilators, serotonin antagonists, clonidine, prazosin and diuretics. There is only large clinical experience for beta-blockers. Other agents have powerful portal pressure reducing effects but require parenteral administration and are used in the medical treatment of acute variceal haemorrhage.

Table 1. Drugs with proven portal pressure decreasing effects that may be used in the long-term treatment of portal hypertension.

Vasoconstrictors:
  Beta-blockers:
    Propranolol
    Nadolol
    Timolol
    Atenolol

Vasodilators:
  Long-acting nitrates:
    Isosorbide-5-mononitrate
    Isosorbide dinitrate
  Molsidomine
  Anti-serotoninergics:
    Ketanserine
    Ritanserine
  Alpha-adrenergic agonists and antagonists:
    Clonidine
    Prazosin

Diuretics
  Spironolactone

Other
  Nipradilol

Combination therapies:
  Propranolol or nadolol + isosorbide-5-mononitrate
  Propranolol + isosorbide dinitrate
  Propranolol + clonidine
  Propranolol + prazosin
  Propranolol + ketanserin
  Propranolol + ritanserin
  Propranolol + spironolactone

Haemodynamic effects of beta-blockers

Non-selective beta-blockers, such as propranolol and nadolol, reduce portal pressure by reducing the portal inflow and hence, the portal and collateral blood flows. Reduction of portal inflow is the result of a decrease in cardiac output caused by the blockade of cardiac beta-1 adrenoceptors, and of splanchnic vasoconstriction because of the blockade of vasodilating beta-2 adrenoceptors in the splanchnic vasculature (Bosch et al, 1984; Mastai et al, 1987). This explains why cardioselective beta-blockers have less effect on reducing portal pressure. The decrease in portal pressure is accompanied by a significant reduction in the pressure of the oesophageal varices (Feu et al, 1993). Measurements of azygos blood flow suggest that another beneficial effect of propranolol in portal hypertension is a marked reduction in the gastroesophageal collateral blood flow, which is observed in most patients (Bosch et al, 1984).

Propranolol is given orally. B.i.d. administration is recommended. Adjustment of the dose is done by stepwise increases by carefully looking at clinical tolerance, heart rate and arterial blood pressure. In general, the dose is increased every 2 days until heart rate decreases by 25%, but not below 55 beats per minute and a systolic blood pressure of above 90 mmHg is maintained. Once the maintenance dose is reached, it is possible to give the total dose in a single administration of a long-acting preparation. If nadolol is used, only the breakfast dose is required since the biological half-life is long enough for once a day administration.

A major inconvenience of propranolol therapy is that over one-third of the patients do not exhibit any decrease in portal pressure despite adequate beta-blockade (Garcia-Tsao et al, 1986; García-Pagán et al, 1990b). The mechanism of non-response is not well understood but it is not related to inadequate dose, aetiology or severity of portal hyper-tension, circulating levels of adrenaline and noradrenaline, nor to down-regulation of beta-2 adrenoceptors (García-Pagán et al, 1992). It is likely that non-response is in part because of the fact that an increase in portal-collateral resistance attenuates the reduction in portal pressure promoted by the decrease in portal venous inflow (Kroeger and Groszmann, 1985). Such an increase in portal-collateral resistance has been documented in experimental models, and may depend on the extent of the collateral circulation (Pizcueta et al, 1989; Escorsell et al, 1997). Thus, there is a wide individual variation in the reduction of portal pressure achieved with propranolol. The portal pressure response to propranolol on a given patient cannot be predicted on clinical grounds or by using non-invasive investigations. This makes it convenient to schedule follow-up measure-ments of HVPG during propranolol therapy. This is especially important since it has been demonstrated that the protection afforded by propranolol depends on the degree of portal pressure reduction (Groszmann et al, 1990; Feu et al, 1995).

The more frequently encountered contra-indications to beta-blockers in patients with cirrhosis are chronic obstructive lung disease, psychosis, A-V heart blocks, aortic valve disease and insulin-dependent diabetes with a past history of hypoglycaemia. Side effects are reported in about 15% of the patients, but severe events (bronchospasm, etc.) are rare. The more frequent complaints are fatigue, shortness of breath (often associated with marked bradycardia, with heart rates below 50 bpm) and sleep disorders. Although complications from propranolol therapy in cirrhosis have never been lethal, side effects are important inasmuch as they detract from compliance. Nadolol is easier to administer because of more prolonged half-life (allowing once a day administration) and is eliminated by the kidneys, which makes its dosage easier than that of propranolol. Also, it has been suggested that since it does not cross the blood–brain barrier it is less likely to cause central effects and side effects. However, this has not been adequately investigated in cirrhosis.

Adequate protection from the risk of bleeding is only achieved when the HVPG is decreased below 12 mmHg (Groszmann et al, 1990) or at least, by more than 20% of baseline values (Feu et al, 1995). This is possible only in a small percentage of patients treated with propranolol. It appears that in order to improve the results of propranolol therapy we have to develop alternative therapies that can offer effective reductions in HVPG in a greater proportion of patients. This is the rationale for looking for new, powerful agents, that alone or in combination with propranolol, may enhance the portal pressure reduction and decrease the number of non-responders (Bosch et al, 1993).

Other pharmacological approaches

Vasodilators

Vasodilators have been investigated in recent years as a possible alternative to beta-blockers in the pharmacological treatment of portal hypertension. These drugs may reduce portal pressure by decreasing the vascular resistance to portal-collateral blood flow, and also, by promoting reflex splanchnic vasoconstriction as a response to reduced mean arterial and cardiac filling pressures (Blei and Gottstein, 1986; Navasa et al, 1989). A further advantage of vasodilators over beta-blockers is that the former may allow a reduction in portal pressure without further impairing liver perfusion (and liver function).

Long-acting nitrovasodilators

Long-acting nitrovasodilators, such as isosorbide dinitrate (Blei et al, 1987; Merkel et al, 1987) or isosorbide-5-mononitrate (Hayes et al, 1988; Navasa et al, 1989; García-Pagán et al, 1990a), have been shown to markedly reduce HVPG (hepatic venous pressure gradient) in acute administration but significantly less after chronic administration, probably because of the development of partial tolerance (García-Pagán et al, 1990a). Isosorbide-5-mononitrate has also been shown to reduce oesophageal variceal pressure (Escorsell et al, 1996). Isosorbide-5-mononitrate, unlike isosorbide dinitrate, has minimal first-pass metabolism, which facilitate dosage in patients with liver failure and portal systemic shunting. Indeed, this is the only vasodilator that has been evaluated in randomized controlled trials for the prevention of variceal haemorrhage.

The major concern with the use of vasodilators in patients with advanced cirrhosis is that they can reduce arterial blood pressure and thus promote the activation of endogenous vasoactive systems that may lead to water and sodium retention as well as to the worsening of renal function in patients with ascites (Salmeron et al, 1993). However, recent studies have shown that long-term treatment with isosorbide-5-mononitrate is safe in compensated cirrhotic patients, without affecting renal function or sodium handling. In a few patients with ascites, hypotension and transient sodium retention was observed, but without need to increase the dose of diuretics (Salerno et al, 1996).

Molsidomine

Molsidomine is a prodrug that is metabolized in the liver to its active metabolite SIN-1. This will then promote relaxation of the vascular smooth muscle cells by the same mechanisms as nitrovasodilators (stimulation of guanylate cyclase and GMPc formation) (Kukovetz and Holzmann, 1985). The acute effects of molsidomine on the splanchnic and systemic haemodynamics are similar to those of long-acting nitrates (Vinel et al, 1990; Ruiz del Arbol et al, 1991). Its long-term effects have only been assessed in a short series of patients suggesting that the reduction in portal pressure is maintained on a long-term basis (Huppe, 1992). Although molsidomine has been suggested to cause little pharmacological tolerance (Stewart et al, 1986), in our experience, long-term treatment with molsidomine caused no greater reductions in portal pressure than long-term isosorbide-5-mononitrate administration (unpublished observations).

Serotonin S2-receptor blockers

These were introduced following the observation that mesenteric veins from portal hypertensive animals are hypersensitive to the venoconstrictor effects of serotonin (Cummings et al, 1986). Ketanserin, a serotonin S_2-receptor blocker, has been shown to reduce portal pressure in patients with cirrhosis (Hadengue et al, 1987; Vorobioff et al, 1989). However, ketanserin administration has been associated with encephalopathy and arterial hypotension (Vorobioff et al, 1989), which might be related to the fact that in addition to be a serotonin-blocker, ketanserin has also an alpha-adrenergic antagonistic effect. New selective S_2-antagonists, such as ritanserin, decrease portal pressure but do not reduce arterial blood pressure in experimental models of portal hypertension (Fernández et al, 1993). Still, the potential for the use of these drugs, either alone or in combination with other agents, requires further investigation.

Clonidine

Clonidine is a centrally acting alpha-2 adrenergic agonist, which results in reduced adrenergic output. Its haemodynamic effects are thus reminiscent of both beta- and alpha-adrenergic blockade. In the systemic circulation clonidine causes reductions in heart rate, cardiac index and arterial blood pressure, while in the splanchnic circulation clonidine reduces portal pressure by decreasing portal resistance and splanchnic inflow (Willet et al, 1986; Moreau et al, 1987; Albillos et al, 1992; Esler et al, 1992; Roulot et al, 1992). The decrease in HVPG is observed both in acute and long-term therapy, and is associated with an increase in FHVP and central venous pressure. The hepatic blood flow and liver function are maintained. Despite the marked fall in arterial pressure, renal function and sodium handling do not appear to be altered following clonidine administration. The magnitude of the fall in portal pressure is slightly greater than that achieved with propranolol (Albillos et al, 1992), but no study has evaluated its efficacy in preventing variceal haemorrhage.

Prazosin

Prazosin is an alpha-1 adrenergic antagonist that markedly reduces HVPG in patients with cirrhosis. This reduction is associated with an increased hepatic blood flow suggesting a reduction in the hepatic vascular resistance (Albillos et al, 1994, 1995). However, chronic prazosin administration was associated with a significant reduction in arterial pressure and systemic vascular resistance, and with an activation of neurohumoral vasoactive systems, leading to sodium retention and plasma volume expansion (Albillos et al, 1995). These data suggest that prazosin should not be used, at least as a single agent, in the pharmacological treatment of portal hypertension. Recent data suggest that some of these adverse effects on renal function may be attenuated by the association of propranolol (Albillos et al, 1995, 1996).

Diuretics

Diuretics have been tested because of the known relationship between plasma volume and portal pressure (Zimmon and Kessler, 1974). Spironolactone has been shown to reduce HVPG in patients with cirrhosis (Okumura et al, 1991; García-Pagán et al, 1994b). By preventing the increase in plasma volume, these agents may attenuate the increase in cardiac output, and therefore the hyperkinetic circulation observed in cirrhosis. In addition, the reduction in plasma volume may trigger vasoactive mechanisms further decreasing the splanchnic blood flow and portal pressure. There is some evidence that suggests that spironolactone may also have a direct effect on the vascular system that is not mediated by anti-aldosteronic mechanisms (Dacquet et al, 1987). In that regard, a recent study in an experimental model of portal hypertension, has shown that the administration of small doses of spironolactone reduce portal pressure without changes in plasma volume or systemic haemodynamics (Van de Casteele et al, 1996). Whatever its mechanisms of action, it is clear that the use of diuretics may be a variable that may have inadvertently influenced portal pressure in some studies. This may explain, in part, some of the conflicting results of previous studies in which the possible use of spirono-lactone was not taken in account.

Calcium channel blockers

Experimental studies in isolated perfused liver suggested that calcium channel blockers will be able to decrease portal pressure in cirrhosis by reducing the hepatic vascular resistance (Reichen and Le, 1986). However, several studies conducted with patients with cirrhosis who were prescribed verapamil (Navasa et al, 1988), nifedipine (Koshy et al, 1987) or nicardipine (García-Pagán et al, 1994a) have failed to provide any evidence for a reduction in portal pressure. In fact, nifedipine administration increases portal pressure (Koshy et al, 1987). Nicardipine improved hepatic perfusion without changing HVPG but increased portocollateral blood flow, an effect that may be dangerous in patients with oesophageal varices (García-Pagán et al, 1994a). Overall, these data suggest that calcium channel blockers do not have a role in the treatment of portal hypertension. Potassium channel blockers are currently under investigation.

Combination therapy

It is unlikely that any single agent will decrease portal pressure enough to protect patients completely from the risk of variceal bleeding or rebleeding. This is probably easier to achieve using combinations of drugs acting through different mechanisms. Again, this is a situation in which the strategy for the treatment of portal hypertension may profit from the experience gained in the treatment of systemic hypertension.

The first approach to combination therapy in portal hypertension was the association of nitroglycerin to vasopressin infusion (Groszmann et al, 1984). This was proven to be more effective and safer than vasopressin alone in double-blind randomized controlled trials (Bosch et al, 1989). More recently we introduced a new drug combination for the continued treatment of portal hypertension, the association of oral *propranolol (or nadolol) and isosorbide-5-mononitrate*, which has been shown to cause a greater reduction in HVPG than either drug alone. Acute (García-Pagán et al, 1990b) and long-term (García-Pagán et al, 1991) haemodynamic studies have shown that this drug association decreases the number of patients who do not have reduced portal pressure, while increases the proportion of cases in whom HVPG is markedly reduced. This is because of the fact that isosorbide-5-mononitrate decreases hepatic resistance and prevents the increase in portal-collateral resistance caused by propranolol. Because of this, the association is also superior to propranolol alone in maintaining liver perfusion and hepatic function, while the beneficial effect of propranolol in reducing azygos blood flow is unchanged (García-Pagán et al, 1991). It is important to remark that the long-term administration of isosorbide-5-mononitrate associated with propranolol (García-Pagán et al,

1991; Morillas et al, 1994) or nadolol (Merkel et al, 1995) did not produce any deleterious effect on renal function or sodium handling either in patients with or without ascites. This is different from what has been shown with the association of propranolol plus isosorbide dinitrate (Vorobioff et al, 1993). Propranolol associated with isosorbide dinitrate produced a greater reduction in HVPG than propranolol alone but this was accompanied by a significant impairment in renal function. This is probably because of the fact that this drug combination produces a greater reduction on arterial pressure than the association of the beta-blocker and isosorbide-5-mononitrate. The lack of deleterious effects on renal function makes isosorbide-5-mononitrate the nitrate of choice to combine with propranolol or nadolol.

Nipradilol is a drug that combines in the same molecule, the action of a non-selective beta-blockade with a nitrate-like vasodilating activity. Two studies in different experimental models of portal hypertension have suggested that nipradilol may achieve a greater reduction in portal pressure than propranolol (Oshuga et al, 1993; Um et al, 1993). However, this has not been confirmed in patients with liver cirrhosis in whom the effects of nipradilol were similar to those of propranolol (Arakami et al, 1992). There is still not enough information on *carvedilol*, a non-selective beta-blocker with alpha-adrenergic antagonistic capacity.

Other drug combinations have been shown to potentiate the portal pressure reducing effect of propranolol either in experimental models of portal hypertension or in patients with liver cirrhosis. These include the association of propranolol and serotonin antagonists (Hadengue et al, 1989; Pomier-Layrargues et al, 1992), that of propranolol and a diuretic like spironolactone (García-Pagán et al, 1992), but not furosemide (Sogni et al, 1994), that of propranolol and clonidine (Roulot et al, 1989; Lin et al, 1995) and that of propranolol and prazosin (Albillos et al, 1995). Indeed, a recent haemodynamic study in patients with cirrhosis has shown that the last combination has a greater portal pressure reducing effect than propranolol plus isosorbide-5-mononitrate (Albillos et al, 1996). However, the combination of propranolol plus prazosin was less well tolerated and caused more side effects than propranolol plus isosorbide-5-mononitrate. Propranolol plus molsidomine has also been tested; although it was able to prevent some of the deleterious effects of propranolol on the systemic haemodynamics, there was no advantage in terms of portal pressure reduction, which was even lower than that caused by propranolol alone (García-Pagán et al, 1996). In patients with cirrhosis receiving prazosin the association of furosemide did not further reduce portal pressure (Albillos et al, 1995). Finally, in an experimental model of portal hypertension, the combination of spironolactone plus isosorbide-5-mononitrate did not increase the portal pressure reducing effect of these agents administered separately (Van de Casteele et al, 1996).

Obviously, these and other possible combinations should be further evaluated. Whether the greater haemodynamic effects achieved with some of these combinations translate into better clinical results should be verified in randomized controlled studies.

CLINICAL USE OF BETA-BLOCKERS: PROPHYLAXIS OF FIRST BLEEDING AND PREVENTION OF REBLEEDING. RESULTS OF RANDOMIZED CONTROLLED TRIALS AND META-ANALYSIS

Prophylactic therapy

The aim of prophylactic therapy is to prevent variceal bleeding and bleeding-related deaths. When considering the results of prophylactic trials meta-analysis provides a more stable and reliable estimate of treatment effects overcoming problems of low power in excessively small trials.

The utility of beta-blockers, such as propranolol or nadolol, in the prevention of the first variceal bleeding is one of those rare clinical situations in that most of the randomized trials have shown similar results. Recent meta-analysis of the nine published trials comparing beta-blockers with non-active treatment and including a total of 996 patients, shows not only a significant benefit of beta-blockers in relation to bleeding, but also a marked trend of reduced mortality that approaches statistical significance (D'Amico et al, 1995). The beneficial effect of beta-blockers was found in patients with and without ascites, and with small or large varices (Poynard et al, 1991). Propranolol was assessed in seven studies and nadolol in two. Side effects of beta-blockers were reported in less than 15% of patients and were usually minor (mainly weakness), and withdrawal of therapy was required less than half of them. No mortality from treatment has been reported. Efficacy of therapy is limited to the time of drug administration. After stopping propranolol therapy, bleeding occurred in one trial (Grace et al, 1990), suggesting that therapy should be maintained for life. Thus, beta-blockers are recommended for the prevention of variceal bleeding in patients with cirrhosis and oesophageal varices without contraindications to beta-blockers.

Pharmacological alternatives to beta-blockers

One randomized study compared isosorbide-5-mononitrate with propranolol in the prevention of first bleeding (Angelico et al, 1993). Both were found equally effective. Although the power of this study was too low to detect a clinically relevant difference between the two drugs and its design was not double-blind, its results indeed suggest that isosorbide-5-mononitrate can be an alternative treatment for patients at high risk of bleeding and who do not tolerate beta-blockers. Further studies are needed to clarify this issue.

Prevention of rebleeding

Eleven controlled trials that have included a total of 755 patients, and have evaluated beta-blockers versus no specific therapy have been reported as full papers or abstracts. Propranolol was assessed in 10 studies and nadolol in one. None was double-blind. Meta-analysis of these studies have shown that beta-blockers significantly reduce the risk of recurrent bleeding and slightly improves survival (approaching statistical significance) (D'Amico et al, 1995). It is important to remark that in none of these studies has there been a single patient with a fatal complication caused by treatment with beta-blockers. Thus, side effects of beta-blockers were not frequent and mild. In addition, nine studies, that included a total of 787 patients, compared beta-blockers with long-term sclerotherapy. The rebleeding rate was very heterogeneous between studies. Because of this, although meta-analyses of these studies have shown that sclerotherapy is slightly better than propranolol in preventing recurrent variceal bleeding, this should not be considered as definite evidence of superiority of sclerotherapy over propranolol (D'Amico et al, 1995). Moreover, despite the small reduction in rebleeding, no trial showed that differences in survival and sclerotherapy was associated with more severe and more frequent complications than beta-blockers. Therefore, the benefit for sclerotherapy is only marginal. The conclusions of two recent consensus meetings, one held in Europe (De Franchis et al, 1992) and the other in the USA, was to include pharmacological treatment among the therapeutic options to prevent rebleeding, which is mandatory in these patients. We usually begin treatment with pharmacological agents, and reserve sclerotherapy, surgery or transjugular intrahepatic portosystemic shunt (TIPS) until after failure of drug therapy or when there is a contraindication for its use.

Beta-blockers have also been used in association with sclerotherapy to reduce the risk of rebleeding during the first months prior to eradication of varices, when most episodes of rebleeding occur (D'Amico et al, 1995). Meta-analysis of nine studies, that included 459 patients, compared sclerotherapy alone versus sclerotherapy associated to propranolol, and showed that there was a trend favouring the combination, but no significant differences were detected. In addition, no significant difference in mortality was observed in any of the trials. On the contrary, two trials, that included 193 patients, compared the efficacy of propranolol administered alone versus propranolol associated with sclerotherapy, and showed a reduction in rebleeding and death-risk with the combined therapy (D'Amico et al, 1995). Clearly more studies are needed to better define the advantages and potential candidates for such a treatment option.

Combination therapy: beta-blockers associated with isosorbide-5-mononitrate

There are now several studies that indicate that the greater reduction in portal pressure achieved with the combination of beta-blockers plus isosorbide-5-mononitrate (as compared with propranolol alone) translates into better clinical results. A prospective randomized, not blinded study showed that nadolol plus isosorbide-5-mononitrate is more effective than nadolol alone in preventing the first variceal bleeding in patients with cirrhosis and oesophageal varices (Merkel et al, 1996). In addition, nadolol plus isosorbide-5-mononitrate has been shown to be more effective than sclerotherapy in preventing oesophageal rebleeding and has less complications related to treatment (Villanueva et al, 1996). In another study, propranolol plus isosorbide-5-mononitrate was found as effective as invasive procedures, such as shunt-surgery or sclerotherapy in good or poor surgical risk patients, respectively, and prevented oesophageal rebleeding (Feu et al, 1995). All these studies strongly suggest that the combination of beta-blockers with isosorbide-5-mononitrate represents the most effective pharmacological treatment that has been evaluated so far.

CLINICAL HAEMODYNAMIC CORRELATIONS DURING PHARMACOLOGICAL THERAPY

Several cross-sectional studies (Viallet et al, 1975; Lebrec et al, 1980; Garcia-Tsao et al, 1985) have shown that there is a threshold portal pressure gradient (HVPG of about 12 mmHg) for varices to bleed. This has been prospectively validated in a placebo-controlled trial of prophylactic propranolol (Groszmann et al, 1990). In this trial no bleeding occurred in those patients in whom the HVPG decreased to 12 mmHg or below during the study, either with propranolol or spontaneously. Moreover, these patients had significantly longer survival. This has been recently confirmed by Vorobioff et al (1994) showing that the actuarial probability of first bleeding was significantly lower in those patients in whom PPG decreased more than 15% than in those who did not. This study confirmed that no patient bled who had a decreased PPG (portal pressure gradient) below 12 mmHg. This important relationship between haemodynamic and clinic events are also reinforced by data from studies performed to prevent rebleeding. Sacerdoti et al (1991) showed that no patient exhibiting a reduction in PPG greater than 12% after 1 month of beta-blockade rebled. However, these results should be taken with caution, because of the small number of patients studied and the small number of events (four rebleeds). A study performed in our unit in a large series of patients (Feu et al, 1995) showed that a fall in the PPG of more than 20% of the baseline values or below 12 mmHg (after 3 months of treatment), is associated with a very low risk of rebleeding on long-term follow-up: 8% versus 55% in patients failing to exhibit such a decrease in PPG. On a multivariate analysis on a Cox's model (including demographic, clinical and endoscopic data) only a reduction in PPG greater than 20% had independent prognostic value for rebleeding. This study again confirmed that decreasing PPG below the 12 mmHg threshold value is associated with a complete protection from the risk of rebleeding. These findings have been corroborated in a recent study by Villanueva et al (1996) that compared pharmacological treatment versus sclerotherapy for the prevention of variceal rebleeding. The study showed that patients who had a reduction in PPG greater or equal to 20% had an actuarial probability of rebleeding that was significantly lower than patients with no or less than 20% reduction in PPG. The protective effect of a PPG reduction greater than 20% was observed either in patients treated with drugs or with sclerotherapy. All these findings demonstrate that the occurrence of clinical events during pharmacological treatment is related to haemodynamic changes, and suggest that portal pressure measurements can be useful in identifying patients who are likely to have a good clinical response to treatment.

NEW CLINICAL SCENARIOS FOR PHARMACOLOGICAL TREATMENT: PREVENTION OF VARICES

Patients with liver cirrhosis and no oesophageal varices at endoscopy will develop oesophageal varices at a rate of about 8% per each year (Christiensen et al, 1981). Several studies have demonstrated that for varices to develop, the PPG shall increase above 10 or 12 mmHg (Viallet et al, 1975; Lebrec et al, 1980; Garcia-Tsao et al, 1985). This observation suggests that it could be possible to prevent the development of gastro-oesophageal varices by an early pharmacological intervention and prevent a sustained increase of PPG above this threshold value. Actually, there is experimental evidence that indicates that development of portal-systemic collaterals can be prevented by portal pressure reducing agents (Lin et al, 1991a,b; Sarin et al, 1991). Furthermore, it is likely that reduction of PPG below this value in patients with varices will cause these gradually to disappear, as demonstrated in a recent study showing that patients with varices in whom the PPG was reduced below threshold values had a significant reduction in the size of the varices (Groszmann et al, 1990). Therefore, it is conceivable that in patients with cirrhosis, early treatment with portal pressure reducing agents may prevent the development of oesophageal varices This is now being evaluated, in a wide series of patients, in a prospective multicentre randomized clinical trial.

REFERENCES

Albillos A, Bañares R, Barrios C et al (1992) Long-term oral administration of clonidine in patients with alcoholic cirrhosis. Hemodynamic and liver function effects. *Gastroenterology* **102:** 248–254.

Albillos A, Lledo JL, Bañares R et al (1994) Hemodynamic effects of alpha-adrenergic blockade with prazosin in cirrhotic patients with portal hypertension. *Hepatology* **20:** 611–617.

*Albillos A, Lledo JL, Rossi I et al (1995) Continous prazosin administration in cirrhotic patients: effects on portal hemodynamics and on liver and renal function. *Gastroenterology* **109:** 1257–1265.

Albillos A, García-Pagán JC, Iborra J et al (1996) Propranolol plus Prazosin vs propranolol plus isosorbide-5-mononitrate in the treatment of portal hypertension. *Hepatology* **24:** 206A.

*D'Amico G, Pagliaro L & Bosch J (1995) The treatment of portal hypertension: a meta-analytic review. *Hepatology* **22:** 332–354.

Angelico M, Carli L, Piat C et al (1993) Isosorbide-5-monorate versus propranolol in the prevention of first bleeding in cirrhosis. *Gastroenterology* **104:** 1460–1465.

Arakami T, Sekiyama T, Katsuta Y et al (1992) Long-term haemodynamic effects of a 4-week regimen of nipradilol, a new beta-blocker with nitrovasodilating properties, in patients with portal hypertension due to cirrhosis. A comparative study with propranolol. *Journal of Hepatology* **15:** 48–53.

Ballet F, Chretien Y, Rey C et al (1988) Differential response of normal and cirrhotic liver to vasoactive agents. A study in the isolated perfused rat liver. *Journal of Pharmacological Experimental Therapy* **244:** 233–235.

*Bathal PS & Grossmann HJ (1985) Reduction of the increased portal vascular resistance of the isolated perfused cirrhotic rat liver by vasodilators. *Journal of Hepatology* **1**: 325–329.

Blei AT & Gottstein J (1986) Isosorbide dinitrate in experimental portal hypertension: a study of factors that modulate the hemodynamic response. *Hepatology* **6**: 107–111.

Blei AT, Garcia-Tsao G, Groszmann RJ et al (1987) Hemodynamic evaluation of isosorbide dinitrate in alcoholic cirrhosis. Pharmacokinetic–hemodynamic interactions. *Gastroenterology* **93**: 576–583.

*Bosch J, Mastai R, Kravetz D et al (1984) Effects of propranolol on azygos blood flow and hepatic and systemic hemodynamics in cirrhosis. *Hepatology* **4**: 1200–1205.

Bosch J, Groszmann RJ, García-Pagán JC et al (1989) Association of transdermal nitroglycerin to vasopressin infusion in the treatment of variceal hemorrhage: a placebo controlled clinical trial. *Hepatology* **10**: 962–968.

Bosch J, Pizcueta P, Feu F et al (1992) Pathophysiology of portal hypertension. *Gastroenterolology Clinics of North America* **21**: 1–14.

Bosch J, García-Pagán JC, Feu F et al (1993) New approaches in the pharmacologic treatment of portal hypertension. *Journal of Hepatology* **17(S2)**: S41–S45.

Van de Casteele M, Van Roey G, Nevens F & Fevery J (1996) Effects of varying doses of spironolactone without and with nitrates on portal vein pressure and kidney function in partial portal vein ligated rats. *Hepatology* **24**: 1492–1496.

Christensen E, Faverholdt L, Schlichting P et al (1981) Aspects of natural history of gastrointestinal bleeding in cirrhosis and the effect of prednisolone. *Gastroenterology* **81**: 944–952.

*Cummings SA, Groszmann RJ & Kaumann AJ (1986) Hypersensitivity of mesenteric veins to 5-hydroxytryptamine and ketanserin-induced reduction of portal pressure in portal hypertensive rats. *British Journal of Pharmacology* **89**: 501–513.

Dacquet C, Loirand G, Mironneau C et al (1987) Spironolactone inhibition of contraction and calcium channels in rat portal vein. *British Journal of Pharmacology* **92**: 535–544.

Escorsell A, Feu F, Bordas JM et al (1996) Effects of Isosorbide-5-mononitrate on variceal pressure and systemic and splanchnic hemodynamics in patients with cirrhosis. *Journal of Hepatology* **24**: 423–434.

Escorsell A, Ferayorni L, Bosch J et al (1997) The portal pressure response to β-blockade is greater in cirrhotic patients without varices than in those with varices. *Gastroenterology* **112**: 2012–2016.

Esler M, Dudley F, Jennings G et al (1992) Increased sympathetic activity and the effects of its inhibition with clonidine in alcoholic cirrhosis. *Annals of Internal Medicine* **116**: 446–455.

Fernandez M, Pizcueta P, García-Pagán JC et al (1993) Effects of ritanserin, a selective and specific S2-serotonergic antagonist, on portal pressure and splanchnic hemodynamics in rats with long-term bile duct ligation. *Hepatology* **18**: 389–393.

Feu F, Bordas JM, Luca A et al (1993) Reduction of variceal pressure by propranolol: comparison of the effects on portal pressure and azygos blood flow in patients with cirrhosis. *Hepatology* **18**: 1082–1089.

Feu F, García-Pagán JC, Bosch J et al (1995) Relation between portal pressure response to pharmacotherapy and risk of recurrent variceal haemorrhage in patients with cirrhosis. *Lancet* **346**: 1056–1059

De Franchis R, Pascal JP, Ancona E et al (1992) Definitions, methodology and therapeutic strategies in portal hypertension. A consensus development workshop. *Journal of Hepatology* **15**: 256–261.

*García-Pagán JC, Feu F, Bosch J & Rodés J (1991) Propanolol compared with propanolol plus isosorbide-5-mononitrate for portal hypertension in cirrhosis. A randomized controlled study. *Annals of Internal Medicine* **114**: 869–873.

García-Pagán JC, Terés J, Calvet X et al (1989) Factors which influence the prognosis of the first episode of variceal hemorrhage in patients with cirrhosis. In J Bosch & J Rodés (eds) *Recent Advances in the Pathophysiology and Therapy of Portal Hypertension*, pp 287–302. Serono, Symposia Review No 22.

García-Pagán JC, Feu F, Navasa M et al (1990a) Long-term haemodynamic effects of isosorbide-5-mononitrate in patients with cirrhosis and portal hypertension. *Journal of Hepatology* **11**: 189–195.

García-Pagán JC, Navasa M, Bosch J et al (1990b) Enhancement of portal pressure reduction by the association of isosorbide-5-mononitrate to propranolol administration in patients with cirrhosis. *Hepatology* **11**: 230–238.

García-Pagán JC, Navasa M, Rivera F et al (1992) Lymphocyte β-2-adrenoceptors and plasma catecholamines in patients with cirrhosis. Relationship with the hemodynamic response to propranolol. *Gastroenterology* **102:** 2015–2023.

García-Pagán JC, Feu F, Luca A et al (1994a) Nicardipine increases hepatic blood flow and the hepatic clearance of indocyanine green in patients with cirrhosis. *Journal of Hepatology* **20:** 792–796.

García-Pagán JC, Salmeron JM, Feu F et al (1994b) Effects of low-sodium diet and spironolactone on portal pressure in patients with compensated cirrhosis. *Hepatology* **19:** 1095–1099.

García-Pagán JC, Escorsell A, Feu F et al (1996) Propranonol plus molsidomine vs propranolol alone in the treatment of portal hypertension in patients with cirrhosis. *Journal of Hepatology* **24:** 430–435.

Garcia-Tsao G, Groszmann RJ, Fisher RL et al (1985) Portal pressure presence of gastroesophageal varices and variceal bleeding. *Hepatology* **5:** 419–424.

Garcia-Tsao G, Grace ND, Groszmann RJ et al (1986) Short term effects of propranolol on portal venous pressure. *Hepatology* **6:** 101–106.

Grace ND, Conn HO, Groszmann RJ et al (1990) Propranolol for prevention of first esophageal variceal hemorrhage: A lifetime commitment? *Hepatology* **12:** 407.

Groszmann RJ, Kravetz D, Bosch J et al (1984) Nitroglycerin improves the hemodynamic response to vasopressin in portal hypertension. *Hepatology,* **2:** 757–762.

*Groszmann RJ, Bosch J, Grace ND et al (1990) Hemodynamic events in a prospective randomized trial of propranolol versus placebo in the prevention of a first variceal hemorrhage. *Gastroenterology* **99:** 1401–1407.

Hadengue A, Lee SS, Moreau R et al (1987) Beneficial hemodynamic effects of ketanserin in patients with cirrhosis: possible role of serotonergic mechanisms in portal hypertension. *Hepatology* **7:** 644–647.

Hadengue A, Moreuar R, Cerini R et al (1989) Combination of ketanserin and verapamil or propranolol in patients with alcoholic cirrhosis: search for an additive effect. *Hepatology* **9:** 83–87.

Hayes DC, Westaby D & Williams R (1988) Effect and mechanism of action of isosorbide-5-mononitrate. *Gut* **29:** 752–755.

Huppe D, Jager D, Tromm A et al (1992) Acute and long-term effects of Molsidomine on portal and cardiac hemodynamics in patients with cirrhosis of the liver. *European Journal of Gastroenterology and Hepatology* **4:** 849–855.

Koshy A, Hadengue A, Lee SS et al (1987) Possible deleterious hemodynamic effect of nifedipine on portal hypertension in patients with cirrhosis. *Clinical Pharmacological Therapy* **42:** 295–298.

*Kroeger R & Groszmann RJ (1985) Increased portal venous resistance hinders portal pressure reduction during the administration of beta-adrenergic blocking agents in a portal hypertensive model. *Hepatology* **5:** 97–101.

Kukovetz WR & Holzmann S (1985) Mechanisms of vasodilation by molsidomine. *American Heart Journal* **109:** 637–640.

Lebrec D, DeFleury P, Rueff B et al (1980) Portal hypertension, size of esophageal varices and risk of gastrointestinal bleeding in alcoholic cirrhosis. *Gastroenterology* **79:** 1139–1144.

Lin HC, Soubrane O, Cailmail S & Lebrec D (1991a) Early chronic administration of propranolol reduces the severity of portal hypertension and portal systemic shunting in conscious portal vein stenosed rats. *Journal of Hepatology* **13:** 213–219.

Lin HC, Soubrane O & Lebrec D (1991b) Prevention of portal hypertension and portosystemic shunting by early chronic administration of clonidine in conscious portal vein stenosed rats. *Hepatology* **14:** 325–330.

Lin HC, Tsai YT, Yang MC et al (1995) Haemodynamic effects of combination of propranolol and clonidine in patients with post-hepatitic cirrhosis. *Journal of Gastroenterology and Hepatology* **10:** 281–286.

Mastai R, Bosch J, Navasa M et al (1987) Effects of alpha-adrenergic stimulation and beta-adrenergic blockade on azygos blood flow and splanchnic haemodynamics in patients with cirrhosis. *Journal of Hepatology* **4:** 71–79.

Merkel C, Gatta A, Donada C et al (1995) Long-term effect of nadolol or nadolol plus isosorbide-5-mononitrate on renal function and ascites formation in patients with cirrhosis. *Hepatology* **22:** 808–813.

Merkel C, Marin R, Enzo E et al (1996) Randomised trial of nadolol alone or with isosorbide mononitrate for primary prophylaxis of variceal bleeding in cirrhosis. Gruppo-triveneto per l'ipertensione portale (GTIP). *Lancet* **348:** 1677–1681.

Mittal MK, Gupta TK, Lee FY et al (1994) Nitric oxide modulates hepatic vascular tone in normal rat liver. *American Journal of Physiology* **267**: G416–422.

Moreau R, Lee SS, Hadengue A et al (1987) Hemodynamic effects of a clonidine-induced decrease in sympathetic tone in patients with cirrhosis. *Hepatology* **7**: 147–154.

Morillas RM, Planas R, Cabre E et al (1994) Propranolol plus isosorbide-5-mononitrate for portal hypertension in cirrhosis: long-term hemodynamic and renal effects. Hepatology **20**: 1502–1508.

*Navasa M, Chesta J, Bosch J & Rodés J (1989) Reduction of portal pressure by isosorbide-5-mononitrate in patients with cirrhosis. Effects on splanchnic and systemic hemodynamics and liver function. *Gastroenterology* **96**: 1110–1118.

Navasa M, Bosch J, Reichen J et al (1988) Effects of verapamil on hepatic and systemic hemodynamics and liver function in patients with cirrhosis and portal hypertension. *Hepatology* **8**: 850–854.

Oshuga M, Cailmail S & Lebrec D (1993) Hemodynamic effects of nipradilol, a new beta-adrenergic antagonist combined with a nitroxy base, in rats with intra- or extra-hepatic portal hypertension. *Journal of Hepatology* **17**: 236–240.

Okumura H, Arakami T, Katsuta Y et al (1991) Reduction in hepatic venous pressure gradient as a consequence of volume contraction due to chronic administration of spironolactone in patients with cirrhosis and no ascites. *American Journal of Gastroenterology* **86**: 46–52.

Pizcueta MP, De Lacy AM, Kravetz D et al (1989) Propranolol decreases portal pressure without changing portocollateral resistance in cirrhotic rats. *Hepatology* **10**: 953–957.

Pizcueta MP, Pique JM, Fernandez M et al (1992), Modulation of the hyperdynamic circulation of cirrhotic rats by nitric oxide inhibition. *Gastroenterology* **103**: 1909–1915.

Pomier-Layrargues G, Giroux L, Rocheleau B & Huet PM (1992) Combined treatment of portal hypertension with ritanserin and propranolol in conscious and unrestrained cirrhotic rats. *Hepatology* **15**: 878–882.

Poynard T, Calès P, Pasta L et al (1991) Beta-adrenergic antagonist drugs in the prevention of gastrointestinal bleeding in patients with cirrhosis and esophageal varices. *New England Journal of Medicine* **324**: 1532–1538.

Reichen J & Lee M (1986) Verapamil favorably influences hepatic microvascular exchange and functions in rats with cirrhosis of the liver. *Journal of Clinical Investigation* **78**: 448–455.

Roulot D, Gaudin C, Braillon A et al (1989) Hemodynamic effects of combination of clonidine and propranolol in conscious cirrhotic rats. *Canadian Journal of Physiological Pharmacology* **67**: 1369–1372.

Roulot D, Moreau R, Gaudin C et al (1992) Long-term sympathetic and hemodynamic responses to clonidine in patients with cirrhosis and ascites. *Gastroenterology* **102**: 1309–1318.

Ruiz del Arbol L, García-Pagán JC, Feu F et al (1991) Effects of molsidomine, a long acting venous dilator, on portal hypertension. A hemodynamic study in patients with cirrhosis. *Journal of Hepatology* **13**: 179–186.

Sacerdoti D, Merkel C & Gatta A (1991) Importance of the 1-month-effect of nadolol on portal pressure in predicting failure of prevention of rebleeding in cirrhosis. *Journal of Hepatology* **12**: 124–125.

Salerno F, Borroni G, Lorenzano E et al (1996) Long-term administration of isosorbide-5-mononitrate does not impair renal function in cirrhotic patients. *Hepatology* **23**: 1135–1140.

Salmeron JM, Ruiz del Arbol L, Gines A et al (1993) Renal effects of acute isosorbide-5-mononitrate administration in cirrhosis. *Hepatology* **17**: 800–806.

Sarin SK, Groszmann RJ, Mosca PG et al (1991) Propranolol ameliorates the development of portal-systemic shunting in a chronic murine schistosomiasis model of portal hypertension. *Journal of Clinical Investigation* **87**: 1032–1036.

Sogni P, Soupison T, Moureau R et al (1994) Hemodynamic effects of acute administration of furosemide in patients with cirrhosis receiving beta-adrenergic antagonists. *Journal of Hepatology* **20**: 548–552.

Stewart DJ, Elsner D, Sommer O et al (1986) Altered spectrum of nitroglycerin-specific venous tolerance with maintenance of arterial vasodepressor potency. *Circulation* **74**: 573–582.

Um S, Nishida O, Tokubayashi M et al (1993) Nipradilol, a new beta-blocker with vasodilatory properties, in experimental portal hypertension: a comparative haemodynamic study with propranolol. *Journal of Gastroenterology and Hepatology* **8**: 414–419.

Viallet A, Marleau D, Huet M et al (1975) Hemodynamic evaluation of patients with intrahepatic portal hypertension: relationship between bleeding varices and the portohepatic gradient. *Gastroenterology* **69**: 1297–1300.

*Villanueva C, Balanzo J, Novella MT et al (1996) Nadolol plus isosorbide-5-mononitrate compared with sclerotherapy for the prevention of variceal rebleeding. *New England Journal of Medicine* **334:** 1624–1629.

Vinel JP, Monnin JL, Combis JM et al (1990) Hemodynamic evaluation of molsidomine: a vasodilator with antianginal properties in patients with alcoholic cirrhosis. *Hepatology* **11:** 239–242

Vorobioff J, Bredfeldt JE & Groszmann RJ (1983) Hyperdynamic splanchnic circulation in portal hypertensive rat model: a primary factor for maintenance of chronic portal hypertension. *American Journal of Physiology* **244:** G52–G57.

Vorobioff J, Garcia-Tsao G, Groszmann RJ et al (1989) Long-term hemodynamic effects of ketanserin, a 5-hydroxytryptamine blocker, in portal hypertensive patients. *Hepatology* **9:** 88–91.

Vorobioff J, Picabea E, Gamen et al (1993) Propranolol compared with propranolol plus isosorbide dinitrate in portal hypertensive patients: long term hemodynamic and renal effects. *Hepatology* **18:** 477–484.

Vorobioff J, Groszmann RJ, Picabea E et al (1994) Prognostic value of sequential measurement of portal pressure in alcoholic cirrhotic patients. Hepatology **20:** 103A

Willett IR, Jennings G, Esler M & Dudley FJ (1986) Sympathetic tone modulates portal venous pressure in alcoholic cirrhosis. *Lancet* **ii:** 939–942.

Zimmon DS & Kessler RE (1974) The portal pressure–blood volume relationship in cirrhosis. *Gut* **15:** 99–101.

6

Endoscopic treatments for portal hypertension

ROBERTO DE FRANCHIS MD

Associate Professor of Medicine and Head of Department

MASSIMO PRIMIGNANI MD

Senior Lecturer

Gastroenterology and Gastrointestinal Endoscopy Service, Istituto di Medicina Interna, University of Milan, IRCCS Ospedale Policlinico, Via Pace 9, 20122 Milan, Italy

Endoscopic treatments for bleeding gastro-oesophageal varices include injection sclerotherapy, variceal obturation with tissue adhesives and variceal rubber band ligation. Today, endoscopic treatments are not recommended for the primary prophylaxis of variceal bleeding. Acute injection sclerotherapy remains a quick and simple technique for the control of active bleeding from oesophageal varices. Its efficacy may be improved by the early administration of vasoactive drugs. Banding ligation is the optimal endoscopic treatment for the prevention of rebleeding from oesophageal varices. The use of tissue adhesives and thrombin as injectates to treat bleeding fundal gastric varices and oesophageal varices not responding to vasoactive drugs or sclerotherapy is promising but needs further assessment by means of randomized controlled trials.

Key words: oesophageal varices; bleeding; endoscopic treatment; sclerotherapy; rubber band ligation; rebleeding; mortality; controlled trials; meta-analysis.

About 30% of patients with cirrhosis and portal hypertension bleed from ruptured oesophageal varices (NIEC, 1988), with a mortality for the initial bleed that may exceed 50% (Pagliaro et al, 1992). After a first bleed, untreated patients have a risk of rebleeding as high as 60% (Pagliaro et al, 1994). The risk decreases with time, returning to baseline values by the 6th week after the variceal bleeding episode (Graham and Smith, 1981). Although gastric varices also bleed, little information is available on their natural history and their fate after endoscopic sclerotherapy of oesophageal varices (Hosking and Johnson, 1988; Watanabe et al, 1988; Mathur et al, 1990; Sarin et al, 1992; Zanasi et al, 1996).

Injection sclerotherapy controls active haemorrhage from oesophageal varices in approximately 90% of cases (Westaby et al, 1989), but rebleeding may occur in as many as 55% (MacDougall et al, 1982) and complication rates of up to 40% have been reported, with mortality rates reaching 2% in some studies (Infante-Rivard et al, 1989).

Baillière's Clinical Gastroenterology —
Vol. 11, No. 2, June 1997
ISBN 0–7020–2339–6
0950–3528/97/020289 + 21 $12.00/00

Because of these limitations of injection sclerotherapy, alternative endoscopic treatments for the management of variceal haemorrhage have been developed. Rubber band ligation (Stiegmann et al, 1989) has been extensively applied in clinical practice. Variceal obturation with tissue adhesives has recently been introduced. This technique is mostly used to treat gastric varices, but is also advocated for uncontrolled bleeding from oesophageal varices (Soehendra et al, 1986; Ramond et al, 1989). However, very little controlled data exists. Other endoscopic devices, such as detachable snares (Lee et al, 1996) and haemostatic clips (Koutsomanis et al, 1995) are in the experimental phase.

In this chapter, we will describe the techniques of injection sclerotherapy, variceal obturation and rubber band ligation, and analyse the results of their application in different clinical situations.

ENDOSCOPIC METHODS

Injection sclerotherapy

Endoscopic injection sclerotherapy has been used to treat variceal haemorrhage for over 50 years (Crafoord and Freckner 1939).

Principle

Sclerotherapy consists of the injection of one of a variety of substances into the variceal lumen or adjacent to the varix. In the acute situation, the goal of sclerotherapy is to achieve haemostasis by inducing thrombosis of the bleeding vessel and/or by external compression of the vessel by tissue oedema or mass effect resulting from the injected sclerosant. In the long-term, the inflammation of the variceal wall and/or of the oesophageal mucosa and submucosa leads to fibrosis of both the vessel and the oesophageal wall, resulting in variceal obliteration.

Technique

Nowadays, sclerotherapy is always performed with flexible endoscopes, using no special equipment other than the endoscope and injection needle ('free hand' technique). Disposable single-use injectors with 23- and 25-gauge needles, 3.6 to 5.6 mm in length, are commonly used. In most cases, sclerotherapy is performed under light i.v. sedation. Disorientated, actively bleeding patients may require deep sedation with endotracheal intubation to prevent aspiration of blood in the airway during the procedure. When active bleeding is present, the use of an endoscope with a large bore working channel is desirable to facilitate removal of blood, clots and secretions. A complete examination of the oesophagus, stomach and duodenum is always performed in all bleeding patients, since the presence of oesophageal varices does not exclude other non-variceal sources of bleeding. If a site of active variceal bleeding is identified at the beginning of the examination, the bleeding is treated immediately, and the examination of the upper gastrointestinal tract is completed after bleeding has been controlled. Injections are initiated at or just above the gastro-oesophageal junction, starting with the most gravity dependent varix, and proceeding in a circumferential fashion. After injecting all varices at the gastro-oesophageal junction, the injections are repeated 2 to 5 cm more cranially. Aliquots of 1 to 5 ml of sclerosant is injected at each site. Injections in the mid or proximal oesophagus should be avoided, since the sclerosant may escape from a varix into the azygos vein and into the pulmonary circulation, where untoward effects may result (Kitano et al, 1988).

After control of bleeding, patients usually enter long-term programmes to prevent rebleeding: these may be based on pharmacological or endoscopic treatments or both. When long-term endoscopic sclerotherapy is chosen, most workers use a 1-week interval between sessions. The aim of long-term sclerotherapy is to achieve variceal obliteration, i.e. the disappearance of all varices from the lower 5 cm of the oesophagus or their reduction to small fibrous cords. Three to six sclerotherapy sessions may be necessary to achieve variceal obliteration (Laine and Cook, 1995).

After variceal obliteration, follow-up endoscopies are carried out at 3-monthly intervals during the first year, and at 6- to 12-month intervals thereafter, to detect and treat recurrent varices.

Sclerosing agents. A number of different sclerosing agents have been proposed: the most widely used are Polidocanol 1–3% and Ethanolamine oleate 5% in Europe, Na Tetradecilsulphate 1–2% and Na Morrhuate 5% in the United States. When used in experienced hands, all sclerosants have given good results and have shown similar safety profiles (Westaby, 1992).

Site of injections. Although some authors advocate direct injection into the variceal lumen, with the aim of obliterating the varix; others suggest that multiple small-volume injections be performed in the vicinity of the varix to produce a protective covering of fibrous tissue over intact vessels; it has been shown that a substantial proportion of intended intravariceal injections end up in the paravariceal tissue, and vice versa. Therefore, the two techniques produce very similar histological changes in the oesophagus.

Timing of injection sclerotherapy. It is generally accepted (Westaby et al, 1996) that endoscopic sclerotherapy should be performed at the moment of diagnostic endoscopy.

Complications of injection sclerotherapy

The reported frequency of complications of sclerotherapy varies greatly between series, and is critically related to the experience of operators as well as the frequency and completeness of follow-up examinations. Minor complications that occur within the first 24–48 hours and do not require treatment, such as low-grade fever, retrosternal chest pain, temporary dysphagia, asymptomatic pleural effusions and other non-specific transient chest radiographic changes, are very common (Schuman et al, 1987). Table 1 illustrates the incidence of clinically significant oesophageal complications (i.e. requiring treatment or changes in planned treatment schedule) observed in a large series of consecutive patients treated in the centres of the North Italian Endoscopic Club (Zambelli et al, 1993). Mucosal ulceration is the most common oesophageal complication, and occurs in up to 90% of patients within 24 hours of injection, and heals rapidly in most cases. Many authors question whether ulceration should be regarded as a complication, or, rather, as a desired effect of sclerotherapy. Nevertheless, ulcerated variceal columns found at follow-up endoscopy should not be injected. Mucosal ulcerations may cause recurrent bleeding in up to 20% of patients (Westaby, 1992). The usefulness of sucralfate in healing oesophageal ulcers and preventing rebleeding is controversial (Burroughs and McCormick, 1992). Chronic deep ulcers are relatively rare: they tend to develop more frequently in patients with more severe liver disease and if large volumes of sclerosant and/or short intervals between sessions are used (Singal et al, 1990). They usually heal with omeprazole. Oesophageal stenoses have been reported with a frequency varying between 2 and 10% (6.5% in the NIEC series, Table 1), and are usually easily dilated. Oesophageal perforation is a rare but severe complication that may occur either by direct traumatic rupture, or by full-thickness oesophageal wall necrosis secondary to excessive injection of sclerosant. The former presents shortly after the procedure, and may be accompanied by subcutaneous emphysema, while the latter may produce insidious symptoms over a few days before free perforation becomes manifest. Management is usually by conservative means including mediastinal drainage, antibiotics and parenteral nutrition. The mortality for oesophageal perforation is in excess of 50%. Rare regional complications include adult respiratory distress syndrome, broncho-oesophageal fistula, chylothorax, pneumothorax and mediastinitis. Bacteraemia following sclerotherapy has been demonstrated, but the incidence of sepsis is low, as is that of remote complications such as distant abscesses and bacterial peritonitis.

Table 1 Clinically significant oesophageal complications of endoscopic sclerotherapy and rubber band ligation observed in patients consecutively treated in the centres of the North Italian Endoscopic Club (NIEC).

	Sclerotherapy No. (%) of patients	Band ligation No. (%) of patients
Total	1192 (100.00)	167 (100.00)
Patients with complications, No. (%)	222 (18.60)	23 (13.80)
Patients with fatal complications, No. (%)	11 (0.92)	2 (1.19)
Confluent/deep oesophageal ulcers, No. (%)	108 (8.60)	2 (1.19)
Bleeding ulcers/early sloughing of bands	56 (4.70)	4 (2.39)
Oesophageal stenosis	78 (6.50)	—
Bleeding at injection site	35 (2.90)	—
Oesophageal wall necrosis	3 (0.30)	—
Oesophageal mucosal tear	—	2 (1.19)

Variceal obturation

The tissue adhesives N-butyl-2-cyanoacrylate (Histoacryl) and isobutyl-2-cyanoacrylate (Bucrylate) have been used to treat oesophageal as well as gastric varices (Soehendra et al, 1986; Ramond et al, 1989).

Principle

Variceal obturation consists of the injection of tissue adhesives into the variceal lumen. The adhesives harden within seconds of coming into contact with blood, forming a solid cast of the injected vessel. Thus their injection, if executed correctly, should result in almost immediate control of bleeding as the lumen of the varix is occluded.

Technique

The rapid hardening of the adhesives makes their application less simple than that of conventional sclerosants. The technique requires care to ensure that the adhesive does not come into contact with the endoscope since this might result in permanent damage to the working channels of the instrument. This risk can be minimized by applying silicone oil to the tip of the endoscope and by mixing the adhesive with a radiographic contrast agent (Lipiodol), in a ratio of 1:1, to delay premature hardening (Soehendra et al, 1986). The latter modification allows the localization of the injected adhesive on a radiograph and may allow the monitoring of injections (Stiegmann and Yamamoto, 1992). A further modification of the technique is to ensure that the needle is correctly placed within the varix by employing a trial injection of distilled water. Once correct placement has been confirmed the tissue adhesive is injected in 0.5 to 1.0 ml aliquots.

Several weeks later (2 weeks to 3 months) the overlying mucosa sloughs off and a glue cast is extruded into the lumen of the gastrointestinal tract. The ulceration subsequently re-epithelializes.

Complications

Mediastinitis caused by the adhesive (Ramond et al, 1986) and cerebrovascular accidents directly attributable to dissemination of the tissue adhesive into the cerebral circulation (See et al, 1986) are the most worrying complications attributed to this technique.

Endoscopic banding ligation

Banding ligation was first reported in humans in 1989 (Stiegmann et al, 1989) and represents an important development in the endoscopic treatment of varices.

Principle

Banding ligation consists of the placement of rubber O-rings on variceal columns, which are sucked into a hollow cylinder attached to the tip of the endoscope (Figure 1). In the acute situation, haemostasis is achieved by physical constriction of the varix at or near the bleeding site, thus interrupting blood flow. In the following days, ischaemic necrosis of mucosa and submucosa develops, followed by granulation tissue formation and sloughing of the O-rings and of the necrotic tissue, which leave shallow mucosal ulcerations. Complete re-epithelialization takes place in 14–21 days, with full-thickness replacement of the vascular structures with maturing scar tissue (Stiegmann et al, 1988).

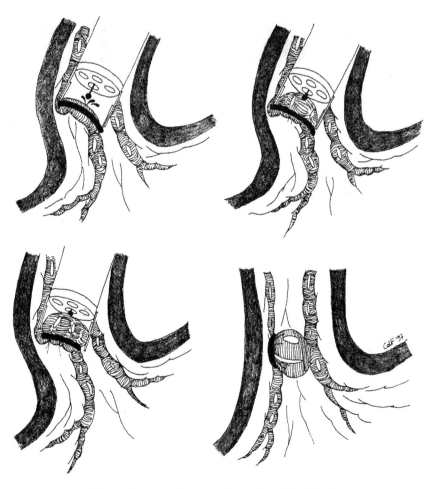

Figure 1. Technique of endoscopic oesophageal band ligation.

Technique

The technique is an adaptation of that applied to banding ligation of internal haemorrhoids. The original endoscopic ligating device consists of an outer cylinder, an inner cylinder, a trip wire and a latex O-ring. The outer cylinder is fitted to the end of a standard gastroscope by a friction mount. The inner, smaller cylinder is fitted with an inner clasp that allows connection with the trip wire, and carries a pre-stressed O-ring at the distal end of its outer surface. After fitting the outer cylinder to the gastroscope, the trip wire is passed through vacuum lock of the biopsy channel and advanced until it exits the distal end of the endoscope. The trip wire is secured to the clasp in the inner cylinder, and the inner cylinder is backed in the outer cylinder.

The endoscope with the ligating device in place is inserted into the oesophagus, the device is closely apposed to the variceal cord, suction is applied through the endoscope, and the band is released over the entrapped varix by pulling the trip wire (Figure 1). This device allows the delivery of only one rubber band at a time. Since several bands are usually placed at each ligating session, an overtube is used to allow multiple insertions and removals of the endoscope. The overtube is preloaded on the endoscope before intubation; after reaching the stomach with the tip of the endoscope, the overtube is advanced into the oesophagus using the endoscope as an obturator. Application of the bands is commenced at the gastro-oesophageal junction and then worked proximally in a helical fashion for approximately 5 cm until six to eight bands have been applied.

While the technique is simple, the need to reload the ligating device several times and the potential difficulties in placing the 27-cm, long over-tube make it relatively cumbersome, with a session of banding ligation taking up to 30 minutes (Stiegmann et al, 1986). Preliminary reports on the use of multiple-shot devices that allow placement of five (Hochberger et al, 1996) or six (Saeed, 1996) bands at a time, and thus do not require the use of an overtube, are encouraging. Banding ligation sessions are repeated at 7- to 14-day intervals until obliteration of varices is achieved. Eradication of varices usually requires two to four band ligation sessions (Laine and Cook, 1995).

Complications

Complications of elastic band ligation can be classified as those resulting from elastic band ligation itself and its tissue effects and those from use of the overtube. Minor complications such as transient dysphagia and chest discomfort are not uncommon. Shallow ulcers at the site of each ligation are the rule, and rarely bleed (Stiegmann et al, 1992). Table 1 reports the complications of banding ligation observed in the first 167 patients con-secutively treated at the centres of the New Italian Endoscopic Club (NIEC) (Battaglia et al, 1996). The most worrisome complication was bleeding because of the untimely sloughing of bands caused by inadvertent contact with the endoscope during follow-up endoscopy. For this reason, we have now adopted a 2-week interval between ligation sessions. Mechanical complications from use of the overtube range from mucosal tear causing bleeding to complete oesophageal perforation. Overtube trauma is usually caused by 'pinching' of the oesophageal wall in the gap between the endoscope and the overtube during insertion of the latter. These complications will probably disappear as the multiple-band ligating devices are increasingly adopted.

PROPHYLAXIS AGAINST THE FIRST VARICEAL HAEMORRHAGE

Today, medical treatment with non-selective beta-blockers is the treatment of choice to prevent the first episode of variceal bleeding in cirrhotics (Pagliaro et al, 1992). However, both endoscopic sclerotherapy and rubber band ligation have been studied in randomized controlled trials for the primary prophylaxis of bleeding from oesophageal varices.

Prophylactic sclerotherapy

Prophylactic sclerotherapy has been studied in 21 trials. In different studies, sclerotherapy was found to be better, equal or worse than no treatment, both for prevention of first bleeding and for survival. In a review of these trials (Pagliaro et al, 1992), an international panel of experts concluded that the heterogeneity of trial results makes meta-analysis meaningless. Therefore, sclerotherapy cannot be recommended as prophylactic treatment of the first variceal bleeding. This conclusion was confirmed at a recent international consensus workshop on portal hypertension (de Franchis, 1996).

Prophylactic rubber band ligation

In the only fully published trial (Sarin et al, 1996) rubber band ligation was compared with no treatment. Over a 1-year follow-up, 8.5% of 35 patients treated with banding and 39% of 33 controls who were followed up with no active prophylactic treatment, bled ($P < 0.01$). Mortality was 11% and 25% respectively ($P = NS$). These data are promising. However, since an effective medical treatment for prevention of first variceal bleeding (i.e. non-elective beta-blockers) does exist (Pagliaro et al, 1992), new treatments such as banding ligation ought to be compared with beta-blockers. Until such comparisons are made, banding cannot be recommended as a routine measure for the primary prophylaxis of bleeding from oesophageal varices.

TREATMENT OF ACUTE VARICEAL BLEEDING

Injection sclerotherapy, rubber band ligation and variceal obturation with tissue adhesives have all been used in the treatment of acute variceal haemorrhage. While randomized controlled trials comparing sclerotherapy and band ligation with alternative treatments abound, controlled data on endoscopic obturation of oesophageal varices are scanty.

Emergency sclerotherapy versus balloon tamponade and/or versus vasoactive drugs

Sclerotherapy has been compared with balloon tamponade in four trials, and with various forms of drug treatment in 10 (Table 2). Two trials in the former group gave data on control of bleeding (Paquet and Feussner, 1985; Moreto et al, 1988), and showed a favourable effect of sclerotherapy. In the latter group, meta-analysis (de Franchis, 1994) shows a significant advantage of sclerotherapy over drug treatment in controlling bleeding (pooled odds ratio (POR) 1.88; 95% confidence intervals (CI) 1.24–2.84) (Figure 2). Meta-analysis of both groups of trials with respect to mortality showed no difference between treatments in the former group, and some advantage for sclerotherapy in the latter (POR 0.69; 95% CI 0.49–0.98) (Figure 2).

Table 2. Randomized controlled trials of treatments for acute variceal bleeding: I.

Trial No.	Author/Treatment Groups	Year	Treatment	Number of patients	% Efficacy	% Mortality
				Bt/Sc	Bt/Sc	Bt/Sc
Balloon tamponade versus sclerotherapy						
1	Barsoum et al	1982	Bt/Sc	50/50	—	42/26
2	EVASP	1984	Bt/Sc	94/93	—	48/48
3	Paquet and Feussner	1985	Bt/Sc	22/21	73/95	27/10
4	Moreto et al	1988	Bt/Sc	20/23	80/100	30/30
1–4	Pooled data			186/187	54/98	42/36
Drugs +/–balloon tamponade versus sclerotherapy				DBt/Sc	DBt/Sc	DBt/Sc
1	Söderlund and Ihre	1985	VB/Sc	50/57	84/95	36/28
2	Larson et al	1986	VB/Sc	38/44	79/95	13/5
3	El-Zayadi et al*	1988	VB/Sc	55/63	—	20/11
4	Westaby et al	1989	VN/Sc	31/33	65/88	39/27
5	Alexandrino et al	1990	VB/Sc	42/41	71/71	40/39
6	Di Febo et al	1990	S/Sc	23/24	78/92	26/21
7	Planas et al	1994	S/Sc	35/35	75/69	23/12
8	Shields et al	1992	S/Sc	39/41	77/83	31/20
9	Jenkins et al	1992	O/Sc	20/20	90/90	25/25
10	Sung et al	1993	O/Sc	49/49	68/78	6/8
1–10	Pooled data			382/407	76/83	26/20

* Patients with schistosomiasis; Bt, balloon tamponade; Sc, sclerotherapy; VB, vasopressin + balloon; VN, vasopressin + nitro-glycerine; S, somatostatin; O, octreotide.

Emergency sclerotherapy versus emergency rubber band ligation

Of 14 randomized controlled trials comparing sclerotherapy with rubber band ligation, nine give separate data for acutely bleeding patients (Table 3). Difference in the control of bleeding between sclerotherapy and band ligation was found in only one of the studies (Lo et al, 1996), which showed a significant advantage for rubber banding. When the results of the nine trials are combined, the difference in control of

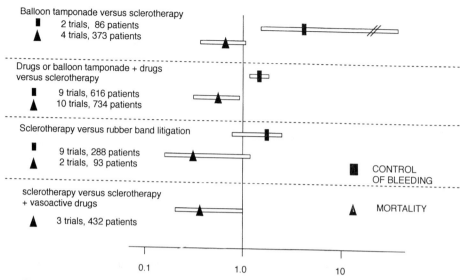

Figure 2. Meta-analysis of treatments of acute variceal bleeding. Pooled odds ratios and 95% confidence intervals.

Table 3. Randomized controlled trials of endoscopic treatments for acute variceal bleeding: II.

Trial No.	Author Treatment groups	Year	Treatment	Number of patients	% Efficacy	% Mortality
Rubber band ligation versus sclerotherapy				L/Sc	L/Sc	L/Sc
1	Stiegmann et al	1992	L/Sc	14/13	86/77	–
2	Laine et al	1993	L/Sc	9/9	89/89	–
3	Gimson et al	1993	L/Sc	21/23	90/91	–
4	Jensen et al	1993	L/Sc	14/11	80/100	–
5	Lo et al	1995	L/Sc	18/15	94/80	–
6	Hou et al	1995	L/Sc	20/16	100/88	–
7	Fakhry et al*	1995	L/Sc	10/12	90/92	10/8
8	Sarin et al	1995	L/Sc	5/7	80/86	–
9	Lo et al	1996	L/Sc	37/34	95/76	19/38
1–9	Pooled data			140/148	84/91	17/30
Combined endoscopic + pharmacological treatment versus endoscopic treatment			EP/E	EP/E	EP/E	EP/E
1	Besson et al	1995	SO/Sc	98/101	87/71[a]	7/10[b]
2	Sung et al	1995	LO/L	47/47	96/94[c]	9/19[c]
					91/62[d]	
3	Avgerinos et al	1996	SS/Sc	75/76	57/33[f]	3/9[b]
4	Brunati et al	1996	SOs/Sc	28/27	80/60[g]	13/15[b]
4b	Brunati et al	1996	ST/Sc	28/27	70/60[g]	13/15[b]
1–4	Pooled data			276/251	–	8/12

[a] Survival without rebleeding at 5 days; [b] 5-day mortality; [c] initial haemostasis; [d] percentage of patients without rebleeding at 2 days; [e] in-hospital mortality; [f] percentage of patients without treatment failure at 5 days; [g] 5-day control of acute bleeding; Sc, sclerotherapy; L, band ligation; EP, endoscopic + pharmacological treatment; E, endoscopic treatments; SO, sclerotherapy + octreotide; SOs, sclerotherapy + subcutaneous octreotide; ST, sclerotherapy + i.v. terlipressin.

bleeding is not statistically significant (POR 1.77; 95% CI 0.88–3.55) (Figure 2). Mortality figures are available from two studies only (Fakhry et al, 1995; Lo et al, 1996) both showing no difference between treatments. From these results, sclerotherapy and band ligation appear to be equally effective in the emergency situation. However, the number of patients on which this conclusion is based is small. In addition, some reports (Veltzke et al, 1996) suggest that emergency banding may be more difficult than sclerotherapy, since the field of vision is reduced by about 30% with the banding device attached. In the acute setting, the reduced field of vision coupled with large volumes of fresh blood refluxing up the oesophagus may hamper the effective placement of the rubber bands. It may be more appropriate, therefore, to use injection sclerotherapy to control haemorrhage in the patient who is actively bleeding at the index endoscopy, and to reserve banding ligation for the patient who has stopped bleeding.

Emergency endoscopic therapy versus emergency endoscopic therapy plus vasoactive drugs

Endoscopic treatments have been recently compared with combined regimens consisting of endoscopic therapy plus vasoactive drugs. The studies compared sclerotherapy versus sclerotherapy plus i.v. octreotide (Besson et al, 1995), rubber banding versus rubber banding plus i.v. octreotide (Sung et al, 1995), sclerotherapy versus sclerotherapy plus i.v. native somatostatin (Avgerinos et al, 1996), while another study had three arms: sclerotherapy alone versus sclerotherapy plus i.v. terlipressin versus sclerotherapy plus subcutaneous octreotide (Brunati et al, 1996) (Table 3). Drug treatment was started before endoscopy (Avgerinos et al, 1996), at endoscopy (Sung et al, 1995; Brunati et al, 1996), or immediately afterwards (Besson et al, 1995). Only the studies by Besson and Avgerinos were double-blind. The definitions of end-points used to evaluate treatment efficacy were so disparate as to make a meaningful meta-analysis impossible (see Table 3). Nevertheless, the efficacy of the combined treatment was equal or superior to that of endoscopic treatment alone in all studies. Meta-analysis of the 5-day mortality could be done for three trials (Besson, Avgerinos, Brunati), and showed no significant difference between treatments (POR 0.59; 95% CI 0.34–1.03) (Figure 2).

Emergency endoscopic sclerotherapy versus sclerotherapy + obturation with tissue adhesive

Two recent randomized studies compared sclerotherapy alone with a combination of sclerotherapy and N-butyl-2-cyanoacrylate for the control of active bleeding from oesophageal (Thakeb et al, 1995) or oesophago-gastric (Feretis et al, 1995) varices. The combined treatment was better than sclerotherapy alone in both studies. If these data are confirmed, variceal obturation may become a useful tool in the rare patients not responding to vasoactive drugs or sclerotherapy.

PREVENTION OF VARICEAL REBLEEDING

Both sclerotherapy and rubber band ligation have been used as long-term treatments to prevent rebleeding from oesophageal varices.

Long-term sclerotherapy versus conservative measures versus long-term beta-blockers versus sclerotherapy + beta-blockers, and versus sclerotherapy + subcutaneous octreotide

Sclerotherapy has been compared with conservative measures (10 trials, 1259 patients; Table 4), with long-term beta-blockers (nine trials, 752 patients, Table 5), and with a combined treatment including sclerotherapy

Table 4. Randomized controlled trials of treatments for the prevention of variceal rebleeding: I. Sclerotherapy versus conservative treatment.

Trial No.	Author/Year	Number of patients C/Sc	% Rebleeding C/Sc	% Mortality C/Sc
1	Barsoum et al 1982	50/50	58/26	42/26
2	Terblanche et al 1983	38/37	53/38	63/62
3	EVASP 1984	94/93	54/48	78/65
4	Westaby et al 1985	60/56	81/55	53/32
5	Korula et al 1985	57/63	54/21	33/33
6	Paquet and Feussner 1985	22/20	32/20	77/33
7	Söderlund and Ihre 1985	50/57	32/28	58/47
8	Burroughs et al 1989	104/102	59/55	59/47
9	Gregory 1990	131/122	60/52	42/52
10	Rossi et al 1991	27/26	63/50	33/23
1–10	Pooled data	633/626	57/43	54/46

C, Control treatments; Sc, sclerotherapy.

Table 5. Randomized controlled trials of treatments for the prevention of variceal rebleeding: II. Beta-blockers versus sclerotherapy.

Trial No.	Author/year	Number of patients β/Sc	% Rebleeding β/Sc	% Mortality β/Sc
1	Fleig et al 1987	34/36	29/28	15/8
2	Terés et al 1993	57/59	51/34	21/30
3	Alexandrino et al 1988	34/31	74/55	32/29
4	Dollet et al 1988	27/28	44/64	44/54
5	Westaby et al 1990	52/56	54/45	42/38
6	Liu et al 1990	58/60	57/33	38/28
7	Rossi et al 1991	27/26	48/50	26/23
8	Martin et al 1991	42/34	55/53	31/24
9	Dasarathy et al 1992	46/45	67/42	41/22
1–9	Pooled data	377/375	54/43	35/29

β, Beta-blockers; Sc, sclerotherapy.

plus beta-blockers (10 trials, 600 patients; Table 6). In a single trial (Primignani et al, 1995) sclerotherapy was compared with sclerotherapy plus subcutaneous octreotide (100 μg t.i.d. for 1 month). In the first group of trials, meta-analysis showed a significant reduction of rebleeding in sclerotherapy-treated patients (POR 0.57; 95% CI 0.45–0.71) (Figure 3). Mortality was also significantly reduced (POR 0.72; 95% CI 0.57–0.90) (Figure 3). It is noteworthy that the complications rate was higher in patients treated by sclerotherapy in all trials. In the group of trials com-

Table 6. Randomized controlled trials of treatments for the prevention of variceal rebleeding: III. Sclerotherapy versus beta-blockers + sclerotherapy.

Trial No.	Author/year	Treatment	Number of patients Sc/Sβ	% Rebleeding Sc/Sβ	% Mortality Sc/Sβ
1	Westaby et al 1986	Sc/SP	27/26	30/27	26/35
2	Jensen and Krorup 1989	Sc/SP	16/15	75/20	7/6
3	Gerunda et al 1990	Sc/SN	30/30	23/20	10/3
4	Lundell et al 1990	Sc/SP	22/19	50/63	NA
5	Bertoni et al 1990	Sc/SN	14/14	28/7	21/7
6	Vinel et al 1992	Sc/SP	35/39	40/18	14/13
7	Acharya et al 1993	Sc/SP	56/58	21/17	12/9
8	Avgerinos et al 1993	Sc/SP	40/45	52/31	18/18
9	Vickers et al 1994	Sc/SP	34/39	53/51	26/23
10	Villanueva et al 1992	Sc/SN	18/22	39/55	0/9
1–10	Pooled data		293/307	39/30	15/13

Sc, Sclerotherapy; Sβ, sclerotherapy + beta-blockers.

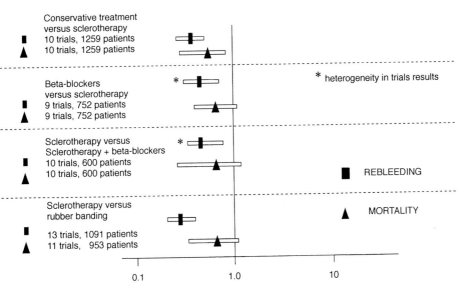

Figure 3. Meta-analysis of treatments for prevention of variceal rebleeding. Pooled odds ratios and 95% confidence intervals.

paring sclerotherapy with beta-blockers, meta-analysis showed a significant reduction of rebleeding in favour of sclerotherapy (POR 0.64; 95% CI 0.48–0.85, Figure 3). However, an important qualitative heterogeneity between trials results has been shown (D'Amico et al, 1995), which approaches significance ($P = 0.07$), and weakens the results of meta-analysis, suggesting that the advantage of sclerotherapy may be small. None of the trials showed a significant difference in mortality in either direction, and this is reflected in the meta-analysis (POR 0.82; 95% CI 0.60–1.11). In trials comparing sclerotherapy alone with sclerotherapy + beta-blockers, the combined treatment was significantly better than sclerotherapy alone in preventing rebleeding (POR 0.65; 95% CI 0.46–0.92), but qualitative heterogeneity in trial results was found (D'Amico et al, 1995), and thus meta-analysis should be interpreted with caution. Mortality was similar with the two treatment regimens (POR 0.81; 95% CI 0.50–1.29). In the trial comparing sclerotherapy alone with sclerotherapy plus subcutaneous octreotide (Primignani et al, 1995), the rebleeding rate was not significantly different in the two treatment groups (34% versus 31%, $P = 0.73$). Mortality was also similar in the two groups.

Long-term sclerotherapy versus long-term beta-blockers + nitrates

A recent trial has compared sclerotherapy with a oral medical treatment consisting of nadolol plus isosorbide-5-mononitrate (Villanueva et al, 1996). Eleven of 43 (25.6%) patients on the medical regimen rebled, as compared with 23 of 43 (53.5%) treated by sclerotherapy ($P < 0.001$). The rebleeding rate of medically treated patients in this study is the lowest ever reported in trials of medical prevention of variceal rebleeding, while that of patients in the sclerotherapy arm is among the highest reported for this kind of treatment. The corresponding figures for mortality were 9.3% and 20.9% ($P = 0.07$). If the data concerning rebleeding are confirmed in other studies, the combination of beta-blockers + nitrates is likely to become the first choice medical therapy to prevent variceal rebleeding, and the standard with which alternative therapies should be compared.

Long-term sclerotherapy versus long-term rubber band ligation

Thirteen trials with a total of 1091 patients have compared sclerotherapy with rubber band ligation (Table 7). Ligation was better than sclerotherapy in preventing rebleeding in all studies, and was significantly so in five trials (Gimson et al, 1993; Hou et al, 1995; Lo et al, 1995; Sarin et al, 1995; Masci et al, 1996). Meta-analysis shows a strong benefit for rubber banding (POR 0.46; 95% CI 0.35–0.60). Only 11 trials give figures for mortality: in two rubber banding was significantly better than sclerotherapy (Laine et al, 1993; Lo et al, 1995) while the other studies showed small, not significant changes in either direction. Meta-analysis confirms that the two treatments are equivalent (POR 0.84; 95% CI 0.62–1.15)

The strong difference in rebleeding rate in favour of rubber banding is probably the consequence of several factors: the number of treatment

Table 7. Randomized controlled trials for treatments for the prevention of variceal rebleeding: IV. Sclerotherapy versus rubber banding.

Trial No.	Author/year	Treatment	Number of patients Sc/L	%Rebleeding Sc/L	%Mortality Sc/L
1	Stiegmann et al 1992	Sc/L	65/64	48/36	45/25
2	Laine et al 1993	Sc/L	39/38	31/24	15/10
3	Gimson et al 1993	Sc/L	49/54	53/30	35/39
4	Young et al 1993	Sc/L	10/13	38/20	31/20
5	Jensen et al 1993	Sc/L	39/37	35/31	24/26
6	Mundo et al 1993	Sc/L	8/11	27/25	36/25
7	Avgerinos et al 1994	Sc/L	40/37	40/27	20/21
8	Lo et al 1995	Sc/L	59/61	44/15	32/16
9	Hou et al 1995	Sc/L	67/67	32/18	16/21
10	Sarin et al 1995	Sc/L	47/48	21/6	6/6
11	Baroncini et al 1995	Sc/L	46/43	9/2	—
12	Fakhry et al 1995	Sc/L	25/24	8/4	—
13	Masci et al 1996	Sc/L	50/50	48/24	14/22
1–13	Pooled data		545/546	36/21	25/22

Sc, Sclerotherapy; L, band ligation.

sessions required to achieve variceal eradication was significantly smaller with banding (2.5 to 4.1 sessions) than with sclerotherapy (2.9 to 6.5 sessions) in all but one of the 12 trials that reported this data (Jensen et al, 1993). In the NIEC series of consecutive patients, eradication was achieved with a mean of 2.5 ± 1.4 band ligation sessions as compared with 3.6 ± 1.9 sessions required with sclerotherapy (Battaglia et al, 1996); the mean time to eradication was 2.8 versus 4.9 months respectively. Decreasing the time required to achieve eradication reduces the 'vulnerable phase' of endoscopic treatments (i.e. the time when the risk of rebleeding is decreased but still exists, owing to the incomplete eradication of varices). In addition, the number of clinically significant complications was generally lower in patients treated with banding (Laine and Cook, 1995): oesophageal stenosis after banding was reported in only one trial (Masci et al, 1996, 2%), while its incidence after sclerotherapy ranged between 0 and 33%; the incidence of bleeding from treatment-induced ulcers was lower with banding in all but one of the studies (Stiegmann et al, 1992). Finally, the incidence of septic complications (pulmonary infections, spontaneous bacterial peritonitis) and of fatal complications was also lower in patients undergoing rubber band ligation, although the difference with sclerotherapy was small (Laine and Cook, 1995). In view of these results, rubber band ligation has become the endoscopic treatment of choice for the prevention of recurrent bleeding from oesophageal varices, (Westaby et al, 1996). Unsolved issues concern the rate of recurrence of varices after obliteration, which was found to be higher after banding than sclerotherapy in at least one study (48% versus 30%, $P = 0.08$) (Hou et al, 1995), and the influence of sclerotherapy and rubber band ligation on the development of portal hypertensive gastropathy (Sarin et al, 1995; Primignani et al, 1996), as well as on the perioesophageal circulation. The value of the association of sclerotherapy and rubber band ligation in comparison with either treatment alone is controversial (Argonz et al, 1996; Jensen et al, 1996; Saeed et al, 1997).

TREATMENT OF GASTRIC VARICES

Injection sclerotherapy with standard sclerosants has been applied to treat active bleeding from fundal/cardia varices, but is associated with a high rate of rebleeding and a frequent need to resort to surgical intervention (Trudeau and Prindiville, 1985; Sarin et al, 1988; Gimson et al, 1991) A randomized controlled trial comparing sodium tetradecilsulphate (STS) with 50% hypertonic glucose-water (HG) has been recently published (Chang et al, 1996). Initial control of bleeding was achieved in 80% of 25 patients treated with STS, and in 92% of 26 patients receiving HG ($P = NS$). Rebleeding occurred in 70% of patients in the former group, as compared with 30% in the latter ($P < 0.05$).

Other substances used to treat acute bleeding from gastric varices in uncontrolled series include thrombin (Williams et al, 1994) and Bucrylate (Ramond et al, 1989). Encouraging, albeit uncontrolled, results have been reported for both substances. In a non-randomized study comparing ethanolamine oleate with Bucrylate (Oho et al, 1995) the latter was significantly more effective in obtaining immediate haemostasis (90% of 23 patients versus 67% of 24 patients, $P < 0.05$), but no significant difference in rebleeding (35% versus 25%), survival (52% versus 33%) and complications rate (52% versus 46%) was detected. Clearly, randomized controlled trials comparing various treatment modalities for gastric varices are needed.

CONCLUSIONS

As of today, endoscopic treatments are not recommended for the primary prophylaxis of variceal bleeding.

Sclerotherapy remains a quick and simple technique for the control of active bleeding from oesophageal varices, and is more effective than drug treatment alone in arresting bleeding, although the difference may be small.

Although few trials have been published so far, there is some evidence suggesting that the early administration of vasoactive drugs (somatostatin, octreotide or terlipressin) is safe and may increase the efficacy of endoscopic treatments. Since, even in the largest Centres, emergency therapeutic endoscopy requires some time to be organized, a sensible strategy could be to start vasoactive drugs when the patient reaches the emergency room, while endoscopy is been organized.

Banding ligation is the optimal endoscopic treatment for the prevention of rebleeding from oesophageal varices. Comparisons of band ligation with long-term beta-blockers have not been made. The value of combining band ligation with long-term pharmacological treatment has not been investigated yet.

The availability of the tissue adhesives and thrombin as injectates for fundal gastric varices provides the option of an initial attempt at endoscopic therapy in this high risk group, but controlled data are needed.

REFERENCES

Acharya SK, Dasarathy S, Saksena S & Pande JN (1993) A prospective randomized study to evaluate propranolol in patients undergoing long-term endoscopic sclerotherapy. *Journal of Hepatology* **19:** 291–300.

Alexandrino PT, Alves MM & Pinto Correia J (1988) Propranolol or endoscopic sclerotherapy in the prevention of recurrence of variceal bleeding. A prospective, randomized controlled trial. *Journal of Hepatology* **7:** 175–185.

Alexandrino P, Alves MM, Fidalgo P et al (1990) Is sclerotherapy the first choice treatment for active oesophageal variceal bleeding in cirrhotic patients? *Journal of Hepatology* **11 (Supplement 2):** SI (Abstract).

*D'Amico G, Pagliaro L & Bosch J (1995) The treatment of portal hypertension: a meta-analytic review. *Hepatology* **22:** 332–354.

Argonz J, Kravetz D, Suarez A et al (1996) Banding plus sclerotherapy is more effective than banding alone in preventing variceal rebleeding. *Hepatology* **24:** 208A (Abstract).

Avgerinos A, Rekoumis G, Klonis C et al (1993) Propranolol in the prevention of recurrent upper gastrointestinal bleeding in patients with cirrhosis undergoing endoscopic sclerotherapy. A randomized controlled trial. *Journal of Hepatology* **19:** 301–311.

Avgerinos A, Armonis A, Manolakopoulos S et al (1994) Endoscopic sclerotherapy (ES) versus endoscopic ligation (EVL) for the prevention of recurrent oesophageal variceal hemorrhage in cirrhotics. A prospective study. *Gastroenterology* **106:** A861 (Abstract).

Avgerinos A, Nevens F, Raptis S et al (1996) Early administration of natural somatostatin increases the efficacy of sclerotherapy in acute bleeding oesophageal variceal episodes. The European ABOVE study. *Hepatology* **24:** 191A (Abstract).

Baroncini D, Piemontese A, Milandri GL et al (1995) Results of mid term follow-up of a prospective, randomized study of comparison of ligation and sclerotherapy for oesophageal varices. *Italian Journal of Gastroenterology* **27:** 24–25.

Barsoum MS, Boulous FI, El-Rooby A et al (1982) Tamponade and injection sclerotherapy in the management of bleeding oesophageal varices. *British Journal of Surgery* **69:** 76–78.

Battaglia G, Capria A, Cestari R et al (1996) One-year outcome following endoscopic band ligation of varices: results in 167 consecutive patients seen at 9 NIEC Centers. *Journal of Hepatology* **25 (Supplement 1):** S93.

Bertoni G, Fornaciari G, Beltrami M et al (1990) Nadolol for prevention of variceal rebleeding during the course of endoscopic injection sclerotherapy: a randomized pilot study. *Journal of Clinical Gastroenterology* **12:** 364–365 (Letter).

*Besson I, Ingrand P, Person B et al (1995) Sclerotherapy with or without octreotide for active variceal bleeding. *New England Journal of Medicine* **333:** 555–560.

Brunati S, Ceriani R, Curioni R et al (1966) Sclerotherapy alone vs sclerotherapy plus terlipressin vs sclerotherapy plus octreotide in the treatment of acute variceal hemorrhage. *Hepatology* **24:** 207A (Abstract).

Burroughs AK & McCormick PA (1992) Prevention of rebleeding. In Groszmann RJ & Grace ND (eds) *Complications of Cirrhosis. Portal Hypertension and Ascites. Gastroenterology Clinics of North America* **20:** pp. 119–147. Philadelphia: WB Saunders.

Burroughs AK, McCormick PA, Siringo S et al (1989) Prospective randomized trial of long term sclerotherapy for variceal rebleeding using the same protocol to treat rebleeding in all patients. Final report. *Journal of Hepatology* **9 (Supplement 1):** S12 (Abstract).

Chang KY, Wu CS & Chen PC (1996) Prospective, randomized trial of hypertonic glucose water and sodium tetradecilsulfate for gastric variceal bleeding in patients with advanced liver cirrhosis. *Endoscopy* **28:** 481–486.

Crafoord C & Freckner P (1939) New surgical treatment of varicose veins of the oesophagus. *Acta Otolaryngologica* (Stockholm) **27:** 422–429.

Dasarathy S, Dwivedi M, Bhargava DK et al (1992) A prospective randomized trial comparing repeated endoscopic sclerotherapy and propranolol in decompensated (Child class B and C) cirrhotic patients. *Hepatology* **16:** 89–94.

Dollet JM, Champigneulle B, Patris A et al (1988) Sclérothérapie endoscopique contre propranolol après hémorrhagie par rupture de varices oesophagiennes chez le cirrhotique. Résultats à 4 ans d'une étude randomisée. *Gastroenterologie Clinique et Biologique* **12:** 234–239.

EVASP (The Copenhagen oesophageal varices sclerotherapy project) (1984) Sclerotherapy after first variceal hemorrhage in cirrhosis. A randomised multicenter trial. *New England Journal of Medicine* **311:** 1594–1600.

Fakhry S, Omer M, Nouh A et al (1995) Endoscopic sclerotherapy versus endoscopic variceal ligation in the management of bleeding esophageal varices: a preliminary report of a prospective randomized study. *Hepatology* **22:** 251A (Abstract).

Di Febo G, Siringo M, Vacirca M et al (1990) Somatostatin (SMS) and urgent sclerotherapy (US) in active oesophageal variceal bleeding. *Gastroenterology* **98:** S583 (Abstract).

Feretis C, Dimopoulos C, Benakis P et al (1995) N-Butyl-2-cyanoacrylate (Histoacryl) plus sclerotherapy alone in the treatment of bleeding esophageal varices: a randomized prospective study. *Endoscopy* **27:** 355–357.

Fleig WE, Stange EF, Hunecke R et al (1987) Prevention of recurrent bleeding in cirrhotics with recent variceal hemorrhage: prospective, randomized comparison of propanolol and sclerotherapy. *Hepatology* **7:** 355–361.

de Franchis R (1994) Treatment of bleeding oesophageal varices: a meta-analysis. *Scandinavian Journal of Gastroenterology* **24 (Supplement 207):** S29–S33.

de Franchis R (1996) Developing consensus in portal hypertension. *Journal of Hepatology* **25:** 390–394.

Gerunda GE, Neri D, Zangrandi F et al (1990) Nadolol does not reduce early rebleeding in cirrhotics undergoing endoscopic variceal sclerotherapy (EVS): a multicenter randomized controlled trial. *Hepatology* **12:** 988 (Abstract).

Gimson AES, Westaby D & Williams R (1991) Endoscopic sclerotherapy in the management of gastric variceal hemorrhage. *Journal of Hepatology* **13:** 274–278.

Gimson AES, Ramage JK, Panos MZ et al (1993) Randomised trial of variceal banding ligation versus injection sclerotherapy for bleeding oesophageal varices. *Lancet* **342:** 391–394.

*Graham DY, & Smith JL (1981) The course of patients after variceal hemorrhage. *Gastroenterology* **80:** 800–806.

Gregory PB (VA Co-operative variceal sclerotherapy group) (1990) Sclerotherapy for male alcoholic cirrhotic patients who have bled from esophageal varices: results of a randomized, multicenter clinical trial. *Hepatology* **20:** 618–625.

Hochberger J, Reh H, Hörning F et al (1996) A new multiple-band ligator (speedband) for the endoscopic treatment of esophageal and gastric varices. Preliminary results in 63 applications of a prospective ongoing study. *Endoscopy* **28:** S14 (Abstract).

Hosking SW & Johnson AG (1988) Gastric varices: a proposed classification and a guide to management. *British Journal of Surgery* **75:** 195–196.

Hou MC, Lin HC, Kuo BIT et al (1995) Comparison of endoscopic variceal injection sclerotherapy and ligation for the treatment of esophageal variceal hemorrhage: a pèrospective randomized trial. *Hepatology* **21:** 1517–1522.

Infante-Rivard C, Esnaola S & Villeneuve JR (1989) Role of endoscopic sclerotherapy in long-term management of variceal bleeding: a meta-analysis. *Gastroenterology* **96:** 1087–1092.

Jenkins SA, Copeland G, Kingsnorth A & Shields R (1992) A prospective randomised controlled clinical trial comparing Sandostatin (SMS) and injection sclerotherapy in the control of acute variceal hemorrhage: an interim report. *Gut* **33:** F221 (Abstract).

Jensen DM, Kovacs TOG, Randall GM et al (1993) Initial results of a randomised prospective study of emergency banding vs sclerotherapy for bleeding gastric or oesophageal varices. *Gastrointestinal Endoscopy* **39:** 279 (Abstract).

Jensen DM, Kovacs TOG, Jutabha R et al (1996) Final results of a randomized prospective trial (RPT) of combination rubber band ligation and sclerotherapy (COMBO) vs. sclerotherapy alone for hemostasis of bleeding esophageal varices (abstract). *Gastroenterology* **110:** 1222A.

Jensen LS & Krarup N (1989) Propranolol in prevention of rebleeding from oesophageal varices during the course of endoscopic sclerotherapy. *Scandinavian Journal of Gastroenterology* **24:** 339–345.

Kitano S, Iso Y, Yamaga H et al (1988) Temporary deterioration of pulmonary functions after injection sclerotherapy for cirrhotic patients with esophageal varices. *European Surgical Research* **20:** 298–303.

Korula J, Balart L, Radvan G et al (1985) A prospective randomized controlled trial of chronic esophageal variceal sclerotherapy. *Hepatology* **5:** 584–589.

Koutsomanis D, Sebti MF & Essaid A (1995) A randomized study of endoscopic hemostatic clipping versus endoscopic variceal ligation. *Gastroenterology* **108:** A630 (Abstract).

Laine L & Cook D (1995) Endoscopic ligation compared with sclerotherapy for treatment of esophageal variceal bleeding. *Annals of Internal Medicine* **123:** 280–287.

*Laine L, El-Newihi HM, Migikowsky B et al (1993) Endoscopic ligation compared with sclerotherapy for the treatment of bleeding oesophageal varices. *Annals of Internal Medicine* **119:** 1–7.

Larson AW, Cohen H, Zweiban B et al (1986) Acute oesophageal variceal sclerotherapy. Results of a prospective randomised controlled trial. *Journal of the American Medical Association* **255:** 497–500.

Lee MS, Bong HK, Kim JO et al (1996) Endoscopic ligation of gastric varices using detachable snares and rubber bands. *Gastroenterology* **110:** A25 (Abstract).

Liu JD, Jeng YS, Chen P et al (1990) *Endoscopic Injection Sclerotherapy and Propranolol in the Prevention of Recurrent Variceal Bleeding.* World Congress of Gastroenterology abstract book: FP1181 (abstract). Abingdon Oxfordshire: The Medical Group (UK).

Lo GH, Lai KH, Cheng JS et al (1995) A prospective, randomised trial of injection sclerotherapy versus banding ligation in the management of bleeding oesophageal varices. *Hepatology* **22:** 466–471.

Lo GH, Lai KH & Huang JS (1996) Emergency sclerotherapy vs banding ligation for arresting of actively bleeding esophageal varices. *Endoscopy* **28:** S50 (Abstract).

Lundell L Leth R, Lind T et al (1990) Evaluation of propranolol for prevention of recurrent bleeding from esophageal varices between sclerotherapy sessions. *Acta Chirurgica Scandinavica* **156:** 711–715.

MacDougall BRD, Westaby D, Theodossi A et al (1982) Increased long-term survival in variceal haemorrhage using injection sclerotherapy. Results of a controlled trial. *Lancet* **i:** 124–127.

Martin T, Taupignon A, Lavignolle A & Perrin D (1991) Prévention des récidives hémorrhagiques chez les malades atteints de cirrhose. Résultats d'une étude controlée comparant propranolol et sclérose endoscopique. *Gastroenterologie Clinique et Biologique* **15:** 833–837.

Masci E, Norberto L, D'Imperio N et al (1996) Prospective multicentric randomized trial comparing banding ligation with sclerotherapy of oesophageal varices. *Italian Journal of Gastroenterology* **28 (Supplement 2):** 170 (Abstract).

Mathur SK, Dalvi AN, Someshwar V et al (1990) Endoscopic and radiological appraisal of gastric varices. *British Journal of Surgery* **77:** 432–435.

Moretò M, Zaballa M, Bernal A et al (1988) A randomised trial of tamponade or sclerotherapy as immediate treatment for bleeding oesophageal varices. *Surgery, Gynaecology and Obstetrics* **167:** 331–334.

Mundo F, Mitrani C, Rodriguez G & Farca A (1993) Endoscopic variceal treatment: is band ligation taking over sclerotherapy? *American Journal of Gastroenterology* **88:** 1493 (Abstract).

NIEC (North-Italian Endoscopic Club for the study and treatment of esophageal varices) (1988) Prediction of the first variceal hemorrhage in patients with cirrhosis of the liver and esophageal varices. A prospective multicenter study. *New England Journal of Medicine* **319:** 983–989.

Oho K, Iwao T, Sumino M et al (1995) Ethanolamine oleate versus butyl-cyanoacrylate for bleeding gastric varices: a non-randomized study. *Endoscopy* **27:** 349–354.

*Pagliaro L, D'Amico G, Soerensen TIA et al (1992) Prevention of first bleeding in cirrhosis. A meta-analysis of randomized trials of nonsurgical treatment. *Annals of Internal Medicine* **11:** 59–70.

Pagliaro L, D'Amico G, Pasta L et al (1994) Portal hypertension in cirrhosis: natural history. In Bosch J & Groszmann RJ (eds) *Portal Hypertension: Pathophysiology and Treatment,* pp 72–92. Oxford: Blackwell Scientific Publications.

Paquet K–J & Feussner H. (1985) Endoscopic sclerosis and oesophageal balloon tamponade in acute haemorrhage from esophago-gastric varices: a prospective controlled randomised trial. *Hepatology* **5:** 580–583.

Planas R, Quer JC, Boix J et al (1994) A prospective randomised trial comparing somatostatin and sclerotherapy in the treatment of acute variceal bleeding. *Hepatology* **20:** 370–375.

Primignani M, Andreoni B, Carpinelli L et al (1995) Sclerotherapy plus octreotide vs sclerotherapy alone in the prevention of early rebleeding from esophageal varices: a randomized, double blind, placebo-controlled, multicenter trial. *Hepatology* **21:** 1322–1327.

Primignani M, Materia M, Bianchi MB et al (1996) Evaluation of changes in portal hypertensive gastropathy following endoscopic treatment of varices with sclerotherapy or band ligation. *Journal of Hepatology* **25 (Supplement 1):** S169.

Ramond MJ, Valla D, Gotlib JP et al (1986) Obturation endoscopique des varices oeso-gastriques par le Bucrylate. *Gastroenterologie Clinique et Biologique* **10:** 575–579.

Ramond M–J, Valla D, Mosnier J–F et al (1989) Successful endoscopic obturation of gastric varices with butyl cyanoacrylate. *Hepatology* **10:** 488–493.

Rossi V, Calés P, Pascal JP et al (1991) Prevention of recurrent bleeding in alcoholic cirrhotic patients: a prospective controlled trial of propranolol and sclerotherapy. *Journal of Hepatology* **12:** 283–289.

Saeed ZA (1996) The Saeed six-shooter: a prospective study of a new endoscopic multiple rubber-band ligator for the treatment of varices. *Gastroenterology* **110:** A1308 (Abstract).

Saeed ZA, Stiegmann GV, Ramirez FC et al (1997) Endoscopic variceal ligation is superior to combined ligation and sclerotherapy for esophageal varices: a multicenter prospective randomized trial. *Hepatology* **25:** 71–74.

Sarin SK, Guptan RC, Jain A & Sundaram KR (1996) Randomised controlled trial of endoscopic variceal band ligation for primary prophylaxis of variceal bleeding. *European Journal of Gastroenterology and Hepatology* **8:** 337–342.

Sarin SK, Sachdev G, Nanda R et al (1988) Endoscopic sclerotherapy in the treatment of gastric varices. *British Journal of Surgery* **75:** 747–750.

Sarin SK, Lahoti D, Saxena SP et al (1992) Prevalence, classification and natural history of gastric varices: long term follow-up study in 568 patients with portal hypertension. *Hepatology* **16:** 1343–1349.

Sarin SK, Goyal A, Jain A et al (1995) Randomized prospective trial of endoscopic sclerotherapy vs variceal ligation for bleeding esophageal varices: influence on gastropathy, gastric varices and recurrences. *Gastroenterology* **108:** A629 (Abstract).

Schuman BM, Beckman JW, Tedesco FJ et al (1987) Complications of injection sclerotherapy: a review. *American Journal of Gastroenterology* **82:** 823–829.

See A, Florent C, Lamy P et al (1986) Accidents vasculaires cerebraux par obturation endoscopique des varices oesophagiennes par l'Isobutyl-2-cyanoacrylate chez deux malades. *Gastro-enterologie Clinique et Biologique* **10:** 604–607.

Shields R, Jenkins SA, Baxter JN et al (1992) Prospective randomised controlled trial comparing somatostatin and injection sclerotherapy in the control of acute variceal hemorrhage. *Journal of Hepatology* **16:** 128–137.

Singal A, Sarin SK, Sood GK & Broor SL (1990) Ulcers after intravariceal sclerotherapy–correlation of symptoms and factors affecting healing. *Journal of Clinical Gastroenterology* **12:** 250–254.

Söderlund C & Ihre T (1985) Endoscopic sclerotherapy vs conservative management of bleeding oesophageal varices. *Acta Chirurgica Scandinavica* **151:** 449–456.

Soehendra N, Nam VC, Grimm H et al (1986) Endoscopic obliteration of large esophago-gastric varices with Bucrylate. *Endoscopy* **18:** 25–26.

Stiegmann GV & Yamamoto M (1992) Endoscopic techniques for the management of active variceal bleeding. In Westaby D (ed.) *Variceal Bleeding. Gastrointestinal Endoscopy Clinics of North America*, pp 59–75. Philadelphia: WB Saunders.

Stiegmann GV, Cambre T & Sun JH (1986) A new endoscopic elastic band ligating device. *Gastrointestinal Endoscopy* **32:** 230–233.

Stiegmann GV, Sun JH & Hammond WS (1988) Results of experimental endoscopic esophageal varix ligation. *American Surgery* **54:** 105–108.

Stiegmann GV, Goff JS, Sun JH et al (1989) Technique and early clinical results of endoscopic variceal ligation (EVL) *Surgical Endoscopy* **3:** 73–78.

*Stiegmann GV, Goff JS, Michaletz-Onody PA et al (1992) Endoscopic sclerotherapy as compared with endoscopic ligation for bleeding oesophageal varices. *New England Journal of Medicine* **326:** 1527–1532.

Sung JJY, Chung SCS, Lai CW et al (1993). Octreotide infusion or emergency sclerotherapy for variceal hemorrhage. *Lancet* **342:** 637–641.

Sung JJY, Chung S, Yung MY et al (1995) Prospective randomised study of effect of octreotide on rebleeding from oesophageal varices after endoscopic ligation. *Lancet* **346:** 1666–1669.

Terblanche J, Bornman PC, Kahn D et al (1983) Failure of repeated injection sclerotherapy to improve long-term survival after oesophageal variceal bleeding. *Lancet* **ii:** 1328–1332.

Terés J, Bosch J, García Pagàn JC et al (1993) Propranolol vs sclerotherapy in the prevention of variceal rebleeding. A randomized controlled trial. *Gastroenterology* **105**: 1508–1514.

Thakeb F, Salama Z, Salama H et al (1995) The value of combined use of N-butyl-2-cyanoacrylate and ethanolamine oleate in the management of esophagogastric varices. *Endoscopy* **27**: 358–364.

Trudeau W & Prindiville T (1985) Endoscopic injection sclerosis in bleeding gastric varices. *Gastrointestinal Endoscopy* **32**: 264–268.

Veltzke W, Adler RE & Hintze RE (1996) Role of endoscopic ligation in active variceal bleeding under emergency conditions. *Endoscopy* **28**: S50 (Abstract).

Vickers C, Rhodes J, Chesner I et al (1994) Prevention of rebleeding from esophageal varices: two-year follow up of a prospective controlled trial of propranolol in addition to sclerotherapy. *Journal of Hepatology* **21**: 81–87.

Villanueva C, Torras X, Tomas A et al (1992) Nadolol como coadyuvante a la scleroterapia en el tratamiento electivo de la hemorragia por varices esofagicas. Estudio randomizado y controlado. *Gastroenterologia y Hepatologia* **15**: 341 (Abstract).

*Villanueva C, Balanzò J, Novella MT et al (1996) Nadolol plus isosorbide mononitrate compared with sclerotherapy for the prevention of variceal rebleeding. *New England Journal of Medicine* **334**: 1624–1629.

Vinel JP, Lamouliatte H, Calés P et al (1992) Propranolol reduces the rebleeding rate during injection sclerotherapy before variceal obliteration. *Gastroenterology* **102**: 1760–1763.

Watanabe K, Kimura K, Matsutani S et al (1988) Portal hemodynamics in patients with gastric varices. A study in 230 patients with oesophageal or gastric varices using portal vein catheterization. *Gastroenterology* **95**: 434–440

Westaby D (1992) Prevention of recurrent variceal bleeding. In Westaby D (ed.) *Variceal Bleeding. Gastrointestinal Endoscopy Clinics of North America*, pp 121–135. Philadelphia: WB Saunders.

Westaby D, MacDougall BRD & Williams R (1985) Improved survival following injection sclerotherapy for oesophageal varices: final analysis of a controlled trial. *Hepatology* **5**: 627–631.

Westaby D, Melia W, Hegarty J et al (1986) Use of propranolol to reduce the rebleeding rate during injection sclerotherapy prior to variceal obliteration. *Hepatology* **4**: 673–675.

Westaby D, Hayes P, Gimson AE et al (1989) Controlled trial of injection sclerotherapy for active variceal bleeding. *Hepatology* **9**: 274–277.

Westaby D, Polson RJ, Gimson AES et al (1990) A controlled trial of oral propranolol compared with injection sclerotherapy for the long-term management of variceal bleeding. *Hepatology* **11**: 353–359.

*Westaby D, Binmöller K, de Franchis R et al (1996) Baveno II consensus statements: the endoscopic management of variceal bleeding. In de Franchis R (ed.) *Portal Hypertension II. Proceedings of the Second International Consensus Workshop on Definitions, Methodology and Therapeutic Strategies*, p 126. Oxford: Blackwell.

Williams SGJ, Peters RA & Westaby D (1994) Thrombin—an effective treatment for fundal gastric varices? *Gut* **35**: 1287–1289.

Young M, Sanowski R & Rasche R (1993) Comparison and characterization of ulcerations induced by endoscopic ligation of esophageal varices versus endoscopic sclerotherapy. *Gastrointestinal Endoscopy* **39**: 119–122.

Zambelli A, Arcidiacono PG, Arcidiacono R et al (1993) Complications of endoscopic variceal sclerotherapy: a multicenter study of 1192 patients. *Gastroenterology* **104**: A 1023 (Abstract).

Zanasi G, Rossi A, Grosso C et al (1996) The effect of endoscopic sclerotherapy of oesophageal varices on the development of gastric varices. *Endoscopy* **28**: 234–238.

El Zayadi A, El Din S & Kabil M (1988) Endoscopic sclerotherapy versus medical treatment for bleeding esophageal varices in patients with schistosomal liver disease. *Gastrointestinal Endoscopy* **34**: 314–317.

7

Advances in drug therapy for acute variceal haemorrhage

D. PATCH MBBS, MRCP

Senior Registrar

A. K. BURROUGHS MBChB(Hons), FRCP

Consultant Physician and Hepatologist

Department of Liver Transplantation and Hepato-Biliary Medicine, The Royal Free Hampstead NHS Trust, Pond Street, Hampstead, London NW3 2QG, UK

Recent advances in the pharmacology of portal hypertension are reviewed, against the background of existing knowledge and current clinical research. The most recent trials are analysed, and conclusions made about the use of drugs in acute variceal haemorrhage, as well as directions for further clinical trials and research.

Key words: portal hypertension; variceal bleeding; pharmacology.

Bleeding from varices remains one of the most feared complications of cirrhosis, with mortality continuing to be in the range of 30–50% (Christensen et al, 1981; Graham and Smith, 1981). A particular characteristic is that bleeding often recurs within days of admission (DeDombal et al, 1986; Burroughs et al, 1989). This, along with severity of the bleed and the severity of underlying liver disease, represent major predictive factors for death.

ADVANTAGES OF PHARMACOLOGICAL THERAPY

Patients suffering from bleeding from varices will often present to accident and emergency departments hypotensive, encephalopathic, oliguric and septic. In addition, the majority will initially be cared for in general hospitals, where expertise in the management of portal hypertensive bleeding may not be readily to hand. There is therefore a need for easily administered, safe, effective drug therapy that may either stop bleeding, or may 'buy time' in order to allow a skilled endoscopist to be called in, or to facilitate safe transfer. In addition, if a drug is effective in reducing or stopping variceal bleeding, it may allow the endoscopist an unimpaired view of the oesophagus, facilitating effective (as opposed to blind) sclerotherapy, as well as reducing the risk of aspiration. Finally, prolonged drug therapy may prevent early rebleeding.

The rationale for drug therapy is based on the factors that influence pressure in a column of fluid—these are resistance and flow. Ohm's law states that pressure = flow × resistance. Thus, it is possible to reduce portal and consequently variceal pressure by reducing the portal collateral blood flow (by splanchnic vasoconstriction), and by decreasing the vascular resistance of the intrahepatic and portal circulation (by means of vasodilators), or a combination of the two. Finally agents that constrict the physiological lower oesophageal sphincter could reduce variceal blood flow by constricting the palisade zone, where the collaterals feed the varices.

REVIEW OF PHARMACOLOGICAL AGENTS

Vasopressin

Vasopressin is a non-selective vasoconstrictor that reduces portal pressure secondary to a reduction in splanchnic flow. It acts on receptors found in the splanchnic circulation, and (unfortunately) throughout the systemic circulation. It has now fallen from favour as a consequence of its questionable efficacy (of 417 episodes of variceal bleeding treated with vasopressin in over 15 randomized clinical trials published to date, control of haemorrhage was only achieved in about 50%) (Patch and Burroughs, 1995), and its high incidence of side effects, seen in up to 45% of patients. These include colicky abdominal pain, angina, cutaneous gangrene and even stroke, resulting in cessation of therapy in up to 25% of cases. In order to minimize the systemic side effects of vasopressin, nitroglycerine has been added to the regime. This reduces the extra-splanchnic effects of vasopressin by its vasodilatory action (particularly on the coronary circulation) as well as reducing portal vascular resistance.

Terlipressin

This synthetic analogue of vasopressin (triglycyl lysine vasopressin) has intrinsic vasoconstrictor activity and is also slowly cleaved in vivo into vasopressin by enzymatic cleavage of the triglycyl residue. Because of its longer biological half-life, it has the advantage of 4-hourly bolus administration, and unlike vasopressin has no effect on haemostasis as it does not increase the plasma concentration of plasminogen activator. In five unblinded trials (Freeman et al, 1982; Desaint et al, 1987; Lee et al, 1990) comparing glypressin with vasopressin, the former agent had a significantly lower complication rate, even when vasopressin was associated with nitroglycerine (Chiu et al, 1990; D'Amico et al, 1994).

Terlipressin is the only vasoconstrictor that has been shown to reduce mortality in placebo-controlled trials of acute variceal bleeding (Walker et al, 1986; Freeman et al, 1989; Söderlund et al, 1990), with a pooled odds ratio for failure to control bleeding of 0.31 (0.15–0.61) compared with placebo. Because of these studies, it is the only drug licensed in Europe for the management of acute variceal bleeding. Recent data (Nevens et al, 1996) has provided further evidence that this agent is, to date, probably the most effective in reducing variceal pressure. In an elegant study using the Varipress non-invasive variceal pressure gauge in 30 patients, glypressin produced a mean reduction of variceal pressure of 27%. Octreotide produced a variable effect, with no overall change in variceal pressure. Saline injection resulted in no change in variceal pressure. A similar study (Monescillo et al, 1995) compared the effects of somatostatin and glypressin on variceal pressure during acute bleeding. At 15 minutes, glypressin maintained a reduction in variceal pressure, whereas the effect of a somatostatin bolus had worn off.

Somatostatin

Somatostatin is a 14-amino acid peptide that has been widely used in the pharmacological treatment of variceal bleeding because of its ability to decrease splanchnic blood flow (Tyden et al, 1979; Sonnenburg et al, 1981), without significant side effects. This is against a background of a wealth of data derived from animal models of portal hypertension and cirrhosis. It was therefore a logical alternative to drugs such as vasopressin or its analogue. Subsequent studies have demonstrated variable effects. In some studies, hepatic blood flow (Merkel et al, 1985), hepatic venous pressure gradient and portal pressure (Bories et al, 1980; Bosch et al, 1981), azygous blood flow (Mastai et al, 1986) and variceal pressure have been shown to fall. However, except for the reduction in azygous blood flow, these findings have not been consistent and others have found no effect on gastric mucosal flow (Sonnenberg et al, 1983) or intravariceal pressure (Kleber et al, 1988), therefore putting its potential clinical use in doubt.

Somatostatin is usually administered as an infusion; however, this may not be the best method as suggested in recent studies (Cirera et al, 1995). Nineteen patients were given either somatostatin as a bolus followed by an infusion, or saline as a placebo followed by a saline infusion. Bolus injection of somatostatin had a significant effect on hepatic venous pressure gradient (HVPG), falling from a mean of 17.4 ± 0.8 to 8.4 ± 0.9 at 1 minute ($P < 0.001$). This effect began to wear off at 3 minutes. Even the high dose somatostatin infusion (500 μg/hour) only reduced HVPG from 20.4 ± 1.5 to 18.2 ± 1.7 ($P < 0.01$).

Octreotide

Octreotide is a synthetic octapeptide of somatostatin that shares four amino acids with the native compound, which are responsible for its biological activity. Its principal advantage is its longer half-life, achieved by the addition of a phenylalanine residue at the N-terminal end, and the elongation of the C-terminal end with threonine. As with somatostatin, octreotide can significantly reduce portal pressure (Jenkins et al, 1988; Mckee et al, 1989), collateral (Jenkins et al, 1985) and azygous blood flow (Navasa et al, 1988), surrogate markers of variceal blood flow, but like somatostatin there are some studies that show no haemodynamic effect.

Precisely how these two agents work is unclear. The putative action is as an indirect vasoconstrictor, by inhibiting the release of vasodilatory peptides such as glucagon, vaso-active intestinal peptide and substance P. It is, however, clear that these effects are not confined to the splanchnic circulation. McCormick clearly demonstrated that an octreotide bolus causes an increase in mean arterial pressure and systemic vascular resistance, with a compensatory fall in pulse and cardiac output (McCormick et al, 1995). These changes were seen within 3 minutes of the bolus, suggesting that octreotide may also act directly on the human vasculature. These effects were not seen with an infusion. Further evidence for the variable of pharmacological efficacy of octreotide infusions may have come from the Barcelona Group. In a study published in abstract, transient but significant reductions in HVPG were seen in 24 patients. Unfortunately, these effects lasted <5 minutes, and the addition of an octreotide infusion failed to prolong or maintain these effects (Escorsell et al, 1996).

It is clear that somatostatin and octreotide have potential as vasoconstrictors in variceal bleeding. In practice, they seem to have fewer side effects than glypressin. Nonetheless not all patients have reduced portal pressures with these drugs, and nor has the mode of administration been resolved (bolus appears to be more effective than infusion). When one reviews the clinical data in terms of effectiveness in stopping variceal bleeding, it is unclear whether they are comparable in efficacy, or if they work at all.

Metoclopramide and domperidone

By constricting the lower oesophageal sphincter, these drugs could reduce variceal blood flow. Metoclopramide has been shown to reduce transmural oesophageal variceal pressure, but has no effect on portal haemodynamics (Taranto et al, 1990; Stanciu et al, 1993). A single small study suggested that metoclopramide could reduce bleeding at the time of endoscopy (Hosking et al, 1990) but this was not confirmed in another preliminary trial (Feu et al, 1988). There is currently no role for these agents in the management of variceal bleeding, except in the context of a clinical trial.

RESULTS OF CLINICAL TRIALS

Vasopressin

Results of clinical trials for vasopressin are shown in Table 1. Only four trials compared the efficacy of vasopressin with a placebo (Merigan et al,

Table 1. Randomized trials of vasopressin versus placebo or no treatment.

Author	Date	Patient admissions	Dose units	Length of infusion	Efficacy (percentage of bleeding episode controlled)		
					Control	:	Vasopressin
Merigan et al	1962	53	20 μ	20 minutes	0%	:	55%
Conn et al	1975	33	<0.4 μ/minute	7–74 hours	25%	:	71%
Mallory et al	1980	12	0.2–0.4 μ/minute	1–196 hours	15%	:	44%
Fogel et al	1982	33	0.6–0.3 μ/minute	24 hours	37%	:	29%

1962; Conn et al, 1975; Mallory et al, 1980; Fogel et al, 1982), and two of these studies used an intra-arterial route of administration (Conn et al, 1975; Mallory et al, 1980). Using meta-analysis, there was a significant reduction in failure to control bleeding (Pooled Odds Ratio 0.22, 95% CI.12–0.43), but no benefit in terms of mortality.

Three randomized controlled clinical trials have compared vasopressin alone with vasopressin plus nitroglycerin (transdermally, Bosch et al, 1989; intravenously, Gimson et al, 1986 and sublingually, Tsai et al, 1986), and all three showed the combination therapy to be more effective in controlling bleeding, with a pooled estimate of treatment effect of 0.51, 95% CI 0.4–0.96. There was a reduction in mortality that was not significantly different. In two of the trials, side effects were significantly reduced (Gimson et al, 1986; Tsai et al, 1986). Despite this, it is the authors' opinion that there is no longer a role for this drug in variceal bleeding.

Terlipressin

The trials for terlipressin are shown in Table 2. There have been criticisms of these studies. The trial by Walker et al (1986) included other

Table 2. Randomized controlled trials of triglycyl vasopressin.

Author	Date	Patient number	Glypressin	:	Efficacy other therapy (percentage of bleeding episodes controlled)
Walker et al	1986	34	100	:	80 (placebo)
Freeman et al	1989	31	60	:	37 (placebo)
Soderlund et al	1990	60	84	:	55 (placebo)
Aracidiacono et al	1992	217	82	:	72 (sclerotherapy)
Desaint et al	1987	19	80	:	83 (vasopressin)
Freeman et al	1982	19	70	:	9 (vasopressin)
Chiu et al	1990	54	50	:	54 (vasopressin)
Walker et al	1992	50	88	:	76 (somatostatin)
D'Amico et al	1994	165	83	:	75 (vasopressin + NG)
Colin	1997*	54	88	:	88 (tamponade)
Fort et al	1990†	47	61	:	72 (tamponade)
VBSG	1994	161	80	:	84 (somatostatin)
Silvain et al	1993+	87	59	:	78 (octreotide)

* With nitroglycerin.
† Included a third group, glypressin and tamponade combined, 96% effective.

therapies, the timing of which is unclear, and the other two trials (glypressin versus placebo) are hampered by insufficient patient numbers to avoid a type 2 error. These issues will be addressed in forthcoming trials.

A recent study (Levacher et al, 1995) in which terlipressin or placebo was administered before arriving at hospital, based on reasonable evidence of bleeding varices, also showed a reduced mortality of glypressin in grade C patients. However, the drug was only given at three doses, with no difference in transfusion requirements at 12 hours. The potential benefit of a vasoactive drug maintaing vital organ perfusion appeared to be nullified by the fact that there was no significant difference in blood pressure between the two groups on arrival at hospital. It remains to be seen whether these data can be reproduced, and whether terlipressin is the gold standard drug for acute variceal bleeding (Burroughs et al, 1996).

Somatostatin/octreotide

The results of randomized controlled studies that evaluate efficacy versus placebo or compare their effects with other drugs are summarized in Table 3. The first two placebo controlled trials came to opposite conclusions. The trial by Valenzuela et al (1989) suggested that somatostatin is no more effective than placebo. Unfortunately, only 84 patients who could be evaluated were recruited over 14 months in 11 centres, suggesting marked patient selection, and the end point was a bleed-free period of 4 hours. Furthermore, the 83% placebo rate is the highest reported in the literature. In contrast, the trial by Burroughs et al (1990) reported a statistically significant benefit for somatostatin in controlling variceal bleeding over a 5-day treatment period, with failure to control bleeding seen in 36% of patients receiving somatostatin, compared with 59% of patients receiving placebo. This emphasizes the problem of differences in end point selection, making meaningful comparisons difficult. The third study (Gotzche et al, 1995) also showed no effect of somatostatin, but it took 5 years to recruit 86 patients, again raising concerns regarding selection.

The trials comparing somatostatin or octreotide versus vasopressin or terlipressin show virtually identical results with no statistical difference in either efficacy or mortality (Kravetz et al, 1984; Jenkins et al, 1985; Caradona et al, 1989; Hsia et al, 1990; Saari et al, 1990; Hwang et al, 1992; Walker et al, 1992; Silvain et al, 1993). However, a statistically significant reduction in side effects and complication rate was observed in the group receiving somatostatin or octreotide. Whilst this is also true in the latest study that compared somatostatin and terlipressin (Feu et al, 1996), there was no difference between the two groups in terms of *serious* side effects, and no patient required specific treatment or stopped their medication. Interestingly, somatostatin was given not only as an infusion, but also as an initial bolus, and up to three additional boluses during the study period.

Table 3. Somatostatin and octreotide* for variceal bleeding.

Authors	Date	Patient(s) admissions	Duration of treatment	Efficacy of somatostatin or octreotide; percentage episodes controlled of bleeding	Other therapy (%)
Kravetz et al	1984	61	48 hours	53	58 (vasopressin)
Jenkins et al	1985	22	25 hours	100	33 (vasopressin)
Bagarani et al	1987	50	48 hours	67	32 (vasopressin)
Saari et al	1990	54	72 hours	66	52 (vasopressin)
Hsia et al	1990	46	24 hours	55	38 (vasopressin)
Walker et al	1992	50	24 hours	76	88 (glypressin)
VBSG	1994	161	24 hours	84	80 (glypressin)
Feu et al	1996	161	48 hours	84	80 (glypressin)
Hwang et al*	1992	48	24 hours	63	46 (vasopressin)
Cardona et al	1989	38	24 hours	45	55 (vasopressin/ nitroglycerin)
Silvain et al*	1993	87	24 hours	78	59 (glypressin/ nitroglycerin)
McKee[a]	1990	40	48 hours	50	70 (tamponade)
Avgerinos et al*	1991	92	24 hours	71	80 (tamponade)
Jaramillo et al	1991	39	< 24 hours	58	50 (tamponade)
Valenzuela et al	1989	84	30 hours	65	83 (placebo)
Burroughs et al	1990	120	5 days	64	41 (placebo)
Gotzsche et al	1995	86	24 hours	30	59 (placebo)
Burroughs*	1996	383	5 days	58	60 (placebo)
DiFebo et al	1990	47	48 hours	78	92 (sclerotherapy)
Jenkins et al*	1992	40	48 hours	90	90 (sclerotherapy)
Shields et al	1992	80	5 days	77	80 (sclerotherapy)
Planas et al	1994	70	48 hours	80	83 (sclerotherapy)
Sung et al*	1993	65	48 hours	72	58 (sclerotherapy)
VBSG	1994	170	5 days	81	83 (sclerotherapy)

* Efficacy was also assessed in a third group given combined somatostatin and balloon tamponade.

   In the four fully published trials where drug treatment was compared with sclerotherapy (Shields et al, 1992; Sung et al, 1993; Planas et al, 1994; VBSG, 1994), no statistical differences were observed between somatostatin/octreotide and injection sclerotherapy. There was no difference in the control of bleeding, blood product usage or mortality in any of the studies, which confirms the potential importance of drug therapy for variceal bleeding.

   Two recent studies have suggested that the addition of octreotide is beneficial to injection sclerotherapy or banding compared with sclerotherapy alone plus placebo (Besson et al, 1995; Sung et al, 1995). A similar study using somatostatin for 5 days, that showed enhancement of the effect of acute injection, has been published as an abstract (Avgerinos et al, 1996). However, in the largest study to date (recently published in abstract) involving 383 patients, octreotide or placebo given double-blind as soon as possible after hospital admission and continued for 5 days resulted in no difference in efficacy, regardless of whether or not injection sclerotherapy was needed for active bleeding at endoscopy or drug failure (Burroughs et al, 1996).

RANDOMIZED TRIALS OF DRUGS VERSUS BALLOON TAMPONADE

There are eight studies in the literature that compare the use of drugs with balloon tamponade (Pinto-Correia et al, 1984; Colin et al, 1987; Fort et al, 1990; McKee, 1990; Teres et al, 1990; Avgerinos et al, 1991; Jaramillo et al, 1991; Blanc et al, 1994) (Table 4). However, comparing them is difficult, because of end-point definition.

Table 4. Drugs versus balloon tamponade.

Author	Year	Drug type	Total number patients (p) or episodes (e)	% Child–Pugh patients	Efficacy % drug: tamponade	Death % drug: tamponade
Pinto-Correia et al	1984	vasopressin	37e	13	65:70	12:20
Colin et al	1987	terlipressin	54e	22	74:74	15:22
Teres et al	1990	vasopressin + nitroglycerin	108p	—	66:87	30:31
Fort et al	1990	terlipressin + nitroglycerin	47e	55	78:79	0:8
McKee	1990	octreotide	40e	7	0:25*	50:70
Avgerinos et al	1991	somatostatin	61p	26	55:33	23:33
Jaramillo et al	1991	somatostatin	39p	41	58:50*	26:25
Blanc et al	1994	terlipressin	40e	—	70:95	35:35

* No information on blood transfusion requirements.

Tamponade, if used properly, provides good control of bleeding. However, the balloons should not be inflated for more than 24 hours and preferably for less, and bleeding frequently occurs when the balloons are deflated. From the trial reports it is not always clear when efficacy is being assessed, e.g. during therapy or at the end of an interval of 24 hours after termination of drug therapy or tamponade. Despite these problems, significant differences in mortality or efficacy have not been demonstrated between tamponade and drugs.

This conclusion is supported by a meta-analysis performed by D'Amico et al (1995) that also demonstrated no difference in efficacy or mortality between balloon tamponade and vasoactive therapy. Furthermore, there were no differences related to the type of drug used.

Complication rates are poorly documented, and in particular it is difficult to differentiate serious side effects from minor ones. A higher complication rate would be expected from balloon tamponade, especially in unskilled hands, yet no statistical difference was reported when this was compared with drug therapy in these trials. Nonetheless, it is clear that balloon tamponade has poor patient acceptability, a high complication rate, including potentially fatal ones, and cannot be recommended as first line treatment except in massive haemorrhage where bleeding cannot otherwise be controlled. Comparisons can only be made with drugs in a selected group of patients who have the same severity of bleeding, and the available trials do not address this question. Furthermore, it is difficult to justify such studies today. Thus balloon tamponade should be reserved for exsanguinating bleeding, emergency management during the transport of the patient, and for failures of drug or endoscopic therapy while awaiting other therapies.

RANDOMIZED TRIALS OF DRUGS VERSUS ENDOSCOPIC SCLEROTHERAPY

All except one of the early studies (Westaby et al, 1989) compared a vasoactive drug and balloon tamponade with sclerotherapy (Table 5). Differences between treatments are hard to evaluate because the time point of assessment is not clearly defined. Nonetheless, there was no significant difference in efficacy or mortality.

Table 5. Drugs and balloon tamponade versus endoscopic sclerotherapy.*

Author	Year	Drug type	Total number patients	% Child–Pugh patients	Efficacy % drugs/T: sclerotherapy	Death % drugs/T: sclerotherapy
Larson et al	1986	vasopressin	82	57	13:5	79:95
COVSP	1984	vasopressin	187	—	—	48:48
Soderlund et al	1985	vasopressin	107	72	84:95	36:28
Alexandrino et al	1990	vasopressin + nitroglycerin	83	49	71:71	40:39

* In these trials sclerotherapy was given if necessary to the group initially treated with drugs and balloon tamponade.

In the trials in which a simple comparison was made between vasoactive drugs and sclerotherapy (Table 6), all but one trial (Westaby et al, 1989) compared somatostatin or octreotide, and no statistically significant difference was found for efficacy or mortality (DiFebo et al, 1990; Jenkins et al, 1992; Shields et al, 1992; Sung et al, 1993; Planas et al, 1994; VBSG et al, 1994).

Table 6. Drugs versus endoscopic sclerotherapy.

Author	Year	Drug type	Duration of treatment	Total number of patients (p) or episodes (e)	% Child–Pugh C	Efficacy % drug: sclerotherapy	Death % drug: sclerotherapy
Westaby et al	1989	vasopressin nitroglycerin	12 hours	64e	34	65:88	39:27
DiFebo et al	1990	somatostatin	48 hours	47p	—	78:92	26:21
Shields et al	1992	somatostatin	5 days	80p	54	77:83	31:20
Jenkins et al	1992	octreotide	48 hours	40p	70	90:90	25:25
Sung et al	1993	octreotide	48 hours	98p	45	72:58	29:41
Planas et al	1994	somatostatin	48 hours	70p	—	80:83	29:23
VSBG	1994*	somatostatin	5 days	170p	—	81:83	11:9

* Randomized 24 hours after admission.

If both groups of trials are taken together (the use of sclerotherapy versus the standard therapy of drugs with or without balloon tamponade, by combining the studies shown in Tables 5 and 6): then there is a statistically significant difference in favour of sclerotherapy for both efficacy ($P < 0.0008$) and mortality ($P < 0.02$). However, when analysed by year of publication, the more recent the study, the less the difference between treatment groups, reflecting either different end-point definitions, or reduced effectiveness of sclerotherapy. The latter is unlikely, so one must re-evaluate what is meant by success of sclerotherapy. More studies are needed in order to define efficacy precisely and the complications that occur between regimens using drugs and those using endoscopic measures.

New advances in the management of acute variceal bleeding

The explosion in knowledge of the mechanisms by which portal hypertension develops and is perpetuated is already beginning to result in the development of new agents. It is now clear that portal pressure is a dynamic process, potentially regulated by a number of cytokines. Many of these act through stellate cells. These are activated in cirrhosis, and appear to be contractile, functioning as regulators of intrahepatic blood flow and thus portal pressure (Rockey and Weisinger, 1996). Endothelins, acting both on ET_A and ET_B receptors, are powerful stellate cell contractors (Zhang et al, 1994; Pinzani et al, 1996), resulting in a rise in portal pressure. ET receptor antagonists have already been shown to reduce portal pressure, and are currently undergoing clinical trials (Rockey and Weisinger, 1996). Conversely, nitric oxide has been shown to cause stellate cell relaxation, resulting in a fall in portal pressure (Rockey and Chung, 1995). Logically, some form of intrahepatic NO donors may be beneficial at the time of bleeding, but these would have to avoid any systemic hypotensive effect.

Whilst much of this should be regarded as potential future developments, there is already good evidence for the use of a 'new' agent in the management of acute variceal bleeding—antibiotics. Variceal bleeding has clearly been shown to be associated with a high incidence of bacterial infection (Bleichner et al, 1986). Furthermore, bacterial infection has been shown to increase the risk of early rebleeding (Bernard et al, 1995). In a meta-analysis published in abstract involving 414 patients, antibiotic prophylaxis was shown to significantly reduce the incidence of bacterial infection, and significantly increase short-term survival (Bernard et al, 1996). It seems clear that the presence of infection, and the use of antibiotics, should be established as part of any clinical trial examining therapies in variceal bleeding, and that there is now a strong argument for the routine use of antibiotic prophylaxis.

REFERENCES

Acharya SK, Dasarthy S, Saksena S & Pando JN (1993) A prospective randomised study to evaluate propranolol in patients undergoing longterm endoscopic sclerotherapy. *Journal of Hepatology* **19:** 291–300.

Alexandrino PT, Alves MM & Pinto Correia J (1988) Propranolol or endoscopic sclerotherapy in the prevention of recurrence of variceal bleeding. A prospective randominized controlled trial. *Journal of Hepatology* **7:** 175–178.

Alexandrino P, Alves MM, Fidalgo P et al (1990) Is sclerotherapy the first choice treatment for active oesophageal varical bleeding in cirrhotic patients? *Journal of Hepatology* **11:** S1.

*D'Amico G, Pagliaro L & Bosch J (1995) The treatment of portal hypertension: a meta analytical review. *Hepatology* **22:** 332–354.

D'Amico G, Traina M, Vizzini G et al (1994) Terlipressin or vasopressin plus transdermal nitroglycerin in a treatment strategy for digestive bleeding in cirrhosis. A randomized clinical trial. *Journal of Hepatology* **20:** 206–212.

Andreani T, Poupon RE, Balbour BJ et al (1990) Prevention therapy of first gastrointestinal bleeding in patients with cirrhosis, results of a controlled trial comparing propranolol, endoscopic sclerotherapy and placebo. *Hepatology* **126:** 1413–1419.

Aracidiacono R, Biraghi M, Bonomo GM & Fiaccadori F (1992) Randomised controlled trial with terlipressin in cirrhotic patients with bleeding oesophageal varices: effects on precocious rebleeding and mortality rates. *Current Therapeutic Research* **52(1):** 186–194.

Avgerinos A, Klonis C, Rekoumis G et al (1991) A prospective randomized trial comparing somatostatin, balloon tamponade and the combination of both methods in the management of acute variceal haemorrhage. *Journal of Hepatology* **13:** 78–83.

Avgeninos A, Rekounis G, Klonis O et al (1993) Propranolol in the prevention of recurrent upper gastrointestional bleeding in patients with cirrhosis undergoing endoscopic sclerotherapy. *Hepatology* **19:** 301–311.

Avgerinos A, Nevens F, Raptis S et al (1996) Early administration of natural somatostatin increases the efficacy of sclerotherapy in acute bleeding oesophageal variceal episodes. The European ABOVE study. *Gut* **39 (supplement 3).**

Bagarani M, Albertini V, Anza M et al (1987) Effect of somatostatin in controlling bleeding from esophageal varices. *Italian Journal of Surgical Science* **17:** 21–26.

Besson I, Ingrand P, Person B et al (1995) Sclerotherapy with or without octreotide for acute variceal bleeding. *New England Journal of Medicine* **333:** 555–560.

*Bernard B, Cadranel J, Valla D et al (1995) Prognostic significance of bacterial infections in bleeding cirrhotic patients: A prospective study. *Gastroenterology* **108:** 1828–1834.

*Bernard B, Grange JD, Nguyen Khac E et al (1996). Antibiotic prophylaxis for the prevention of bacterial infections in cirrhotic patients with gastrointestinal bleeding: a meta-analysis. *Hepatology* **24(2):** A1271.

Bernard B, Lebrec D, Mathurin P et al (1997) Beta adrenergic antagonists in the prevention of gastrointestinal re-bleeding in patients with cirrhosis: a beta-analysis. *Hepatology* **25:** 63–70.

Bertoni G, Fornaciari G, Beltrami M et al (1990) Nadolol does not improve the result of sclerotherapy in prevention of variceal rebleeding. *Gut* **34 (supplement):** S5.

Blanc P, Bories J, Desperez D et al (1994) Balloon tamponade with Linton–Michel tube versus terlipressin in the treatment of acute oesophageal and gastric variceal bleeding. *Journal of Hepatology* **21:** Si33.

Bleichner G, Boulanger R, Squara P et al (1986) Frequency of infections in cirrhotic patients with acute gastrointestinal haemorrhage. *British Journal of Surgery* **73(9):** 724–726.

Bories P, Pomler-Layrargues G, Chotard JP et al (1980) Somatostatin reduces portal hypertension in cirrhotic patients. *Gastroenterology and Clinical Biology* **4:** 616–617.

Bosch J, Kravetz D & Rodes J (1981) Effects of somatostatin on hepatic and systemic haemodynamics in patients with cirrhosis of the liver: comparison with vasopressin. *Gastroenterology* **80:** 518–525.

Bosch J, Groszman RJ, Garcia-Pagan JC et al (1989) Association of transdermal nitroglycerin to vasopressin infusion in the treatment of variceal haemorrhage: a placebo controlled clinical trial. *Hepatology* **10:** 962–968.

Burroughs AK & Patch D (1996) Hepatology elsewhere. Therapeutic benefit of vasoactive drugs for acute variceal bleeding: a real pharmacological effect or a side effect of definition in trials. *Hepatology* **22:** 737–739.

Burroughs AK, Jenkins WJ, Sherlock S et al (1983) Controlled trial of propranolol for the prevention of recurrent variceal haemorrhage in patients with cirrhosis. *New England Journal of Medicine* **309:** 1539–1542.

Burroughs AK, Mezzanotte G, Phillips A et al (1989) Cirrhotic with variceal haemorrhage: the importance of the time interval between admission and the start of analysis for survival and rebleeding rates. *Hepatology* **9:** 801–807.

Burroughs AK, McCormick PA, Hughes MD et al (1990) Randomized, double blind, placebo controlled trial of somatostatin for variceal bleeding. Emergency control and prevention of early variceal rebleeding. *Gastroenterology* **99**: 1388–1395.

*Burroughs AK (for the International Octreotide Varices Group) (1996) Double-blind RCT of 5 day octreotide versus placebo associated with sclerotherapy for trial failures. *Hepatology* **24**: 901 A (abstract)

Cardona C, Vida F, Balanzo J et al (1989) Eficacia terapetica de la somatostatina versus vasopresina mas nitroglicerina en la hemorragia activa por varices esofagogastricas. *Gastroenterologia Y Hepatologia* **12**: 30–34.

Cerebelaud P, Langiolie A, Perain D et al (1986) Propranolol et prevention des recidives des ruptures de varice oesophagienne du cirrhotique. *Gastroenterologie Clinique Biologie* **10**: 18 (Abstract).

Chiu WK, Sheen IS & Liaw YF (1990) A controlled study of glypressin versus vasopressin in the control of acute oesophageal variceal haemorrhage. *Journal of Gastroenterology and Hepatology* **5**: 549–553.

Christensen E, Fauerholdt L, Schlichting P et al (1981) Aspects of the natural history of gastrointestinal bleeding in cirrhosis and the effects of prednisolone. *Gastroenterology* **81**: 944–952.

*Cirera I, Feu F, Luca A et al (1995) Effects of bolus injections and continuous infusions of somatostatin and placebo in patients with cirrhosis: a double blind hemodynamic investigation. *Hepatology* **22**: 106–111.

Colin R, Giuli N, Czernichow P et al (1987) Prospective comparison of Glypressin, tamponade and their association in the treatment of bleeding esophageal varices. In Lebrec D & Blei AT (eds) *Vasopressin Analogs and Portal Hypertension*, pp 149–153. Paris: John Libbey Eurotext.

Colman J, Jones P, Finch C & Dudley F (1990) Propranolol in the prevention of variceal hemorrhage in alcoholic cirrhotic patients. *Hepatology* **12**: 851 (abstract).

Colombo M, De Franchis R, Rommasni M et al (1989) Beta blockade prevents recurrent gastrointestinal bleeding in well decompensated patients with alcoholic cirrhosis. A multicentre randomized controlled trial. *Hepatology* **9**: 433–438.

Conn HO, Ramsby GR, Storer EH et al (1975) Intra arterial vasopressin in the treatment of upper gastrointestinal haemorrhage: a prospective, controlled clinical trial. *Gastroenterology* **68**: 211–221.

Conn HO, Grace ND, Bosch J et al (1991) Propanolol in the prevention of the first hemorrhage from esophagogastric varices. A multicentre randomized clinical trial. *Hepatology* **13**: 902–912.

COVSP (Copenhagen Oesphageal Varices Sclerotherapy Project) (1984) Sclerotherapy after first variceal haemorrhage in cirrhosis. A randomized multicenter trial. *New England Journal of Medicine* **311**: 1594–1600.

Dasarathy S, Buivedi M, Bhargua DK et al (1992) A prospective randomized trial comparing repeated endoscopic sclerotherapy and propranolol in decompensated (Child class B and C) cirrhotic patients. *Hepatology* **16**: 89–94.

Desaint B, Florent C & Levy VG (1987) A randomized trial of triglycyl-lysine vasopressin versus lysine vasopressin in active cirrhotic variceal haemorrhage. In Lebrec D & Blei AT (eds) *Vasopressin Analogs and Portal Hypertension*. Paris: John Libbey Eurotext, 987: pp 155–157.

Dollet JM, Champigneulle B, Patris MA & Gaucher P (1988) Sclerotherapie endoscopique contre propranolol après le monagie par rupture de varices oesophagiennes cher le cirrhotique. Results a 4 ans d'une étude randomisée. *Gastroenterologie Clinique Biologie* **12**: 239.

DeDombal FT, Clarke JR, Clamp SE et al (1986) Prognostic factors in upper GI bleeding. *Endoscopy* **18 (supplement)**: 6–10.

Elsayed S, Shiha G, Hamid M et al (1996) Sclerotherapy versus sclerotherapy and propranolol in the prevention of recurrent bleeding in patients with severe cirrhosis? A prospective randomised trial. *Gut* **38**: 770–774.

Escorsell A, Bandi JC, Francois E et al (1996) Desensitisation to the effects of intravenous octreotide in cirrhotic patients with portal hypertension. *Hepatology* **24(2)**: A322.

Di Febo G, Siringo S, Vacirca M et al (1990) Somatostatin (SMS) and urgent sclerotherapy (US) in active oesophageal variceal bleeding. *Gastroenterology* **99**: A583.

Feu F, Mas A, Bosch J et al (1988) Domperidone or metoclopramide versus placebo in the prevention of early variceal re-bleeding in cirrhosis. A prospective randomized trial. *Hepatology* **7 (supplement 1)**: 531 (Abstract).

*Feu F, Del Arbol LR, Banares R et al (1996) Double-blind randomized controlled trial comparing terlipressin and somatostatin for acute variceal haemorrhage. *Gastroenterology* **111**: 1291–1299.

Fleig W, Strange EF, Binecke R et al (1987) Prevention of recurrent bleeding in cirrhotics with recent variceal haemorrhage. Prospective randominized comparison of propranolol and sclerotherapy. *Hepatology* **7**: 355–361.

Fogel MR, Knauer CM & Andress LL (1982) Continuous intravenous vasopressin in active upper gastrointestinal bleeding. A placebo controlled trial. *Annals of Internal Medicine* **96**: 565–569.

Fort E, Sautereau D, Silvain C et al (1990) A randomized trial of terlipressin plus nitroglycerin vs balloon tamponade in the control of acute variceal hemorrhage. *Hepatology* **11**: 678–681.

Freeman JG, Cobden I & Record CO (1989) Placebo controlled trial of terlipressin (glypressin) in the management of acute variceal bleeding. *Journal of Clinical Gastroenterology* **11**: 58–60.

Freeman JG, Cobden I, Lishman AH & Record CO (1982) Controlled trial of terlipressin (glypressin) versus vasopressin in the early treatment of oesophageal varices. *Lancet* **ii**: 66–68.

Garden OJ, Mills PR, Birnie CG et al (1990) Propranolol in prevention and recurrent variceal haemorrhage in cirrhotic patients. A controlled trial. *Gastroenterology* **98**: 185–190.

Gatta A, Merkel C, Sacerdoti D et al (1987) Nadolol for the prevention of variceal rebleeding in cirrhosis. A controlled clinical trial. *Digestion* **37**: 22–28.

Gerunda GE, Neri D, Zangraundi F et al (1990) Nadolol does not reduce early rebleeding in cirrhotics undergoing endoscopic variceal sclerotherapy: a multicentre randomized controlled trial. *Hepatology* **12**: 988 (abstract).

Gimson AES, Westaby D, Hegarty J et al (1986) A randomized trial of vasopressin plus nitroglycerin in the control of acute variceal haemorrhage. *Hepatology* **6**: 410–413.

*Goetzche P, Gjorup I, Bonnen H et al (1995) Somatostatin versus placebo in bleeding oesophageal varices: randomized trial and meta-analysis. *British Journal of Medicine* **310**: 1495–1498.

Graham DY & Smith JL (1981) The course of patients after variceal haemorrhage. *Gastroenterology* **80**: 800–809.

Hosking SW, Doss W, El-einy H et al (1990) Pharmacological constriction of the lower esophageal sphincter: a simple method of arresting variceal haemorrhage. *Gut* **29**: 1098–1102.

Hsia H-C, Lee F-Y, Tsai Y-T et al (1990) Comparison of somatostatin and vasopressin in the control of acute esophageal variceal haemorrhage: a randomized controlled study. *Chinese Journal of Gastroenterology* **7**: 71–78.

Hwang S-J, Lin H-C, Chang C-F et al (1992) A randomized controlled trial comparing octreotide and vasopressin in the control of acute esophageal variceal bleeding. *Journal of Hepatology* **16**: 320–325.

Ideo G, Bellah S, Fesce F & Grimoldi D (1988) Nadolol for prophylaxis of gastrointestinal bleeding in patients with cirrhosis. A randomised trial. *Hepatology* **6**: 6–9.

Jaramillo JL, de la Mata M, Mino G et al (1991) Somatostatin versus Sengstaken balloon tamponade for primary haemostasia of bleeding esophageal varices. *Journal of Hepatology* **12**: 100–105.

Jenkins SA, Baxter JN, Corbett WA et al (1985a) Effects of somatostatin analogue SMS 201–995 on hepatic haemodynamics in the pig and on intravariceal pressure in man. *British Journal of Surgery* **72**: 1009–1012.

Jenkins SA, Baxter JN, Corbett W et al (1985b) A prospective randomized controlled clinical trial comparing somatostatin and vasopressin in controlling acute variceal haemorrhage. *British Medical Journal* **290**: 275–278.

Jenkins SA, Baxter JN & Snowden S (1988) The effects of somatostatin and SMS 201–995 on hepatic and systemic haemodynamics in patients with cirrhosis and portal hypertension. *Fibrinolysis* **2**: 48–50.

Jenkins SA, Yates J, Baxter JN et al (1992) A prospective randomized controlled clinical trial comparing somatostatin and injection sclerotherapy in the control of acute variceal haemorrhage: an interim report. *Gut* **23 (supplement 1)**: F233.

Jensen LS & Krarup N (1989) Propranolol in prevention of rebleeding from oesophageal varices during the course of endoscopic sclerotherapy. *Scandinivian Journal of Gastroenterology* **24**: 213–222.

Kleber G, Sauerbruch T, Fischer G & Paumgartner G (1988) Somatostatin does not reduce oesophageal variceal pressure in liver cirrhosis. *Gut* **29**: 153–156.

Kobe van E, Zipprich B, Schentre KU & Millus R (1990) Prophylactic endoscopic sclerotherapy of esophageal varices: a prospective randomized trial. *Endoscopy* **22**: 245–248.

Kravetz D, Bosch J, Teres J et al (1984) Comparison of intravenous somatostatin and vasopressin infusions in treatment of acute variceal haemorrhage. *Hepatology* **4**: 442–446.

Larson AW, Cohen H, Zweilan B et al (1986) Acute oesophageal variceal sclerotherapy. Results of a prospective randomized controlled trial. *Journal of the American Medical Association* **255**: 497–500.

Lebrec D, Poynard T, Benamou J et al (1984) A randomized controlled study of propranolol for prevention of recurrent gastrointestinal bleeding in patients with cirrhosis. A final report. *Journal of Hepatology* **4:** 355–358.

Lebrec D, Poynard T, Capron JP et al (1988) Nadolol can prevent the first gastrointestinal bleeding in cirrhosis: a prospective randominised study. *Journal of Hepatology* **7:** 118–126.

Lee YF, Tsay YT, Lai KH et al (1990) A randomized controlled study of triglycyl-vasopressin and vasopressin in the control of bleeding from oesophageal varices. *Journal of Gastroenterology and Hepatology* **5:** 549–553.

Levacher S, Letoumelin P, Pateron D et al (1995) Early administration of terlipressin plus glyceryl trinitrate to control active upper gastrointestinal bleeding in cirrhotic patients. *Lancet* **346:** 865–868.

Liu JD, Yeng YS, Chen PB et al (199) Endoscopic injection sclerotherapy and propranolol in the prevention of recurrent variceal bleeding. World Congress of Gastroenterology, Sydney: BP118 (abstract).

Lundell L, Leth R, Lind T et al (1990) Evaluation of propranolol for prevention of recurrent bleeding from oesophageal varices between sclerotherapy sessions. *Acta Chirurgia Scandinavica* **156:** 711–715.

McCormick PA, Chin J, Greenslade L et al (1995) Cardiovascular effects of octreotide in patients with hepatic cirrhosis. *Hepatology* **21:** 1255–1260.

McKee R (1990) A study of octreotide in oesophageal varices. *Digestion* **45 (Supplement 1):** S60–S65.

McKee RK, Pringle SD, Garden OJ et al (1989) SMS 201–995 in the management of variceal bleeding. *Gut* **28(A):** 1380.

Mallory A, Schaefer JE & Cohen JR (1980) Selective intra arterial vasopressin infusion for upper gastrointestinal tract haemorrhage. A controlled trial. *Archives of Surgery* **115:** 30–32.

Martin TH, Taupignon A, Lauignolle A et al (1991) Prevention des redicues hemorragiques du cirrhotique: resultats d'une etude controlée comparant propranolol et sclerose endoscopie. *Gastroenterologie Clinique Biologie* **15:** 833–837.

Mastai R, Bosch J, Navasa M et al (1986) Effects of continuous infusion and bolus injections of somatostatin on azygous blood flow and hepatic and systemic haemodynamics in patients with portal hypertension; comparison with vasopressin. *Journal of Hepatology* **3 (Supplement 1):** S53 (Abstract).

Merigan TC Jr, Poltkin JR & Davidson CS (1962) Effect of intravenously administered posterior pituitary extract on haemorrhage from bleeding esophageal varices. *New England Journal of Medicine* **266:** 134–135.

Merkel C, Gatta A, Zuin R et al (1985) Effect of somatostatin on splanchnic haemodynamics in patients with liver cirrhosis and portal hypertension. *Digestion* **32:** 92–98.

Monescillo A, Arocena C, Lafuente C et al (1995) Effects of vasoactive drug therapy on variceal pressure during acute variceal haemorrhage. *Journal of Hepatology* **23 (Supplement 1):** p/C2/101.

Navasa M, Bosch J, Chesta J et al (1988) Haemodynamic effects of subcutaneous administration of SMS 201–995, a long acting somatostatin analogue, in patients with cirrhosis and portal hypertension. *Hepatology* **7:** 123.

*Nevens F, Van Steenbergen W, Yap S & Fevery J (1996) Assessment of variceal pressure by continuous non-invasive endoscopic registration: a placebo controlled evaluation of the effect of terlipressin and octreotide. *Gut* **38:** 129–134.

Pascal JP, Cales P and a Multicentre Study Group (1987) Propranolol in the prevention of the first upper gastrointestinal tract haemorrhage in patients with cirrhosis. *New England Journal of Medicine* **317:** 856–861.

Patch D & Burroughs AK (1995) Pharmacological treatment of portal hypertension. *Progress in Liver Diseases* **13:** 269–292.

Pinto Correia J, Malies M, Alexandrino P & Silveira J (1984) Controlled trial of vasopressin and balloon tamponade in bleeding oesophageal varices. *Hepatology* **4:** 885–888.

Pinzani M, Milani S, De Frnco R et al (1996) Endothelin-1 is overexpressed in human cirrhotic liver and exerts multiple effects on activated hepatic stellate cells. *Gastroenterology* **110:** 534–548.

Planas R, Quer JC, Boix J et al (1994) A prospective randomized trial comparing somatostatin and sclerotherapy in the treatment of acute variceal bleeding. *Hepatology* **20:** 370–375.

Queuniet AM, Czenichow P, Lerebroug E et al (1987) Etude controlée du propranolol dans la prevention des recidives hemorragiques des les patients cirrhotiques. *Gastroenterologie Clinique Biologie* **11:** 41–47.

Rockey D & Chung J (1995) Inducible nitric oxide synthase in rat hepatic lipocytes and the effect of nitric oxide on lipocyte contractility. *Journal of Clinical Investigation* **95:** 1199–1206.

*Rockey DC & Weisinger R (1996) Endothelin induced contractility of stellate cells from normal and cirrhotic rat liver: implications for the regulation of portal pressure and resistance. *Hepatology* **24:** 233–240.

Rossi VV, Cales P, Barbi P et al (1991) Prevention of recurrent variceal bleeding in alcoholic cirrhotic patients: prospective controlled trial of propranolol and sclerotherapy. *Journal of Hepatology* **12:** 283–289.

Saari A, Elvilaakso E, Inberg M et al (1990) Comparison of somatostatin and vasopressin bleeding esophageal varices. *American Journal of Gastroenterology* **85:** 804–807.

Sheen JS, Chen Y & Liaw YF (1989) Randomized controlled study of propranolol for prevention of recurrent oesophageal varices bleeding in patients with cirrhosis. *Liver* **9:** 1–5.

Sheilds R, Jenkins SA, Kingsworth AN et al (1992) A prospective randomized controlled trial comparing the efficacy of somatostatin with injection sclerotherapy in the control of bleeding oesophageal varices. *Journal of Hepatology* **16:** 128–137.

Silvain C, Carpenter S, Savereau D et al (1993) Terlipressin plus transdermal nitroglycerin vs octreotide in the control of acute bleeding from esophageal varices: a multicenter randomized trial. *Hepatology* **18:** 61–65.

Smith JL & Graham DY (1982) Variceal haemorrhage: a critical evaluation of survival analysis. *Gastroenterology* **82:** 968–973.

Söderlund C & Hue T (1985) Endoscopic sclerotherapy vs conservative management of bleeding oesophageal varices. A 5-year prospective controlled trial of emergency and long term treatment. *Acta Chirugica Scandinavica* **151:** 499–456.

Söderlund C, Magnusson I, Torngren S et al (1990) Terlipressin (triglycyl-lysine vasopressin) controls acute bleeding oesophageal varices. A double blind, randomized, placebo-controlled trial. *Scandinavian Journal of Gastroenterology* **25:** 622–630.

Sonnenberg A & West C (1983) Somatostatin reduced gastric mucosal flow in normal subjects but not in patients with cirrhosis of the liver. *Gut* **24:** 148–153.

Sonnenburg GE, Keller U, Perruchud A et al (1981) Effect of somatostatin on splanchnic haemodynamics. *Gastroenterology* **80:** 5226–5232.

Spence RAJ (1992) Surgical measures for active variceal bleeding. *Gastrointestinal Endoscopy* (Clinics of North America) **2:** 77–94.

Stanciu C, Cijevschi C, Stan M & Sandalulescu E (1993) Endoscopic intravascular oesophageal pressure measurements in cirrhotic patients: response to metaclopramide. *Hepato-Gastroenterology* **40:** 173–175.

Strauss E, de Sa MFG, Albano A et al (1988) A randomized controlled trial for the prevention of the first upper gastrointestinal bleeding due to portal hypertension in cirrhosis. Sclerotherapy or propranolol versus control groups. *Hepatology* **8:** 1395 (abstract).

Sung JY, Chung S, Lai CW et al (1993) Octreotide infusion or emergency sclerotherapy for variceal haemorrhage. *Lancet* **342:** 637–641.

Sung JYC, Chung SCS, Yung MY et al (1995) Prospective randomised study of effect of octreotide on rebleeding from oesophageal varices after endoscopic ligation. *Lancet* **346:** 1666–1669.

Taranto D, Suozzo R, de Sio I et al (1990) Effect of metoclopramide on transmural oesophageal variceal pressure and portal blood flow in cirrhotic patients. *Digestion* **47:** 56–60.

Teres J, Planas R, Panes J et al (1990) Vasopressin/nitroglycerin infusion vs oesophageal tamponade in the treatment of acute variceal bleeding. A randomized controlled trial. *Hepatology* **11:** 964–968.

Teres J, Bosch J, Bordas JM et al (1993) Propranolol versus sclerotherapy in preventing variceal rebleeding: a randomized controlled trial. *Gastroenterology* **105:** 1508–1514.

The Italian Multicentre Project for Propranolol in Prevention of Bleeding (1991) Propranolol prevents first gastrointestional bleeding in non-ascitic cirrhotid patients. Final report of a multicentre randomized trial. *Journal of Hepatology* **9:** 75–83.

The Prova Study Group (1991) Prophylaxis of first haemhorrage from eosophageal varices by sclerotherapy, propranolol or both in cirrhotic patients. A randomized multicentre trial. *Hepatology* **14:** 1016–1024.

Thomson BL, Moller S, Sorensen T and the Copenhagen Esophageal Varices Sclerotherapy Project (1994) Optimized analysis of recurrent bleeding and death in patients with cirrhosis and esophageal varices. *Hepatology* **21:** 367–375.

Tsai YT, Lay CS, Lai KH et al (1986) Controlled trial of vasopressin plus nitroglycerin vs vasopressin alone in the treatment of bleeding oesophageal varices. *Hepatology* **6:** 406–409.

Tyden G, Samnegaard H, Thulin L et al (1979) Circulatory effects of somatostatin in anaesthetized man. *Acta Chirugica Scandinavica* **145:** 443–446.

Valenzuela JE, Schubert T, Fogel MR et al (1989) A multicenter, randomized, double-blind trial of somatostatin in the management of acute haemorrhage from esophageal varices. *Hepatology* **10:** 958–961.

VBSG (Variceal bleeding study group) (1994) Randomized controlled trial of sclerotherapy versus somatostatin infusion in the prevention of early rebleeding following variceal haemorrhage in patients with cirrhosis. *Hepatology* **19:** 1361 (A395).

Vickers C, Rhodes J, Hillenbrand P et al (1987) Prospective controlled trial of propranolol and sclerotherapy for prevention of re-bleeding from oesophageal varices. *Gut* **28:** A1359 (abstract).

Villanueva C, Balanzo J, Novella MT et al (1996) Nadolol plus isosorbide mononitrate compared with sclerotherapy for the prevention of variceal rebleeding. *New England Journal of Medicine* **334:** 1624–1629.

Villeneuve JP, Pomer-Layrargues G, Infante Rivard C et al (1986) Propranolol for the prevention of recurrent variceal haemorrhage: a controlled trial. *Hepatology* **6:** 1239–1243.

Vinel JP, Lamouliatte U, Cales P et al (1992) Propranolol reduced the rebleeding rate during endoscopic sclerotherapy for prevention of rebleeding from oesophageal varices. *Gut* **28:** A1359 (Abstract).

Walker S, Stiehl A, Raedseh R et al (1986) Terlipressin in bleeding oesopheal varices: a placebo controlled double blind study. *Hepatology* **6:** 112–115.

Walker S, Kreichgauer H-P, Bode JC et al (1992) Terlipressin vs somatostatin in bleeding esophageal varices: a controlled, double-blind study. *Hepatology* **15:** 1023–1030.

Westaby D, Melia W, Hegarty J et al (1986) Use of propranolol to reduce the rebleeding rate during injection sclerotherapy prior to variceal obliteration. *Hepatology* **6:** 673–675.

Westaby D, Hayes PC, Gimson AES et al (1989) Controlled trial of injection sclerotherapy for active variceal bleeding. *Hepatology* **9:** 274–277.

Westaby D, Polson RJJ, Grimson AES et al (1990) A controlled trial of oral propranolol compared with injection sclerotherapy for long term management of variceal bleeding. *Hepatology* **11:** 353–359.

Zhang JX, Pegoli WJ & Clemens MG (1994) Endothelin-1 induces direct constrictions of hepatic sinusoids. *American Journal of Physiology* **266:** G624–G632.

8

Transjugular intrahepatic portosystemic shunts (TIPS)

PATRICK S. KAMATH* MD

Assistant Professor of Medicine, Consultant
Department of Gastroenterology and Internal Medicine, Mayo Clinic and Mayo Medical School, 200 First Street Southwest, Rochester, MN 55905, USA

MICHAEL A. McKUSICK MD

Assistant Professor of Radiology, Consultant
Department of Diagnostic Radiology, Mayo Clinic and Mayo Medical School, 200 First Street Southwest, Rochester, MN 55905, USA

Transjugular intrahepatic portosystemic shunt (TIPS) is a procedure recently introduced for the management of complications of portal hypertension. TIPS can be placed in the liver with relative ease by a skilled radiologist with a low risk of mortality. The major complications following the procedure are infection, especially in patients undergoing emergency TIPS, intra-abdominal haemorrhage from capsular punctures, and long-term problems related to encephalopathy and stenosis of the shunt. Encephalopathy is more of a problem in older patients with wide diameter shunts. Stenosis of the shunt is related to pseudo-intimal hyperplasia, probably related to transection of bile ductules during placement of the shunt. In view of the high rate of encephalopathy and stenosis following the shunt, a careful follow-up of all patients, including ultrasonographic and angiographic examination of the shunt, is mandatory. TIPS is used predominantly for the control of acute variceal haemorrhage, prevention of recurrent variceal bleeding, and refractory ascites when conventional treatment has failed. However, the role of TIPS in the management of complications of portal hypertension still awaits the outcome of clinical trials.

Key words: portosystemic shunts; portal hypertension; variceal haemorrhage; ascites.

Though transjugular intrahepatic portosystemic shunts (TIPS) can be placed in the liver with relative ease by a skilled radiologist, the role of this type of portosystemic shunt in the management of complications of portal hypertension is far from clear. TIPS has been widely used for the treatment of variceal haemorrhage (Rossle et al, 1994b; LaBerge et al, 1995), intractable ascites (Ochs et al, 1995b; Somberg et al, 1995a; Crenshaw et

*Address for correspondence.
The authors thank Ms Linda Veer for expert secretarial assistance.

al, 1996), hepatic hydrothorax (Strauss et al, 1994), Budd–Chiari syndrome (Ochs et al, 1993), chylous fistulae (Rosser et al, 1996), and hepato-pulmonary syndrome (Riegler et al, 1995). We review here the technique, complications, and potential indications of TIPS, a procedure introduced within the past decade to treat complications of portal hypertension.

TERMINOLOGY

Several terms have been used to describe the procedure. The term most commonly used is transjugular intrahepatic portosystemic shunt (TIPS). Alternative terms are intrahepatic portosystemic shunt (IPS) or transjugular intrahepatic portosystemic stent shunt (TIPSS). TIPS is the most commonly used term, even though the transjugular route may on occasion not be used, the femoral vein being another approach to insertion of intrahepatic porto-systemic shunts. A broad term that might be used is 'transvenous intra-hepatic portosystemic shunt', and the procedure is still designated TIPS.

HISTORICAL ASPECTS

Even though TIPS was carried out in humans only recently (Richter et al, 1990), the concept has been around for close to three decades. Rösch and others successfully placed teflon catheters between the hepatic vein and portal vein branches in dogs (Rösch et al, 1971). Patency of the shunts could not, however, be maintained for more than a few days. The first successful intrahepatic portosystemic shunt in humans was reported in 1983 (Colapinto et al, 1983). A parenchymal tract was created between the hepatic vein and portal vein using balloon catheters. Creation of the parenchymal shunt in patients with variceal bleeding resulted in a fall in portal pressure, but the parenchymatous tract collapsed rapidly and the shunts occluded. Patients thus had recurrence of variceal bleeding and the procedure lost some of its appeal. The introduction of an expandable metal stent to keep the parenchymal tract open was a welcome addition to the armamentarium of interventional radiologists. Not only could the parenchymal tract be kept open, the stent could be introduced with minimal patient discomfort.

PRE-TIPS EVALUATION

Doppler ultrasonography of the liver is carried out to confirm patency of the portal and hepatic veins. Patients in whom TIPS is carried out for treatment of intractable ascites usually have a shrunken and hard liver. In these patients, a CT scan of the abdomen is recommended (Theoni, 1995), not only to delineate the portal vein and the hepatic vein, but also to give the radiologist an idea of the amount of parenchyma available safely to create a tract. A platelet count $> 60\,000$ mm^{-3} and prothrombin time < 1.8 INR are ideal, but emergency TIPS may be carried out with more advanced coagulopathy. Echocardiography needs to be carried out in a patient in whom cardiac disease or pulmonary hypertension is suspected.

TECHNIQUE

The preferred route of access for TIPS is the right internal jugular vein as this is the most direct route to the hepatic veins. Alternative routes are the left internal jugular vein, the external jugular vein, and even the femoral vein (LaBerge et al, 1991). The TIPS procedure is quite painful with significant discomfort occurring during establishment and dilatation of the intrahepatic tract, and so conscious sedation is mandatory. Sedation for the procedure is a combination of Midazolam and Meperidine or Propofol with fentanyl. We prefer carrying out the procedure using intravenous Propofol (Zeneca, Inc., Wilmington, DE, USA).

A wedge hepatic venogram (Uflacker et al, 1994) is performed before the shunt is created to outline the hepatic venous anatomy. Most often, the right hepatic vein is used for the shunt because of its relatively large size. However, if the right liver lobe is atrophic and its vein small, the middle or left hepatic veins can be used. The wedge hepatic venogram can also help find a portal vein branch suitable for shunting, as well as delineate the location of the portal vein bifurcation. Some authors utilize real time ultrasound (Longo et al, 1992) or the previous placement of a radio-opaque marker within the liver as guides to find the portal vein (Harman et al, 1992). Once the hepatic vein to be used has been cannulated, the portal vein access needle/catheter is inserted over a wire into the hepatic vein. Passes are then made through the liver with the needle device. The hepatic vein is punctured 1–2 cm from the cava and needle thrusts are restricted to less than 4 cm in length. This helps to prevent liver capsule perforations, which may result in intraperitoneal haemorrhage and contribute to the 1–2% procedure mortality rate (Kerlan et al, 1995a).

A baseline portacaval gradient is obtained by recording pressure measurements from the portal vein and inferior vena cava (*not* the right atrium). A portogram is then performed. A stiff, 180-cm guide-wire is advanced into the portal system and an 8-mm high pressure angioplasty balloon used to dilate the intrahepatic tract. Hepatic and portal venous interfaces with the tract are easily identified by the tight constrictions they cause on the balloon. This enables the operator to determine the approximate length of stent needed.

When the tract has been suitably prepared, a metallic stent is positioned to bridge the hepatic and portal venous system. Several prostheses have been used: Palmaz (Johnson&Johnson, Warren, NJ), Wallstent (Schneider, Minneapolis, MN), nitinol Strecker/(Medi-Tech, Watertown, MA) and Gianturco-Rosch (Cook Inc., Bloomington, IN). The stent is laid down in the tract so that the ends of the stent extend only about 1 cm into the main portal vein and into the hepatic vein. Care is taken to avoid extending the stent either into the right atrium or far into the main portal vein to prevent difficulties with possible future liver transplantation. Additional stents are deployed as needed to cover the tract and to ensure that there are no acute angles between the ends of the stent and the venous system. Pressures are then recorded in the portal vein and inferior vena cava.

A portacaval gradient of 12 mmHg or less is acceptable. If a higher gradient is found, the stent is dilated to achieve an adequate gradient. Occasionally, 'dual TIPS' (a second shunt placed between the contralateral hepatic and portal vein) may be necessary to lower the gradient below 12 mmHg. When the portacaval gradient is acceptable, a portogram is performed to check for residual variceal filling with injection of contrast material in the splenic vein. Roughly one-fourth of patients have residual variceal filling after TIPS placement (Coldwell et al, 1995). If TIPS is being carried out for emergency control of variceal bleeding, these varices may be embolized. Embolization may also be recommended in the patient with poor liver function at risk for encephalopathy. In such patients an 8-mm diameter shunt is preferable. Since this narrow diameter is unlikely to reduce the portacaval gradient below 12 mmHg, embolization of varices might decrease the risk of rebleeding while at the same time allowing some maintenance of portal blood flow. When the TIPS procedure has been completed, the access sheath in the neck is removed and may be replaced with a shorter 8-F sheath. This sheath is sewn in place to enable quick access if needed during the initial post-shunt observation period.

With experience, it is possible to perform a TIPS in most patients in less than 60 minutes. Table 1 deals with technical difficulties usually experienced when one starts doing TIPS for the first time. About 20 procedures are required to advance beyond the steep slope of the learning

Table 1. Technical difficulties with TIPS.

Problem	Solution
Puncture of right internal jugular vein.	Ultrasound to confirm patency and guide puncture. If thrombosed, use right external or left internal jugular vein.
Advancement of portal vein access trocar into hepatic vein.	Remove trocar and bend/shape over wire to fit hepatic venous anatomy.
Portal vein localization.	Wedge hepatic venogram with CO_2 contrast. Pre-procedure localization and marking of portal bifurcation with metalic microcoil using ultrasound guidance.
Main, right, or left portal vein puncture.	Place access trocar in hepatic vein 1–2 cm from origin with IVC.
Advancement of catheter over a wire into portal system.	Place stiffening cannula over a wire through jugular access sheath into hepatic vein; this acts as a strut to prevent catheter buckling and allow passage into portal vein.
Unexpected partial or complete portal vein thrombosis.	Recanalize and stent portal system if possible.
Inability to lower portosystemic pressure gradient below 12 mmHg with 10-mm diameter shunt.	Over-dilate shunt with 12-mm diameter balloon or create a second intrahepatic shunt (dual TIPS).
Massive varices compete with newly created shunt for flow.	Embolize varices.

curve. For this reason, the procedure should be limited to institutions where that kind of experience can be easily accumulated. Further, TIPS is only one modality in the treatment of complications of portal hypertension. Thus, TIPS should only be carried out in centres that are well-experienced in all aspects of treatment of liver disease, including liver transplantation.

POST-TIPS EVALUATION

Ultrasonography is carried out to confirm patency of the shunt within 24 hours following the procedure. Success of thrombolytic therapy if the shunt is thrombosed is dependent on the 'freshness' of the thrombosis. Ultrasonography at 24 hours is optimum since thrombosis detected by ultrasonography a week after TIPS (as is recommended by some authors) may not be amenable to thrombolytic therapy. The sheath in the neck is removed once patency of the shunt is confirmed. If the shunt is thrombosed, the sheath provides quick access to the shunt. Following TIPS, we recommend Doppler ultrasonography of the shunt every 3 months. Angiography with measurements of portal pressure is recommended when shunt stenosis is suspected. This may be on clinical grounds, as when the patient has variceal haemorrhage or has recurrence of ascites, or when Doppler ultrasonography suggests shunt stenosis. Ultrasonography is less accurate in determining stenosis than it is in determining patency or occlusion of the shunt (Shiffman et al, 1995). Therefore, we recommend that angiography of the shunt with pressure measurements be carried out at least on an annual basis, if not more frequently.

POTENTIAL INDICATIONS FOR TIPS

TIPS has been used in the treatment of variceal haemorrhage, ascites, hepatic hydrothorax, and several other complications related to portal hypertension. We review potential indications of TIPS before making recommendations that are based on consensus statements.

Control of acute variceal haemorrhage

About 10% of patients who present with an episode of acute variceal haemorrhage cannot be controlled with two sessions of endoscopic therapy within 24 hours (Burroughs et al, 1989). Such patients are likely to have poor liver function, advanced coagulopathy, as well as a large rent in the varix. Some of these patients have bleeding from gastric varices. TIPS done on an emergency basis is effective in the control of acute variceal haemorrhage in most of these patients. In the San Francisco study, variceal haemorrhage could be controlled in all but one of the 30 patients undergoing the emergency procedure. In the Freiburg study all 10 of the patients had control of the acute bleeding episode following TIPS. The survival of patients following control of the haemorrhage, however, seems to be variable, with some authors reporting reasonably good survival. In our own hands, even though the TIPS can be placed successfully in these patients, survival is poor, with the median survival being only 18 days (Kamath et al, 1994). The cause of death in our patients, as in other series (Coldwell et al, 1995), has invariably been multi-system organ failure resulting from worsening hepatic function and systemic sepsis. While selection bias may account for the difference in results between various studies, the definition of an emergency procedure is also likely to be a variable. Our own definition of an emergency procedure is when the patient is continuing to bleed at the time TIPS is performed: two sessions of endoscopic treatment, pharmacotherapy and balloon tamponade having been unsuccessful in controlling the acute variceal haemorrhage. TIPS is carried out in these emergency situations with a Minnesota tube *in situ* with the balloons inflated.

A retrospective study comparing TIPS with oesophageal transection and devascularization has been published recently (Jalan et al, 1995). Nineteen patients underwent TIPS while 19 other patients underwent the surgical procedure. Mortality and rebleeding were significantly lower in the TIPS group, while encephalopathy and infection were similar. This study suggests that TIPS may be preferred over surgery for therapy of un-controlled variceal haemorrhage.

Prevention of recurrent variceal haemorrhage

In the two largest experiences published, TIPS was effective in prevention of recurrent variceal haemorrhage (Rossle et al, 1994b; La Berge et al, 1995). In these uncontrolled series the risk of rebleeding at the end of 1 year was approximately 20% as compared with historical data of 50% or greater risk of rebleeding with endoscopic therapy. A better index of the utility of TIPS in the prevention of variceal rebleeding can be obtained from trials where TIPS was compared with conventional therapy.

Several studies (Merli et al, 1994; Sanyal et al, 1994a; Cello et al, 1995; Cabrera et al, 1996) have compared TIPS with endoscopic sclerotherapy in the prevention of variceal bleeding (Table 2). TIPS was shown to be superior to endoscopic sclerotherapy in preventing variceal rebleeding in all except one study (Sanyal et al, 1994a). In only Cello et al's study (1995) was randomization completed within 24 hours of control of variceal haemorrhage. Cello et al compared 19 patients undergoing sclerotherapy with 21 other patients undergoing TIPS to prevent variceal rebleeding. All patients underwent emergency sclerotherapy for control of the acute bleed. At the end of the period of follow-up, bleeding was less common in patients undergoing TIPS as compared with sclerotherapy. As expected, encephalopathy was more common in the TIPS group, and survival was unchanged. The only study published in full (Cabrera et al, 1996) again demonstrated a lower rebleeding rate but higher encephalopathy rate with TIPS as compared with endoscopic therapy, and similar survival.

Two studies comparing TIPS with a combination of sclerotherapy and beta-blockers (Rossle et al, 1994a; Group d'Etudes Anastomoses intra-

Table 2a. Randomized trials comparing TIPS with sclerotherapy for variceal rebleeding.

Authors	Sanyal et al (1994a)		Merli et al (1994)		Cello et al (1995)		Cabrera et al (1996)		Garcia-Villareal et al (1996)	
Study groups	TIPS	ES	TIPS	ES	TIPS	ES	TIPS	ES	TIPS	ES
Subjects (n)	40	39	23	23	21	19	31	32	18	19
Rebleed (%)	25	20.5	13	30.4*	0	36.8	22.5	50*	11	47*
Encephalopathy (%)	22.5	NS	NS	NS	52.4	42.1	32.2	12.5	22	26
Deaths (%)	27.5	10.2	13	8.6	19	3	19	15.8	5.6	42*
Bleed to randomization interval	3–21 days		1 week– 6 months		3 days		24 hours		NS	

Table 2b. Randomized trials comparing TIPS with sclerotherapy + beta-blockers for variceal rebleeding.

Authors	Rossle et al (1994a)		GDAIH (1995)	
Study groups	TIPS	ES + BB	TIPS	ES + BB
Subjects (n)	26	27	32	33
Rebleed %	8	26*	41	61
Encephalopathy %	19	NS	NS	NS
Deaths %	4	8	50	42
Bleed to randomization interval	2 weeks		4 days	

Table 2c. Randomized trials comparing TIPS with variceal ligation for variceal rebleeding.

Author	Jalan et al (1996)	
Study groups	TIPS	EVL
Subjects (n)	31	27
Rebleed %	9.8	50.1*
Encephalopathy %	22.2	7.5
Deaths %	19.3	11.1
Bleed to randomized trial	24 hours	

BB, beta-blockers; ES, endoscopic variceal sclerotherapy; EVL, endoscopic variceal ligation; GDAIH, Groupe d'Etude des Anastomoses Intra-hepatiques; NS, not stated. * $P < 0.05$.

hepatique, 1995), and one comparing TIPS and variceal ligation (Jalan et al, 1996) did not conclusively demonstrate a better outcome in the TIPS group. Finally, one study has compared TIPS with surgically created small diameter prosthetic portocaval shunts (Rosemurgy et al, 1996). In this small study, there seemed to be fewer rebleeding episodes, as well as deaths in the surgical group. The final results of the trial are awaited. Thus, present data do not suggest that TIPS is superior to either endoscopic therapy or surgical shunts in the prevention of recurrent variceal bleeding. Larger studies need to be carried out before definite recommendations can be made.

Treatment of refractory ascites

Refractory ascites is defined as ascites that cannot be mobilized, or the early recurrence of which cannot be satisfactorily prevented by medical therapy (Arroyo et al, 1996). Less than 5% of patients with ascites are refractory to conventional medical treatment of large volume paracentesis, sodium restriction and diuretics. TIPS, which acts like a side-to-side porto-caval shunt, decreases sinusoidal hypertension and can alleviate ascites.

In a recently published study of 50 patients who underwent TIPS for refractory ascites (Ochs et al, 1995b), more than two-thirds of the patients had complete response (remission of ascites) within 3 months, while nine patients (18%) had partial response (ascites detected only on ultrasound examination). The mean serum creatinine decreased from 1.5 ± 0.9 mg/dl before TIPS to 0.9 ± 0.3 mg/dl at 6 months. In patients with underlying organic renal disease, kidney function did not improve. Patients who had a complete response and those patients under 60 years of age who had a bilirubin of < 1.3 mg/dl were more likely to survive 1 year. None of the patients went into cardiac failure following TIPS, and this may be related to the fact that before treatment a large volume paracentesis was carried out in all these patients. A large US study demonstrated similar therapeutic responses to TIPS in patients with refractory ascites (Crenshaw et al, 1996). TIPS is followed by an improvement in the glomerular filtration rate and a decrease in the abnormally elevated renin and aldosterone (Quiroga et al, 1995). Natriuresis is often delayed for several weeks after TIPS and this delay may be because of persistent sympathetic hyperactivity. A recent study from Toronto in patients undergoing TIPS for refractory ascites shows that reversal of sinusoidal hypertension and arterial underfilling are necessary to decrease renal Na^+ retention (Wong et al, 1996).

Two studies have been carried out that compare TIPS with large volume paracentesis (LVP) for the treatment of refractory ascites (Ochs et al, 1995a; Lebrec et al, 1996). Only one of these studies has been published in manuscript form (Lebrec et al, 1996). Lebrec et al compared patients under-going TIPS with patients undergoing LVP in a randomized trial. Control of ascites was easier in patients undergoing TIPS as compared with those in the LVP group. Mortality, however, was higher in the TIPS group in Child's Class C patients. Efficacy of TIPS was seen only in patients of Child's Class B, albeit without any survival advantage. Thus, the role of TIPS in the treatment of patients with refractory ascites needs to be established. Since a large number of patients with refractory ascites are candidates for liver transplantation, in the absence of data from controlled trials, our recom-mendations would be to carry out TIPS only if the waiting time to trans-plant is greater than 3–6 months (Kamath and McKusick, 1996). If waiting periods are shorter, repeated large volume paracentesis might be a better option.

TIPS and orthotopic liver transplantation

Precautions should be taken during placement of TIPS not to compromise future orthotopic liver transplantation (OLT). The stent should not extend into the suprahepatic cava as the recipient liver is transected at the level of the suprahepatic cava and the mesh stent extending into this area makes transection both difficult, as well as dangerous to the surgeon. The ends of the wire stent mesh are extremely sharp and can result in finger injuries, while the stent is removed literally one wire at a time. In patients in whom the stents have been malpositioned the transplantation procedure is prolonged because cross clamping at the usual vascular sites is not possible (Wilson et al, 1995). The shunt also should not extend far into the main portal vein, since transection of the vein to remove the liver might be difficult. Further, occlusion within this area would result in portal vein thrombosis, making liver transplantation more challenging.

Patients who have had OLT following TIPS have fewer changes of portal hypertension in the surgical field. However, the requirement for blood transfusions, as well as the operative mortality and morbidity are not significantly reduced as compared with patients without portosystemic shunts (Millis et al, 1995; Somberg et al, 1995b). Thus, TIPS cannot be recommended pre-liver transplant for the sole purpose of reducing portal hypertension. In retrospective studies when patients undergoing OLT following TIPS were compared with patients undergoing OLT following surgical portosystemic shunt procedures, the operative morbidity, mortality and requirement for blood transfusion in the TIPS groups have been similar or less (Menegaux et al, 1994; Abouljoud et al, 1995). Patients who are candidates for liver transplantation in our opinion should have TIPS rather than a surgical portosystemic shunt.

Other indications for TIPS

There have been isolated reports of the successful use of TIPS for the treatment of several other problems related to or resulting in portal hypertension. These include portal vein thrombosis (Radosevich et al, 1993; Blum et al, 1995), hepatic hydrothorax (Strauss et al, 1994), intestinal varices (Haskal et al, 1994; Bernstein et al, 1996), chylous fistula, Budd–Chiari syndrome (BCS), and hepatopulmonary syndrome. TIPS for veno-occlusive disease following bone-marrow transplantation has not generally altered overall survival (Fried et al, 1996).

TIPS can be carried out in patients with portal vein thrombosis, provided the thrombus is not extensive. A transhepatic approach may be used in some patients with portal vein thrombosis to allow for portal vein recanalization before transjugular catheterization and TIPS (Radosevich et al, 1993). While the stent may extend far down in the portal systems, in some cases even into the superior mesenteric vein, it should be realized that injudicious extension of the stent may compromise future liver transplantation. In Budd–Chiari syndrome, TIPS can be placed most easily when there is some patency of the hepatic vein. However, even when the hepatic vein is completely occluded in its entire length, it is usually possible to recanalize the vein sufficiently to allow placement of a stent. The shunt should be placed such that the entire segment of involved hepatic vein is covered by the stent. TIPS is indicated especially in patients in whom pressure on the inferior vena cava from an enlarged caudate lobe causes a pressure gradient greater than 10 mmHg between the infrahepatic and suprahepatic inferior vena cava. When the pressure gradient is > 10 mmHg, a surgical portocaval shunt would not be beneficial because the portal system cannot be adequately decompressed into the high pressure infra-hepatic inferior vena cava. If canalization of the hepatic vein is impossible, TIPS may be placed by creating an intraparenchymal tract between the intrahepatic inferior vena cava and the portal vein. Though TIPS is technically possible in most patients with the Budd–Chiari syndrome, we recommend the procedure only in patients with acute BCS who are at risk of developing hepatic failure. In these patients, TIPS may also serve as a bridge to liver transplantation (Kuo et al, 1996). In patients with chronic BCS, especially if cirrhosis has set in, liver transplantation might be a better approach, with TIPS being reserved for patients with refractory ascites or variceal bleeding.

RECOMMENDED INDICATIONS FOR TIPS

The place of TIPS in the management of complications of portal hyper-tension awaits the results of control trials (Kamath and McKusick, 1994). Till such time, the accepted indications of TIPS, as outlined in a consensus conference sponsored by the United States National Digestive Diseases Advisory Board, are for the 'control of acute variceal haemorrhage after two sessions of endoscopic therapy have failed to control the bleed, and for the prevention of recurrent variceal haemorrhage in patients who have failed endoscopic and pharmacological therapy' (Shiffman et al, 1995). TIPS should be considered particularly if the cause of bleeding is from gastric varices, since in this situation endoscopic and pharmacological options are limited. However, variceal bleeding due to extensive extra-hepatic portal vein thrombosis with thrombosis extending into a significant length of splenic vein or superior mesenteric vein is not an indication for TIPS. Promising indications for TIPS include treatment of refractory ascites, hepatic hydrothorax, and the Budd–Chiari syndrome. TIPS cannot be recommended as the initial therapy of acute variceal haemorhage or as the initial therapy to prevent either the first variceal bleed or recurrent variceal haemorrhage. Similarly, TIPS is not recommended prior to liver transplantation solely as a means of decreasing mortality or the requirement of blood transfusion.

CONTRAINDICATIONS TO TIPS

With increasing expertise, the list of contraindications keeps decreasing. Contraindications to TIPS include right-sided cardiac failure, pulmonary arterial hypertension, polycystic liver disease, hepatic neoplasms within the tract between the hepatic vein and portal vein, and patients with advanced liver failure who are not candidates for liver transplantation. TIPS is also contraindicated in patients with intrinsic renal disease causing renal failure, especially if the procedure is carried out as treatment for refractory ascites. Relative contraindications include systemic sepsis, and Stage III–IV hepatic encephalopathy in a patient who is not a candidate for liver transplantation. Advanced hepatic encephalopathy is not a contraindication if the encephalopathy has been precipitated by gastrointestinal bleeding. If portal hypertension is a result of a hepatic artery–portal vein fistula, TIPS is contraindicated because it creates a large systemic arteriovenous fistula, which may result in high output cardiac failure. Similarly, in a patient with hepatic arterial thrombosis, TIPS would divert portal blood away from the liver. The liver thus loses its sole source of blood supply and thus TIPS is contraindicated in a patient with hepatic arterial thrombosis.

COMPLICATIONS POST-TIPS

Acceptable procedure related mortality is 1–2% (Kerlan et al, 1995a), while other complications are of the order of 10%. Complications following TIPS have been excellently reviewed (Freedman et al, 1993). They may be either procedure related, early (within 30 days of the procedure) or long-term problems related to shunt stenosis and encephalopathy (Table 3). Most of the complications are transient and minor. Only the major procedure-related and long-term complications are discussed. Table 4 summarizes the causes of many procedure related complications and precautions that should be taken for their prevention.

Table 3. Complications post-TIPS*.

Procedure-related life-threatening complications:	Intraperitoneal haemorrhage
	Sepsis
	Cardiopulmonary failure
Early complications (1–30 days post-procedure)	
Minor:	Haematoma at puncture site
	Pain
	Cardiac arrhythmias
	Fever
	Reactions to contrast media
	Haemolytic anaemia
Major:	Shunt thrombosis
	Stent migration
	Portal systemic encephalopathy
	Progressive hepatic failure
	Pulmonary artery hypertension
Late complications (> 30 days)	
	Shunt stenosis
	Portal systemic encephalopathy
	Portal vein thrombosis
	Progressive hepatic failure

* Modified from Kamath and McKusick (1996).

Table 4. Prevention and treatment of TIPS-related complications.

Complication	Prevention	Treatment
Inadvertent carotid artery puncture during jugular vein access.	Ultrasound guide for venous access.	Manual compression of carotid puncture to prevent haematoma.
Hepatic capsular laceration during portal vein access.	To prevent laceration, stay away from atrophic lobes and limit needle passes to 3–4 cm of excursion.	Usually requires no treatment. For severe haemorrhage, transfuse with blood products until stable. Obtain abdominal CT scan and surgical consultation.
Extrahepatic puncture of portal venous system.	Delineate bifurcation of portal vein by pre-procedure CT scan.	Leave catheter in place for porto-gram. Use as guide to gain intra-hepatic portal vein puncture. Work quickly to establish functioning shunt, then remove errant catheter.
Intrahepatic arterial or biliary puncture.	Work centrally within the liver.	Usually no treatment required; remove catheter and continue. If a fistula develops, embolize arterial feeder with steel coils.
Sepsis post-shunt.	Prophylactic antibiotics. Strict sterile technique.	Broad spectrum antibiotic coverage.
Early shunt thrombosis.	Avoid sharp angles when placing stent. Ends should not abut against vein intima.	Shunt venogram and clot lysis using 250 000 units Urokinase delivered pulse-spray technique. Extension of shunt to ensure stent coverage of intrahepatic tract and adequate length in both hepatic and portal veins.
Uncontrollable encephalopathy post-shunt.	Use narrow shunts in high risk patients.	Reduce diameter of shunt with additional concentrically placed stents. Embolize shunt with steel coils.
Shunt stenosis.	Wider stents. Avoid bile duct injury.	Dilatation or atherectomy of shunt. Placement of additional stent if necessary.
Post-shunt liver failure.	Pre-shunt views of celiac axis in elderly patients to detect stenosis.	Angiogram to exclude hepatic artery stenosis with angioplasty as needed.

Mortality

In expert hands, mortality from TIPS is insignificant. Mortality is related to intraperitoneal haemorrhage, systemic sepsis, cardiac tamponade related to right atrial tears and pulmonary oedema, especially in patients with ascites. Sepsis is a problem, seen predominantly in patients undergoing emergency TIPS. Aspiration pneumonia in these patients might be the source of sepsis associated with increased mortality (Sanyal et al, 1996a). Haemobilia resulting from a portobiliary fistula or, less often, an arteriobiliary fistula (Menzel et al, 1995), is also a source for mortality.

PROCEDURE RELATED COMPLICATIONS

Procedure complications are related to the various manoeuvres involving placement of the TIPS, namely percutaneous puncture of the jugular vein, getting access to the portal vein, dilatation of the tract and placement of the TIPS stent.

Shunt dislodgement

This is important since stent dislodgement can predispose to shunt thrombosis or result in migration into the pulmonary vessels. Stent dislodgement is best treated by repositioning the stent in the iliac or femoral vein and, if possible, the stent is extracted through a surgical venotomy.

Shunt thrombosis

Shunt thrombosis occurs shortly after placement of TIPS and is often related to improper placement of the stent where one end of the stent abuts against the wall of the vein. When shunt thrombosis is recognized early, the treatment is infusion of urokinase locally into the thrombus in a dose of 250 000 units over about 20 minutes. The stent also needs to be repositioned if necessary.

Intraperitoneal haemorrhage

Most episodes of intraperitoneal haemorrhage are self-limited and require no specific treatment. They are recognized during the procedure by extravasation of radiographic contrast material into the intraperitoneal cavity. More major bleeding episodes post-procedure are recognized by worsening of the patient's haemodynamic status with a fall in the haematocrit. Bleeding into the intraperitoneal cavity may be detected at the bedside using ultrasonography, but is best confirmed non-invasively by abdominal CT scans. Surgery is rarely required as the bleeding can be controlled by correction of coagulation parameters.

Bleeding is most likely to occur when the liver is small and firm and the capsule is traversed during attempts to puncture the portal vein. Major bleeding may occur when the inferior vena cava is lacerated when the middle hepatic vein is used for creation of the TIPS. The middle hepatic vein lies immediately anterior to the inferior vena cava and is anterior to the left portal vein. Thus, a tract between the middle hepatic vein and left portal vein has to be created by puncturing the middle hepatic vein in a posterior direction, and during this procedure, the inferior vena cava may be punctured. Major intra-abdominal haemorrhage may also occur because of tearing of the portal vein. This situation is more common when the portal vein is extrahepatic, and typically occurs soon after the balloon, which is used to dilate the parenchymous tract, is deflated. Treatment for this situation includes prompt deployment of the shunt, but this may not always work, and this complication, like bleeding from the vena cava, can be fatal.

Infection

Infection following TIPS is more common in patients with impaired liver function and in those who have either a biliary enteric anastomosis, or biliary strictures such as in primary sclerosing cholangitis. Infections in patients with structural biliary abnormalities are predominantly Gram-negative organisms. Overall, the most frequent organism isolated in blood is *Staphylococcus aureus*. Sepsis is usually manifested as fever, which persists beyond the first 24 hours following the procedure. Sepsis is more common in patients undergoing emergency TIPS procedure as a means of controlling acute variceal haemorrhage, and is a major contributing factor to the mortality in these patients (Coldwell et al, 1995; Sanyal et al, 1996). A biliary-shunt fistula following TIPS, which results in recurrent episodes of polymicrobial Gram-negative sepsis, has been described recently (Mallery et al, 1996). Endoscopic sphincterotomy and biliary drainage resulted in rapid closure of the fistula and resolution of the infection. A biliary shunt fistula may need to be considered in the differential diagnosis of a patient with recurrent sepsis. We routinely use antibiotics as prophylactic therapy before a TIPS procedure. Our current recommendations are Piperacillin-Tazabactam, 3.375 grams intravenously 30 minutes before the procedure to provide broad Gram-positive and Gram-negative coverage.

Cardiopulmonary changes

There are impressive cardiovascular changes that occur post TIPS. The hyperdynamic circulation of cirrhosis seems to be at least transiently worsened (Azoulay et al, 1994). Immediately following the procedure there is an increase in cardiac index and a decrease in systemic vascular resistance. Approximately a month later there is evidence of further change in these haemodynamic parameters with increase in cardiac index and a decrease in systemic vascular resistance, while pulmonary artery pressure continues to be elevated (Vanderlinden et al, 1996). Pulmonary artery pressure increases as a result of an increase in pulmonary vascular resistance. The worsening of the haemodynamic status soon after placement of a TIPS can result in cardiac failure in patients with poor myocardial function and, thus, cardiac failure is a contraindication to TIPS placement. There seems to be, however, a beneficial effect of TIPS in patients with hepatopulmonary syndrome. There is improvement in symptoms of dyspnea combined with improvement in arterial oxygenation (Riegler et al, 1995).

Adult respiratory distress syndrome (ARDS), an uncommon complication following TIPS, is seen more often in patients undergoing TIPS for refractory ascites. The conditions predisposing to ARDS are not known; large volume paracentesis shortly before TIPS in patients with refractory ascites may reduce the risk of cardiopulmonary complications.

LONG-TERM COMPLICATIONS

The significant long-term problems following TIPS are shunt stenosis and encephalopathy. Shunt related haemolysis, when it does occur, is usually asymptomatic and most often subsides in 3–4 months (Sanyal et al, 1996b). Changes related to hypersplenism, namely thrombocytopenia and leuko-penia, remain unchanged. Based on data on surgical shunts, there is a predictable relationship between the extent of portal-systemic shunting and portal-systemic encephalopathy (Sarfeh and Rypins, 1994). Moreover, shunt patency can be maintained longer with wide diameter shunts but this is at the expense of a higher risk of encephalopathy. The same is likely to hold good for TIPS. Thus, with present technology, the risk of shunt stenosis has to be weighed against the risk of long-term encephalopathy. Even though stenosis and encephalopathy are problems that are probably going to be long-term issues, most patients who survive longer than 1 month after TIPS have a good quality of life (Nazarian et al, 1996).

Shunt stenosis

The 1-year stenosis rate in the largest series is between 20 and 30% at 1 year, and approximately 50% at 2 years (LaBerge et al, 1995). The reported incidence varies greatly and is related to what one uses as the definition of shunt stenosis. Using standard definitions (Rutherford and Becker, 1991), *primary patency* of the shunt is the duration of patency without inter-vention. *Primary assisted patency* is the duration of patency with or with-out intervention. Primary assisted patency involves situations where the stent is seen to be narrowed but not occluded, and intervention is used for dilatation. *Secondary patency* is the total duration of patency, including patency that is re-established after shunt occlusion. The gold standard for diagnosis of shunt stenosis should be the demonstration of an elevation in portacaval gradient > 12 mmHg, the pressure above which the risk of bleed-ing and development of ascites occurs (Casado et al, 1995). Thus, TIPS venography and pressure measurements are mandatory for documenting the diagnosis of stenosis. Only one study has carefully addressed the issue of stenosis using venography and pressure measurements; Lind and others, however, defined shunt stenosis as an increase in portacaval pressure gradient to above 15 mmHg (Lind et al, 1994). They followed 21 patients undergoing TIPS with venography at 3 months and 1 year post-procedure. In the 12 patients who survived for 1 year and did not require liver trans-plantation, the shunt had stenosed in all but three patients. However, with interventional techniques the shunts can be kept open in more than 90% of patients at 2 years. In Laberge's series, the primary, primary assisted, and secondary patency rates were 66%, 83% and 96% at 1 year; and 42%, 79% and 90% at 2 years, respectively (Laberge et al, 1995).

Causes of shunt stenosis

Shunt occlusion occurring within 30 days following the procedure is usually related to thrombosis. Beyond 30 days, stenosis of the shunt is usually related to narrowing of the lumen by a proliferative pseudo-intima. If the proliferation is excessive, the shunt can be completely occluded. The cause of pseudo-intimal proliferation is not clear and should be the subject of further study. There is some evidence that an inflammatory reaction incited by bile extravasation may contribute to the pseudo-intimal proliferation (Laberge et al, 1993). A recent experimental study in pigs with TIPS confirmed this hypothesis as TIPS stenosis was seen only in those animals with bile duct transection. Studies of coronary stents indicate that thrombosis occurring immediately after the placement of the stents in animals serves as a template for pseudo-intimal proliferation later (Schwartz et al, 1992). Thus, early anti-coagulation, which prevents thrombosis, has been found to be associated with a decreased risk of long-term coronary stent stenosis. However, this has not been the case with TIPS. The long-term risk of stenosis was not decreased with oral anti-coagulation; in fact, there was a questionable benefit, even in terms of preventing short-term stent thrombosis (Sauer et al, 1996). In the only study in humans undergoing TIPS, aspirin was not found to be useful in decreasing shunt stenosis (Theilman et al, 1994). Outside controlled trials, we do not recommend routine use of anti-coagulants. Finally, TIPS using PTFE-coated stents has been associated with longer patency in animal studies (Nishimine et al, 1995), and one hopes to see similar results in humans.

Detection of shunt stenosis

There are clinical, endoscopic, ultrasonographic and angiographic methods to detect shunt stenosis. Shunt stenosis is suspected on clinical grounds if ascites increase or if the patient has recurrent bleeding. In Lind's series, all patients who had recurrent bleeding had shunt stenosis (Lind et al, 1994). A broad generalization would be that any patient with recurrent bleeding following a TIPS is likely to have shunt dysfunction. Shunt stenosis on endoscopy is indicated by an increase in the size of the varices or of portal hypertensive gastropathy. It is important to emphasize that even in the presence of a patent shunt, large oesophageal and gastric varices, as well as portal hypertensive gastropathy, may not completely regress (Kamath et al, 1995). On Doppler ultrasonography, shunt stenosis is suspected when the velocity of shunt flow is < 50 cm per second, or when there is a change from hepatofugal to hepatopetal intraparenchymal portal venous flow (Feldstein et al, 1996). The gold standard for diagnosing shunt stenosis, however, is angiography with pressure measurement, and whenever shunt stenosis is suspected, angiography is mandatory.

Treatment of shunt stenosis

There are several methods of treating shunt stenosis. These include balloon dilatation of the shunt or excision of the hyperproliferative pseudo-intima using atherotomy devices (Gray et al, 1992). If these methods do not decrease the portacaval gradient sufficiently, an additional stent may be placed through the stenosed shunt. Occluded shunts can be treated similarly by placing a second stent through the original shunt. If this is not technically possible, an additional TIPS needs to be placed on the contralateral side.

Encephalopathy

TIPS functions haemodynamically are in effect like a side-to-side porto-systemic shunt that deprives the liver sinusoid of portal blood (Figure 1). Further, because portal hypertension is reduced, putative toxins of intestinal origin gain access to the portal circulation, bypass the liver and enter the systemic circulation. The incidence of hepatic encephalopathy following TIPS depends on the definition of portosystemic encephalopathy, the close-ness of follow-up, and whether lactulose is used prophylactically in all patients or not. New onset encephalopathy following TIPS typically occurs within 1 month, and is easily treatable in most instances (Sanyal et al, 1994b). Hepatic encephalopathy tends to be more common in older patients, those of female gender, and patients with hypoalbuminaemia (Somberg et al, 1995).

Encephalopathy is related both to portosystemic shunting, as well as to altered liver function. New onset encephalopathy following TIPS may, therefore, be attributable to worsening liver function or to increased porto-systemic shunting. A recent study is important in sorting out this issue (Sanyal et al, 1994b). They prospectively studied 30 patients undergoing TIPS and compared them with 25 control patients undergoing sclero-therapy, both study groups being comparable for severity of liver disease. Mental status and asterixis worsened, usually within the first month in patients undergoing TIPS, while there was no change in patients under-going sclerotherapy. In three of the patients undergoing TIPS, there was new onset of encephalopathy. There were 24 episodes of encephalopathy during follow-up in the TIPS group, and only six episodes of encephal-opathy in the sclerotherapy group, clearly demonstrating that portosystemic encephalopathy is higher after TIPS than after sclerotherapy, and is related to increased portosystemic shunting.

Hepatic encephalopathy is treated by conventional methods, including lactulose and protein restriction. When encephalopathy is intractable, such patients are candidates for orthotopic liver transplantation. Balloon occlusion of the shunt (Fenyves et al, 1994), or reduction in diameter of the shunt (Hauenstein et al, 1995), may be used successfully as a means of alleviating the encephalopathy, especially if patients are not candidates for liver transplantation. The shunt can be thrombosed by occluding the shunt with a balloon for longer than 12 hours (Kerlan et al, 1995b). It should be realized that occluding the shunt or reducing the shunt increases the risk of variceal bleeding.

FUTURE DIRECTIONS

The place of TIPS in the management of complications of portal hyper-tension is uncertain. In patients undergoing TIPS to prevent recurrent variceal bleeding, a survival model using bilirubin and creatinine can predict patients who are likely to have a poor outcome (Gordon et al, 1995). When TIPS is performed for refractory ascites, neither pre-procedure

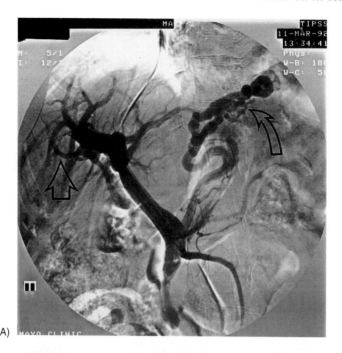

(A)

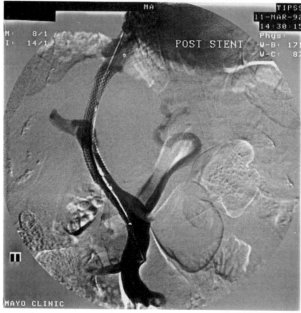

(B)

Figure 1. (A) Portal venogram prior to deployment of stent shows prominent varices (curved arrow), as well as intrahepatic branches of the portal vein (broad arrow). (B) Portal venogram following deployment of the stent. Note that the varices have disappeared; there no longer is significant perfusion of the intrahepatic portal venous system.

serum creatinine nor portal venous pressure gradient predicts response to treatment (Ochs et al, 1995b). Data need to be pooled from several centres and survival models developed so that only the most suitable candidates undergo TIPS. TIPS should not be carried out in high risk candidates whose survival can be measured only in days unless they are candidates for liver transplantation.

The role of TIPS in the management of variceal bleeding is also as yet unclear (D'Amico et al, 1995). Endoscopic variceal ligation has increasingly been used in the management of variceal haemorrhage and, thus, a large multicentre study needs to be carried out comparing variceal ligation with TIPS placement. TIPS needs also to be compared with pharmacological therapy and with surgical shunts for the prevention of recurrent variceal haemorrhage.

There have been no large studies carried out that compare TIPS with standard therapy in the management of intractable ascites, and such studies are urgently called for. Further investigation is also required to address questions related to shunt stenosis, especially since patients with relatively preserved liver function, or children (Berger et al, 1994) might have the stent in for long durations. These questions include the type of material used for the stent, coated stents, and anticoagulant therapy and treatment of trivial stenosis.

TIPS serves as an ideal model to study the relationship between the liver and kidney function (Wong et al, 1995). Patients undergoing liver transplantation cannot be used to address this question because of the effect of immunosuppressive drugs like cyclosporin on the kidney. The TIPS procedure is an ideal model to separate out the effects of portal hypertension on kidney function from those of hepatocyte dysfunction on kidney function. Such studies might also provide insights into the management of hepatorenal syndrome.

TIPS is a novel technique, but close follow-up of patients is mandatory in view of the high incidence of shunt-related problems. It is a useful method of treating difficult problems such as refractory variceal bleeding and refractory ascites. Be that as it may, the role of TIPS in the management of complications of portal hypertension awaits the results of several ongoing trials.

REFERENCES

Abouljoud MS, Levy MF, Rees CR et al (1995) A comparison of treatment with transjugular intra-hepatic portosystemic shunt or distal splenorenal shunt in the management of variceal bleeding prior to liver transplantation. *Transplantation* **59:** 226–229.

D'Amico G, Pagliaro L & Bosch J (1995) The treatment of portal hypertension: a meta-analytic review. *Hepatology* **22:** 332–354.

Arroyo V, Gines P, Gerbes AL et al (1996) Definition and diagnostic criteria of refractory ascites and hepatorenal syndrome in cirrhosis. *Hepatology* **26:** 164–176.

Azoulay D, Castaing D, Dennison A et al (1994) Transjugular intrahepatic portosystemic shunt worsens the hemodynamic circulatory state of the cirrhotic patient: preliminary report of a prospective study.*Hepatology* **19:** 129–132.

LaBerge JM, Ring EJ & Gordon RL (1991) Percutaneous intrahepatic portosystemic shunt created via a femoral approach. *Radiology* **181:** 679–681.

LaBerge JM, Ferrell LD, Ring EJ et al (1993) Histopathological study of stenotic and occluded transjugular intrahepatic portosystemic shunts. *Journal of Vascular and Interventional Radiology* **4:** 779–786.

*LaBerge JM, Somberg KA, Lake JR et al (1995) Two year outcome following transjugular intrahepatic portosystemic shunt for variceal bleeding: results in ninety patients. *Gastroenterology* **108:** 1143–1151.

Berger H, Bugnon F, Goffette P et al (1994) Percutaneous transjugular intrahepatic portosystemic stent shunt for treatment of intractable varicose bleeding in pediatric patients. *European Journal of Pediatrics* **153:** 721–725.

Bernstein D, Yrizarry J, Reddy KR et al (1996) Transjugular intrahepatic portosystemic shunt in the treatment of intermittently bleeding stomal varices. *American Journal of Gastroenterology* **91:** 2237–2238.

Blum U, Haag K, Rossle M et al (1995) Noncavernomatous portal vein thrombosis in hepatic cirrhosis: treatment with transjugular intrahepatic portosystemic shunt and local thrombolysis. *Radiology* **195:** 153–157.

Burroughs AK, Hamilton G, Philips A et al (1989) A comparison of sclerotherapy with staple transection of the esophagus for the emergency control of bleeding from oesophageal varices. *New England Journal of Medicine* **321:** 857–862.

*Cabrera J, Maynar M, Granados R et al (1996) Transjugular intrahepatic portosystemic shunt versus sclerotherapy in the elective treatment of variceal haemorrhage. *Gastroenterology* **110:** 832–839.

Casado M, García Pagàn JC, Banares R et al (1995) Clinical events following TIPS: correlation with hemodynamic findings. *Hepatology* **22:** A296.

Cello JP, Ring EJ, Olcott E et al (1995) Transjugular intrahepatic portosystemic shunt (TIPS) vs sclerotherapy (ES) for variceal haemorrhage (VH). *Gastroenterology* **108:** A1045.

Colapinto RF, Stronell RD, Gildiner M et al (1983) Formation of an intrahepatic portosystemic shunt using balloon dilatation catheter: preliminary clinical experience. *American Journal of Roentgenology* **140:** 709–714.

Coldwell DM, Ring EJ, Rees CR et al (1995) Multicenter investigation of the role of transjugular intrahepatic portosystemic shunt in management of portal hypertension. *Radiology* **196:** 335–340.

Crenshaw WB, Gordon FD, McEniff NJ et al (1996) Severe ascites—efficacy of the transjugular intrahepatic portosystemic shunt in treatment. *Radiology* **200:** 185–192.

Feldstein VA, Patel MD & LaBerge JM (1996) Transjugular intrahepatic portosystemic shunts— accuracy of Doppler ultrasound in determination of patency and detection of stenosis. *Radiology* **201:** 141–147.

Fenyves D, Dufresne MP, Raymond J et al (1994) Successful reversal of chronic incapacitating post-TIPS encephalopathy by balloon occlusion of the stent. *Canadian Journal of Gastroenterology* **8:** 75–80.

Freedman AM, Sanyal AJ, Tisnado J et al (1993) Complications of transjugular intrahepatic porto-systemic shunt: a comprehensive review. *Radiographics* **13:** 1185–1210.

Fried MW, Connaghan DG, Sharma S et al (1996) Transjugular intrahepatic portosystemic shunt for the management of severe renooclusive disease following bone marrow transplantation. *Hepatology* **24:** 588–591.

Garcia Villareal L, Martinez-Lagares F, Sierra A et al (1996) TIPS versus sclerotherapy (SCL) for the prevention of variceal bleeding. Preliminary results of a randomized study. *Hepatology* **24:** A208.

Gordon FD, Malinchoc M, Peine CJ et al (1995) A model for predicting survival in patients under-going elective transjugular intrahepatic portosystemic shunts (TIPS). *Gastroenterology* **108:** A1074.

Gray RJ, Dolmatch BL & Buick MK (1992) Directional atherotomy treatment for hemodialysis access: early results. *Journal of Vascular and Interventional Radiology* **3:** 497–503.

Groupe d'Etude des Anastomoses intra-hepatiques (GDAIH) (1995) TIPS versus sclerotherapy plus Propranolol in the prevention of variceal rebleeding: preliminary results of a multi-center randomized trial. *Hepatology* **22:** A297.

Harman JT, Reed JD & Kopecky KK (1992) Localization of the portal vein for transjugular catheter-ization: percutaneous placement of a metallic marker with real-time US guidance. *Journal of Vascular and Interventional Radiology* **3:** 545–547.

Haskal ZJ, Scott M, Rubin RA et al (1994) Intestinal varices—treatment with a transjugular intra-hepatic portosystemic shunt. *Radiology* **191:** 183–187.

Hauenstein KH, Haag K, Ochs A et al (1995) The reducing stent: treatment for transjugular intra-hepatic portosystemic shunt-induced refractory hepatic encephalopathy and liver failure. *Radiology* **194:** 175–179.

Jalan R, John TG, Redhead DN et al (1995) A comparative study of emergency transjugular intra-hepatic portosystemic stent shunt and oesophageal transection in the management of un-controlled variceal haemorrhage. *American Journal of Gastroenterology* **90:** 1932–1937.

Jalan R, Forest EH, Stanley AJ et al (1996) TIPSS versus variceal band ligation for the prevention of variceal bleeding in cirrhosis: a randomized control study. *Hepatology* **24:** A247.

Kamath PS & McKusick MA (1994) Transjugular intrahepatic portosystemic shunts: a note of caution. *Gastroenterology* **106:** 1384–1387.

*Kamath PS & McKusick MA (1996) Transjugular intrahepatic portosystemic shunts. *Gastro-enterology* **111:** 1700–1705.

Kamath PS, Malinchoc M, Peine CJ et al (1994) Risk factors associated with survival following the TIPS procedure. *Gastroenterology* **106:** A914.

Kamath PS, Lacerda M, Ahlquist DA et al (1995) Endoscopic transitions in patients undergoing transjugular intrahepatic portosystemic shunts. *Gastrointestinal Endoscopy* **41:** A352.

*Kerlan RK Jr, LaBerge JM, Gordon RL et al (1995a) Transjugular intrahepatic portosystemic shunts: current status. *American Journal of Roentgenology* **164:** 1059–1066.

Kerlan RK, LaBerge JM, Baker EL et al (1995b) Successful reversal of hepatic encephalopathy with intentional occlusion of transjugular intrahepatic portosystemic shunts. *Journal of Vascular and Interventional Radiology* **6:** 917–921.

Kuo PC, Johnson LB, Hastings G et al (1996) Fulminant hepatic failure from Budd–Chiari syndrome—a bridge to transplantation with transjugular intrahepatic portosystemic shunt. *Transplantation* **62:** 294–296.

Lebrec D, Giuily N, Hadengue A et al (1996) Transjugular intrahepatic portosystemic shunts—comparison with paracentesis in patients with cirrhosis and refractory ascites—a randomized trial. *Journal of Hepatology* **25:** 135–144.

Lind CD, Malisch TW, Chong WK et al (1994) Incidence of shunt occlusion or stenosis following transjugular intrahepatic portosystemic shunt placement. *Gastroenterology* **106:** 1277–1283.

Longo JM, Bilbao JI & Rousseau HP (1992) Color Doppler US guidance in transjugular intrahepatic portosystemic shunts. *Radiology* **184:** 281–284.

Mallery S, Freeman ML, Peine CJ et al (1996) Biliary-shunt fistula following transjugular intrahepatic portosystemic shunt placement. *Gastroenterology* **111:** 1353–1357.

Menegaux F, Baker E, Keeff EB et al (1994) Impact of transjugular intrahepatic portosystemic shunt on orthotopic liver transplantation. *World Journal of Surgery* **18:** 866–871.

Menzel J, Vestring T, Foerster EC et al (1995) Arterio-biliary fistula after transjugular intrahepatic portosystemic shunt: a life-threatening complication of the new technique for therapy of portal hypertension. *Zeitschrift für Gastroenterology* **33:** 255–259.

Merli M, Riggio O, Capocaccia L et al (1994) Transjugular intrahepatic portosystemic shunt (TIPS) vs endoscopic sclerotherapy (ES) in preventing variceal rebleeding. Preliminary results of a randomized trial. *Hepatology* **20:** A107.

Millis M, Imagawa D, Olthoff K et al (1995) TIPS: impact on liver transplantation. *Transplantation Proceedings* **27:** 1248–1249.

Nazarian GK, Ferral H, Bjarnason H et al (1996) Effect of transjugular intrahepatic portosystemic shunt on quality of life. *American Journal of Roentgenology* **167:** 963–969.

Nishimine K, Saxon RR, Kichikawa K et al (1995) Improved transjugular intrahepatic portosystemic shunt patency with PTFE-covered stent-grafts: experimental results in swine. *Radiology* **196:** 341–347.

Ochs A, Sellinger M, Haag K et al (1993) Transjugular intrahepatic portosystemic stent-shunt (TIPS) in the treatment of Budd–Chiari syndrome. *Journal of Hepatology* **18:** 217–225.

Ochs A, Gerbes AL, Haag K et al (1995a) TIPS and paracentesis for the treatment of refractory ascites (RA). Interim analysis of a randomized control trial. *Hepatology* **22:** A297.

*Ochs A, Rossle M, Haag K et al (1995b) The transjugular intrahepatic portosystemic stent-shunt procedure for refractory ascites. *New England Journal of Medicine* **332:** 1192–1197.

Quiroga J, Sangro B, Nunez M et al (1995) Transjugular intrahepatic portosystemic shunt in the treat-ment of refractory ascites: effect on clinical, renal, humoral, and hemodynamic parameters. *Hepatology* **21:** 986–994.

Radoscvich PM, Ring EJ, LaBerg JM et al (1993) Transjugular intrahepatic portosystemic shunt in patients with portal vein occlusion. *Radiology* **186:** 523–527.

Richter GM, Noldge G & Palmaz JC (1990) The transjugular intrahepatic portosystemic stent shunt (TIPSS): results of a pilot study. *Cardiovascular and Interventional Radiology* **13:** 200–207.

Riegler JL, Lang KA, Johnson SP et al (1995) Transjugular intrahepatic portosystemic shunt improves oxygenation in hepatopulmonary syndrome. *Gastroenterology* **109:** 978–983.

Rosch J, Hanafee WN, Snow H et al (1971) Transjugular intrahepatic portosystemic shunt: an experimental work. *American Journal of Surgery* **121:** 588–592.

Rosemurgy AS, Goode SE, Zwiebel BR et al (1996) A prospective trial of transjugular intrahepatic portosystemic stent shunts versus small diameter prosthetic H-graft portocaval shunts in the treatment of bleeding varices. *Annals of Surgery* **224:** 378–384.

Rosser BG, Poterucha JJ, McKusick MA et al (1996) Thoracic duct cutaneous fistula: successful treatment using transjugular intrahepatic portosystemic shunt. *Mayo Clinic Proceedings* **71:** 793–796.

Rossle M, Deibert P, Haag K et al (1994a) TIPS versus sclerotherapy and beta blockade: preliminary results of a randomized study in patients with recurrent variceal haemorrhage. *Hepatology* **20:** A107.

*Rossle M, Haag K, Ochs A et al (1994b) The transjugular intrahepatic portosystemic stent shunt procedure for variceal bleeding. *New England Journal of Medicine* **330:** 165–171.

Rutherford RB & Becker GB (1991) Standards for evaluating and reporting the results of surgical and percutaneous therapy for peripheral arterial disease. *Journal of Vascular and Interventional Radiology* **2:** 169–174.

Sanyal AJ, Freedman AM, Purdum PP et al (1994a) Transjugular intrahepatic portosystemic shunt (TIPS) vs sclerotherapy for prevention of recurrent variceal haemorrhage. A randomized prospective trial. *Gastroenterology* **106:** A975.

*Sanyal AJ, Freedman AM, Shiffman ML et al (1994b) Portosystemic encephalopathy after transjugular intrahepatic portosystemic shunt—results of a prospective controlled study. *Hepatology* **20:** 46–55.

*Sanyal AJ, Freedman AM, Luketic VA et al (1996a) Transjugular intrahepatic portosystemic shunts for patients with active variceal haemorrhage unresponsive to sclerotherapy. *Gastroenterology* **111:** 138–146.

Sanyal AJ, Freedman AM, Purdum PP et al (1996b) The hematologic consequences of transjugular intrahepatic portosystemic shunts. *Hepatology* **23:** 32–39.

Sarfeh J & Rypins EB (1994) Partial versus total portacaval shunt in alcoholic cirrhosis. Results of a prospective randomized trial. *Annals of Surgery* **219:** 353–361.

Sauer P, Theilmann L, Hermann S et al (1996) Phenprocoumon for prevention of shunt occlusion after transjugular intrahepatic portosystemic stent shunt: a randomized trial. *Hepatology* **24:** 1433–1436.

Schwartz RS, Holmes DR Jr & Topol EJ (1992) The restenosis paradigm revisited: an alternative proposal for cellular mechanisms. *Journal of the American College of Cardiology* **20:** 1284–1293.

Shiffman ML, Jeffers L, Hoofnagle JM et al (1995) The role of transjugular intrahepatic portosystemic shunt (TIPS) for treatment of portal hypertension and its complications. A conference sponsored by the National Digestive Diseases Advisory Board. *Hepatology* **22:** 1591–1597.

Somberg KA, Lake JR, Tomlanovich SJ et al (1995a) Transjugular intrahepatic portosystemic shunts for refractory ascites: assessment of clinical and hormonal response and renal function. *Hepatology* **21:** 709–716.

Somberg KA, Lombardero MS, Lawlor SM et al (1995b) Impact of transjugular intrahepatic portosystemic shunts on liver transplantation: a controlled analysis. NIDDK Liver Transplantation Database. *Transplantation Proceedings* **27:** 1248–1249.

Strauss RM, Martin LG, Kaufman SL et al (1994) Transjugular intrahepatic portosystemic shunt for management of symptomatic cirrhotic hydrothorax. *American Journal of Gastroenterology* **89:** 1520–1522.

Theilmann L, Sauer P, Roeren T et al (1994) Salicylic acid in the prevention of early stenosis and occlusion of transjugular intrahepatic portosystemic stent shunts—a controlled study. *Hepatology* **20:** 592–597.

Theoni RF (1995) The role of imaging in patients with ascites. *American Journal of Roentgenology* **165:** 16–18.

Uflacker R, Reichert P, D'Albuquerque LC et al (1994) Liver anatomy applied to the placement of transjugular intrahepatic portosystemic shunts. *Radiology* **191:** 705–712.

Vanderlinden P, Lemoine O, Ghysels M et al (1996) Pulmonary hypertension after transjugular intra-hepatic portosystemic shunt—effects on right ventricular function. *Hepatology* **23:** 982–987.

Wilson MW, Gordon RL, LaBerge JM et al (1995) Liver transplantation complicated by malposition and transjugular intrahepatic portosystemic shunts. *Journal of Vascular and Interventional Radiology* **6:** 695–699.

*Wong F, Sniderman K, Liu P et al (1995) Transjugular intrahepatic portosystemic stent shunt: effects on hemodynamics and sodium homeostasis in cirrhosis and refractory ascites. *Annals of Internal Medicine* **122:** 816–822.

Wong F, Sniderman K, Liu P et al (1996) The mechanism of the initial two-stage natriuresis follow-ing normalization of portal pressure post TIPS in cirrhotic patients with refractory ascites. *Hepatology* **24:** A190.

the adverse effects of portal diversion in careful animal studies. In 1903 Eugene Vidal performed the first end-to-side portacaval anastomosis successfully in man and observed cessation of bleeding and resolution of ascites. However, the patient subsequently developed encephalopathy, reaccumulation of ascites, and died 3.5 months after surgery. Several historical articles have reviewed these early experiences (Child, 1953; Donovan and Covey, 1978; Chandler, 1993).

A number of procedures were developed in the early 20th century to promote portal-systemic collateralization. These included the omentopexy of Drummond and Morrison (White, 1906), splenic transposition first described by Talma (Holman, 1933), and the visceral abrasion techniques of Madden et al (1954). Enthusiasm for these procedures waned as their results yielded no improvement in patient outcome. In 1945, Allen Whipple reintroduced portasystemic shunting for the management of complications of portal hypertension (Whipple, 1945). He reported a series of portacaval and central splenorenal shunts. Linton (Linton et al, 1961) continued this work and reviewed his experience in 169 patients. He concluded that each type of shunt had equal efficacy in controlling bleeding, end-to-side portacaval shunts did not control ascites and splenorenal shunting resulted in less encephalopathy. The incidence of encephalopathy continued to remain high and progression to hepatic failure was accelerated following total, non-selective shunting procedures. These findings led to the development of selective shunting including the distal splenorenal shunt by Warren (Warren et al, 1967) and the coronary-caval shunt by Inokuchi (1968). These shunting procedures maintain portal hypertension and hepatic perfusion while selectively decompressing gastro-oesophageal varices.

The past two decades have seen major changes in managing patients with cirrhosis and portal hypertension. The greatest advance has been the successful clinical application of liver transplantation, with other advances in pharmacological, endoscopical, radiological and surgical therapies.

The pathophysiology of portal hypertension is now better understood and has led to the use of newer and more efficacious medications to prevent and treat variceal bleeding (Reichen, 1990; Roberts and Kamath, 1996). Medical pharmacotherapy presently includes the use of vasopressin in combination with nitro-glycerine, propranolol, and more recently, octreotide and isosorbide mononitrate (Lebrec, 1994; Morillas et al, 1994; Vorobioff et al, 1994).

Endoscopic sclerotherapy, initially described in 1939, was reintroduced in the 1970s and has become widely accepted. This modality has become the principal means for treating acute bleeding and for attempting obliteration of varices. Sclerotherapy combined with pharmacological reduction of portal hypertension using beta-blockers is the primary treatment for acute bleeding varices and prevention of recurrent bleeding (Johnston and Rodgers, 1973; Lebrec et al, 1980b). Improved endoscopic techniques utilizing elastic band ligation have proven to be more efficacious with fewer procedure-related complications (Steigmann et al, 1992).

Radiological intervention by the transjugular intrahepatic portasystemic shunt (TIPS) has rapidly gained acceptance as a method to create a functional, total side-to-side shunt utilizing a minimally invasive technique (LaBerge et al, 1993; Rossle et al, 1994). TIPS patency rates have improved with aggressive monitoring and radiographic interventional procedures. Presently, the accepted indications for TIPS are acutely bleeding varices that cannot be successfully controlled with medical treatment and recurrent variceal bleeding in patients who are refractory or intolerant to conventional medical management.

Surgical management for portal hypertension has also changed in the last two decades. Surgical shunt procedures now include partial portal-systemic shunts and improved methods for selective shunts (Henderson et al, 1989; Collins et al, 1994). The emergence of liver transplantation in the 1980s as a clinical reality has provided definitive treatment of the underlying liver disease and is the ultimate treatment for portal hypertension (Starzl et al, 1989). Liver transplantation has improved with lower morbidity and mortality, and improved survival, with the development of techniques and the introduction of more effective immunosuppression medications.

Presently, it can be difficult to decide the optimal treatment for a given patient with such options available (Pagliaro et al, 1989). Careful patient evaluation with an understanding of the underlying liver disease, portal anatomy, possible need for transplantation, and availability of appropriate technology and expertise must be considered for the treatment plan (Knechtle et al, 1994; Hermann et al, 1995).

SURGICAL PROCEDURES

Surgical decompression of gastro-oesophageal varices controls bleeding, but has not been widely accepted to treat all patients with variceal bleeding. This is primarily because the first type of shunts were total portal-systemic shunts, and diversion of portal blood flow gave a high rate of encephalopathy and was detrimental to liver function. However, changes in surgical methods in the past two decades with other types of operative shunts, devascularization procedures and liver transplantation, have reintroduced surgical options in portal hypertension. The recent success of TIPS has focused attention back on decompression procedures and re-emphasized the effect of different types of shunts on portal perfusion (Rikkers et al, 1992; Collins and Sarfeh, 1995; D'Amico et al, 1995; Iannitti and Henderson, 1997).

Total portal-systemic shunts

Total portal-systemic shunts divert the entire blood flow of the portal system into the systemic circulation. Total shunts can be achieved in several ways. The classic end-to-side portacaval anastomosis (the Eck fistula) clearly provides complete diversion of all portal flow, but because the hepatic end of the portal vein is ligated this does not provide outflow of the liver sinusoids and as such does not relieve ascites. A side-to-side porta-caval anastomosis of 1.2 cm or greater will also result in a total portal-systemic shunt, but because the portal vein remains intact it acts as an outflow from the liver sinusoids, decompresses the liver and thus controls ascites. Any portacaval shunt requires dissection of the hepatic hilus to free the portal vein and will make subsequent liver transplantation more difficult.

Total portal-systemic shunting can also be accomplished with the use of a large calibre (16–22 mm) interposition graft placed from the portal or superior mesenteric vein to the inferior vena cava, left renal vein or right atrium. Although some of these shunts do require dissection of the hepatic hilus they are more easily divided should liver transplantation be needed. The major disadvantage of an interposition graft is if the primary patency is less than that of a side-to-side portacaval vein-to-vein anastomosis.

Non-selective or total shunts eliminate portal hypertension, effectively control and prevent variceal bleeding, and, with the exception of the end-to-side portacaval shunt, are useful in treating ascites. Disadvantages are related to diversion of all portal flow, which leads to an increased incidence of encephalopathy and accelerated progression of the underlying liver disease.

Partial shunts

These create a side-to-side communication of limited size between the portal and systemic circulation, lower the portal pressure and maintain some hepatic portal perfusion. This concept of partial shunting was begun by Bismuth (Bismuth et al, 1974) who observed an initial gradient across a 15-mm side-to-side portacaval anastomosis. At this size, these eventually became total shunts with reversal of portal flow. Johansen (1989) continued this work by creating smaller 10–12 mm side-to-side portacaval anastomoses, and although significant pressure gradients could be measured initially between the portal and systemic circulations, these shunts became total shunts eventually.

Recently, Sarfeh has popularized the use of small diameter, reinforced PTFE interposition grafts between the portal vein and inferior vena cava (Sarfeh and Rypins, 1986; Collins et al, 1994). The difference in this work is that the fixed diameter of the graft sets a maximum size for these shunts. An 8-mm graft will reduce portal pressure to 12 mmHg, which is low enough to control bleeding, while maintaining hepatic portal perfusion in 80% of subjects. When a 10-mm graft is used, hepatic portal perfusion is only maintained in 20% of subjects (Sarfeh et al, 1986; Rosemurgy et al, 1996a). The coronary vein, gastroepiploic veins, and other collateral vessels can be ligated to decrease inflow to the oesophageal varices, although this is controversial. Partial shunting results in lowered portal pressure while maintaining some prograde hepatic venous flow, and is an effective treatment for bleeding oesophageal varices with a lower rate of encephalopathy than total shunts. The disadvantages include dissection of the hepatic hilus and an early thrombosis rate of 16%, but with modern radiological interventional techniques long-term patency can be maintained.

Selective shunts

Selective shunts provide selective decompression of gastro-oesophageal varices while maintaining portal hypertension and portal venous perfusion. These shunts selectively decompress gastro-oesophageal varices and are not portal-systemic shunts since portal blood flow is not diverted. Generally there are two types of selective shunts, the distal splenorenal shunt devised and popularized by Warren (Warren et al, 1967) and the infrequently used coronary-caval shunt of Inokuchi (1968).

The coronary–caval shunt includes splenectomy, and then involves dissection and disconnection of the portal vein and of the coronary (left gastric) vein, and anastomosis to the inferior vena cava. This procedure is technically difficult, usually requires interposition vein grafting, and is rarely used in present times.

The distal splenorenal shunt, which selectively decompresses the spleen and gastro-oesophageal junction has gained world-wide acceptance. The procedure requires disconnection of the splenic vein from the superior mesenteric vein, dissection of this vein out from the pancreas, and anastomosis to the left renal vein in an end-to-side fashion. This provides a low pressure outflow tract for gastro-oesophageal varices. Portal-systemic collateral vessels including the left gastric vein, gastroepiploic veins, and vessels within the splenocolic ligament are ligated. The distal splenorenal shunt has several advantages over portal-systemic shunting for the decompression of gastro-oesophageal varices. Oesophageal and gastric varices are effectively decompressed and bleeding is controlled. Maintenance of hepatopedal portal vein flow decreases the risk of encephalopathy and accelerated liver failure. Dissection is within the lesser sac, distant to hepatic hilus, and thus does not compromise subsequent liver transplant. Long-term patency is excellent in this high flow vein-to-vein anastomosis (Henderson, 1994). Although portal vein thrombosis has been recorded in 5–10% of patients, hepatic portal perfusion is maintained in 90% of patients early after shunt. In non-alcoholic patients good hepatic portal perfusion is maintained long term, while in alcoholics it is lost in 16–50% depending on how much splenic vein is dissected out of the pancreas. Loss of portal flow occurs through the development of intrapancreatic portal-systemic collateralization known as the 'pancreatic siphon' (Warren et al, 1986). Improved maintenance of portal perfusion in alcoholic patients has been achieved by the addition of splenopancreatic disconnection to the distal splenorenal shunt procedure (Warren et al, 1986; Henderson et al, 1989). In this modification, the splenic vein is completely disconnected from the posterior pancreas to the splenic hilum. Other modifications such as transposition of the splenic vein (Orozco et al, 1993) or interposition grafting to the inferior vena cava can be made in patients with a retro-aortic left renal vein (present in 4% of the population).

Devascularization (non-shunting) procedures

These procedures of the stomach and lower oesophagus were introduced by several groups in the 1950s and 1960s (Crile, 1950), and compromised components of devascularization procedures with the modifications of variceal ligation, oesophageal transection and splenectomy. Sugiura and Futagawa in 1973 reported a two-stage procedure involving both transthoracic and transabdominal approaches for interruption of gastro-oesophageal varices while still maintaining flow through other portal-azygous collaterals. Yammamoto modified this procedure to be performed through the transabdominal approach only (Yammamoto et al, 1976).

The effectiveness of devascularization procedures for the control of variceal bleeding appears to be related to the extent of the procedure. For maximal efficacy, a devascularization procedure usually devascularizes the distal 7–8 cm of the oesophagus, the entire greater curve and two-thirds of the lesser curve of the stomach. The spleen is usually removed, and they may include oesophageal transection and re-anastomosis. This provides interruption of inflow to gastro-oesophageal varices with maintenance of portal hypertension and portal perfusion. Devascularization procedures are effective in controlling actively bleeding gastro-oesophageal varices. In Japan, when used to prevent rebleeding, there is a low operative mortality and rebleeding rate of < 10% (Idezuki et al, 1994). Outside of Japan, most centres report up to a 37% rebleeding rate (Orozco et al, 1992; Dagenais et al, 1994). Most surgeons can perform devascularization procedures, so they remain an acceptable alternative in an emergency and for 'unshuntable' patients (Caps et al, 1996). Splenectomy alone may be curative in patients with bleeding gastric varices from isolated splenic vein thrombosis, but is not indicated in patients with portal hypertension secondary to cirrhosis.

Liver transplantation

Liver transplantation was pioneered by Starzl and Calne in the 1970s and has rapidly expanded worldwide as a clinical reality in the past decade (Starzl et al, 1989). Transplant is the treatment of choice for patients with end-stage liver disease and the complications of such disease, which include oesophageal varices, encephalopathy, ascites, fatigue, and muscle wasting, can all be improved following successful transplantation.

The technical aspects of liver transplantation have advanced significantly in the 1990s, allowing many centres to perform this procedure. Prior surgery involving the hepatic hilum adds to the difficulty of hepatectomy, as have may previous shunt procedures. However, several studies, while documenting increased operative complexity, have not shown different long-term outcomes in this population. Morbidity and mortality of liver transplantation have significantly improved in recent years. Improved perioperative care, surgical techniques, immunosuppression medications, treatment of infection, and nutritional support have had positive impacts on outcome and patient survival.

SURGICAL THERAPY AT SPECIFIC TIMES

Prophylaxis

Surgical management is not indicated to treat gastro-oesophageal varices that have not bled. Therapy for these patients is with a non-cardioselective beta-blocker. Prospective, randomized trials in the 1960s, which compared portacaval shunts to medical management in this population, documented a higher mortality in patients receiving surgery (Jackson et al, 1968; Resnick et al, 1969). The bleeding risk of only 30% in this population is the main factor in defining that an aggressive surgical approach is not indicated (Conn et al, 1972).

A single study of portal non-decompression surgery from multiple centres in Japan has documented increased survival in patients randomized to surgery (Inokuchi et al, 1990). This study included devascularization and selective shunt procedures in the surgical group. However, the data are not sufficiently convincing, nor have they been confirmed, to advocate this therapy.

Acute bleeding

Approximately 30% of patients with cirrhosis and oesophageal varices will experience variceal haemorrhage, usually within 1 year of diagnosis. The first acute bleed carries a mortality of approximately 30% (range 15–50%). Most deaths are in poorer risk patients (Child's C), and are due to progressive liver failure. Early rebleeding occurs in 20–50% of patients in the first 7 to 10 days and is a poor prognostic sign. While these figures have led to Orloff's justification for emergency portacaval shunt for all patients, this aggressive surgical approach has not been taken up by others.

The initial management of a patient with bleeding oesophageal varices consists of adequate volume replacement with blood, blood products, and colloid solutions. Pharmacological portal pressure reduction can be acutely achieved with medications such as vasopressin and nitro-glycerine, or octreotide (Roberts and Kamath, 1996). Early endoscopy is employed to identify and confirm the source of bleeding, and to control bleeding with sclerotherapy or banding. When these measures are carried out, control of variceal haemorrhage can be achieved in about 90% of patients (D'Amico et al, 1995). Pharmacological and endoscopic treatment are the primary management tools to control acute variceal bleeding.

Urgent or emergent shunting may be required in the 10% of patients whose acute bleeding is not controlled by endoscopic measures (Potts et al, 1984; Rikkers and Jin, 1994). At the current time, this will almost always be with a TIPS procedure, because failure to control acute bleeding endoscopically almost always occurs in poor risk patients. In some good risk patients, operative shunting procedures may be utilized (Johansen and Helton, 1992; Rosemurgy et al, 1996a). The unique experience of emergency portacaval shunts for acute variceal bleeding has recently been reported by Orloff (Orloff et al, 1995). He reviewed 340 unselected cirrhotic patients undergoing emergency side-to-side portacaval shunts. All patients had control of bleeding and long-term patency of their shunts. Remarkably the recent group of 220 patients had a 15% incidence of hepatic failure and 9% incidence of encephalopathy. These results represent a single institution's outcomes and may not reflect national results.

Non-shunting, devascularization procedures can be performed in patients whose anatomy precludes portal or variceal decompressive procedures (Caps et al, 1996). Devascularization adequately controls bleeding and can be performed by most surgeons. This procedure is associated with a low rate of encephalopathy and hepatic failure; however, late rebleeding rates remain high at about 40%. Devascularization is a reasonable alternative in an emergency situation.

Prevention of rebleeding

The prevention of rebleeding is based on the following principles:

- First-line therapy: pharmacological and endoscopic methods.
- Second-line therapy: decompression, by surgery or TIPS.
- End-stage liver disease: transplant.

Following the control of acute bleeding, patient evaluation is the key to making definitive treatment choices. Several issues must be addressed in this time period, in order to focus on the varices and the risk of bleeding, and on the status of liver function. Does the patient have end-stage liver disease that can be only managed by transplantation, and if so, is the patient a transplant candidate? Of equal importance is the definition of the patient with normal hepatic function because of extra hepatic portal vein thrombosis, who has normal life expectancy if their bleeding is controlled. Most patients, however, have cirrhosis with mild to moderate functional impairment, and it is important to define the aetiology, severity, activity and likely rate of progress of their disease.

Evaluation of varices involves endoscopy and haemodynamic studies with Doppler ultrasound and angiography to evaluate the patency of the portal venous system and measure portal pressure. Endoscopy evaluates the extent and size of varices, and assesses the presence of risk factors such as red colour signs (Japan classification, NIEC classification) (Lebrec et al, 1980b; NIEC, 1988). Doppler ultrasound is the standard for documenting portal vein patency and flow pattern. Angiography is required to measure hepatic venous pressure gradient, which has increasingly been recognized as a useful measure to assess response to pharmacological therapy. Angiography is also needed to define all anatomic pathways of variceal filling and collateral development in portal hypertension.

Finally, the question must be asked, what resources are available for definitive treatment? These include endoscopists capable of performing sclerotherapy and elastic band ligation, interventional radiologists skilled in TIPS, surgeons familiar with various shunting and non-shunting procedures, and liver transplant capability and availability. The first line of treatment for prevention of recurrent bleeding in patients with portal hypertension is by pharmacological and endoscopic treatment (Lebrec et al, 1980b; Terblanche et al, 1994). When these measures fail to prevent recurrent variceal bleeding, variceal decompression should be considered. TIPS, surgical shunts and liver transplantation are the decompression options.

Transjugular intrahepatic portal systemic shunt (TIPS)

Patients with poor hepatic function who are potential transplant candidates and who have recurrent bleeding not controlled by endoscopy, should be managed by TIPS. Equally, TIPS is an option in patients who fail medical and endoscopic therapy, have poor liver function, and who are not transplant candidates. More controversial is the role of TIPS in patients with preserved liver function who fail first-line treatment. There are currently randomized trials that address this issue. The current data on TIPS demonstrate technical success is achieved in approximately 90% of patients, and results in a portal-systemic pressure gradient of < 12 mmHg. Failure of TIPS is related to shunt stenosis and occlusion. Primary patency at 1 year ranges from 50–65%, and primary assisted patency is about 85% at 1 year. Careful follow-up with Doppler ultrasound and repeat catheterization for shunt monitoring results in a 25–50% re-intervention rate to maintain patency. The 1-year rebleeding rate after TIPS is 18–20% (Helton et al, 1993; LaBerge et al, 1993). Long-term patency and rebleeding rates are now being evaluated. Encephalopathy is the other major complication after TIPS, with a rate of 25–30% over pre-TIPS rates.

Liver transplantation

Transplant is the treatment of choice in patients with advanced liver disease and hepatic dysfunction. Transplant is the ultimate decompressive shunt for portal hypertension, which also restores liver function. In addition to preventing variceal rebleeding, liver transplantation treats the other complications of poor hepatic function, ascites, encephalopathy, fatigue and nutritional status. Transplantation in patients with advanced liver disease results in 1 and 5 year survivals of 80–90% and 60–70%, respectively (Iwatsuki et al, 1988; Ringe et al, 1994). Prior shunt surgery involving the porta hepatis can significantly add to the difficulty and blood loss during a transplant procedure, but overall morbidity and mortality are not adversely affected in these patients (Ringe et al, 1994). Non-operative shunts (TIPS) or shunts not involving the porta hepatis (distal splenorenal shunt) should be favoured over other operative shunts in patients expected to undergo future transplantation.

Surgical shunts

Patients with good or adequate hepatic function who fail medical and endoscopic treatment are candidates for surgical decompression. Recently published uncontrolled trials of surgical shunts for variceal bleeding reveal patients generally do well with any type of decompressive procedure.

Mortality and morbidity, primarily encephalopathy and liver failure, are related to the underlying liver disease and its rate of progression (Orloff et al, 1977; Henderson, 1993; Stipa et al, 1994). Proponents for one type of shunt or another can usually obtain good results with the procedure with which they have most experience.

The distal splenorenal shunt is the most commonly performed selective shunt performed worldwide (Warren et al, 1967; Maffei-Faccioli et al, 1990; Myberg, 1990; Orozco et al, 1990; Spina et al, 1992a). DSRS has been proven to be more efficacious in prevention of rebleeding from gastro-oesophageal varices than endoscopic sclerotherapy in a meta-analysis of four randomized clinical trials (Spina et al, 1992b). Control of bleeding is achieved in over 90% of patients with an encephalopathy rate in the 10–15% range. The rate of encephalopathy appears to correlate primarily with the underlying disease and its progression. Portal perfusion is maintained in more than 90% of patients with non-alcoholic liver disease and 50–84% of patients with alcoholic liver disease. Modifications of selective shunting with increasing degrees of portal-azygous and pancreatic disconnection improve the selectivity of the distal splenorenal shunt (Henderson et al, 1989). The reported operative mortality for distal splenorenal shunting in Child's Class A and B patients has fallen to less than 5% in most series in the 1990s. Distal splenorenal shunting has been compared prospectively with partial portal systemic shunting in a recent study (Mercado et al, 1996). Both shunts are equally efficacious in the control of rebleeding; however, encephalopathy and shunt thrombosis rates were higher in patients who received partial, 10-mm interposition mesocaval shunts. A multi-centre prospective randomized controlled trial is being conducted at the moment, which compares distal splenorenal shunt with TIPS for the prevention of recurrent variceal bleeding in patients with good hepatic function.

Partial portacaval shunts using 8-mm interposition grafts have been popularized in the last decade by Sarfeh et al (1986). Overall, these shunts have shown equivalent control of bleeding to other surgical shunts at about 90%. Shunt stenosis or occlusion has been a documented problem in 10–20% of cases; however, it has been and can be managed with radiological intervention techniques. Studies show maintenance of portal perfusion in up to 80% of patients, and the encephalopathy rate is about 15% in these reported series. Currently, a prospective randomized control trial is being conducted by Rosemurgy et al (1996b) that compares the 8-mm portacaval shunt with TIPS. Preliminary reports of this indicate a more favourable outcome in the surgical as opposed to the radiological group.

Total portal systemic shunts are not being widely used in the 1990s. The largest reported recent experience in the 1990s is that of Orloff et al (1995), who in their total experience with this type of shunt have had an excellent outcome. Much of this success is because of the overall advances in patient care, rehabilitation and follow-up. Another significant recent series of total portal systemic shunts comes from Stipa et al (1994) who have documented a higher encephalopathy and liver failure rate with total shunts than that reported by Orloff. Excellent bleeding control has been achieved with any series of successful total portal systemic shunts.

Devascularization procedures

Recent reviews have looked at the outcome of devascularization procedures in Japan (Idezuki et al, 1994) and in the non-Japanese experience (Dagenais et al, 1994). The data suggest that the extent of devascularization is the key in control of bleeding. Reports from Japan, with extensive procedures, indicate rebleeding as a cause of death in only 6% of patients. The literature from elsewhere report overall rebleeding rates, which run in the 30–40% range. The incidence of encephalopathy is low following devascularization procedures at 10% or less, but again depends on the underlying liver disease and its severity. As with most of the operative approaches in portal hypertension the quality of the outcome is in large part dependent on the surgeon's experience. In this group's view, devascularization procedures should be used for patients who have thrombosed all their major vessels and who continue to have significant gastric or oesophageal variceal bleeding during endoscopic and pharmacological therapy. Extensive devascularization for these patients can reduce the risk of bleeding significantly for several years. Devascularization remains a good alternative in otherwise unshuntable patients.

CONCLUSIONS

The role of surgery in the treatment of portal hypertension continues to evolve. Presently, the clinician has a wide array of treatment options in his armamentarium to treat patients with complications of portal hypertension. Pharmacological therapy is the primary treatment modality for the prophylaxis of variceal bleeding. Current data do not support the use of endoscopy, surgical shunts or TIPS as prophylactic measures for variceal haemorrhage. However, in the emergent setting failure of pharmacological and endoscopic treatment is an indication for invasive interventional decompression such as TIPS or a surgical shunt. Total portacaval, partial portacaval, and selective distal splenorenal shunts are equally effective in controlling variceal haemorrhage. Consideration must be given to maintaining portal perfusion, possibility of future liver transplantation, and technical ability to perform a satisfactory shunt procedure to control haemorrhage. Non-shunting or devascularization procedures are an alternative following failure of first-line and/or decompressive procedures. Surgical shunts are a second-line treatment following failure of pharmacological and endoscopic treatment in patients with good hepatic function. Past data suggests that distal splenorenal shunting provides selective variceal decompression with less encephalopathy and accelerated hepatic failure than portal decompression. The long-term efficacy of TIPS in prevention of variceal rebleeding in patients with good hepatic function remains to be determined. Liver transplantation remains the treatment of choice for patients with poor hepatic function.

Currently, transplantation resolves the complications of end-stage liver disease and portal hypertension, and offers an improved quality of life and survival with acceptable morbidity and mortality rates.

REFERENCES

D'Amico G, Pagliaro L & Bosch J (1995) The treatment of portal hypertension: a meta-analytic review. *Hepatology* **22(1):** 332–354.

Bismuth H, Franco D & Hepp J (1974) Portal-systemic shunt in hepatic cirrhosis: Does the type of shunt decisively influence the clinical result? *Annals of Surgery* **179:** 209.

Caps MT, Helton WS & Johansen K (1996) Left-upper-quadrant devascularization for 'unshuntable' portal hypertension. *Archives of Surgery* **131:** 834.

Chandler JG (1993) The history of surgical treatment of portal hypertension. *Archives of Surgery* **128:** 925.

Child CG (1953) Eck's fistula. *Surgery, Gynecology and Obstetrics* **96:** 375.

Collins JC & Sarfeh IJ (1995) Surgical management of portal hypertension. *Western Journal of Medicine* **162:** 527.

Collins JC, Rypins EB & Sarfeh IJ (1994) Narrow-diameter portacaval shunts for management of variceal bleeding. *World Journal of Surgery* **18(2):** 211.

Conn HO, Lindenmuth WW, May CJ et al (1972) Prophylactic portacaval anastomosis. A tale of two studies. *Medicine* **51:** 27.

Crile G, Jr (1950) Transesophageal ligation of bleeding esophageal varices. *Archives of Surgery* **61:** 654–660.

Dagenais M, Langer B, Taylor BR et al (1994) Experience with radical esophagogastric devascularization procedures (Sugiura) for variceal bleeding outside Japan. *World Journal of Surgery* **18(2):** 222.

Donovan AJ & Covey PC (1978) Early history of portacaval shunt in humans. *Surgery, Gynecology and Obstetrics* **147:** 423.

Helton WS, Belshaw A, Althaus S et al (1993) Critical appraisal of the angiographic portacaval shunt (TIPS). *American Journal of Surgery* **165:** 566.

Henderson JM (1993) Portal hypertension and shunt surgery. *Advances in Surgery* **26:** 233.

Henderson JM (1994) The role of distal splenorenal shunt for long-term management of variceal bleeding. *World Journal of Surgery* **18:** 205.

Henderson JM, Warren WD, Millikan WJ et al (1989) Distal splenorenal shunt with splenopancreatic disconnection: A 4-year assessment. *Annals of Surgery* **210(3):** 332.

Hermann RE, Henderson JM, Vogt DP et al (1995) Fifty years of surgery for portal hypertension at the Cleveland Clinic Foundation. *Annals of Surgery* **221(5):** 459.

Holman E (1933) Implantation of the spleen in the abdominal wall for portal obstruction: A suggested operation for hepatic cirrhosis. *Western Journal of Surgery, Obstetrics and Gynecology* **41:** 255.

Iannitti DA & Henderson JM (1997) The role of surgery in the treatment of portal hypertension. *Clinical Liver Disease* **1:** 99–114.

Idezuki Y, Kokudo N, Sanjo K et al (1994) Sugiura procedure for management of variceal bleeding in Japan. *World Journal of Surgery* **18(2):** 216.

Inokuchi K (1968) A selective portacaval shunt. *Lancet* **ii:** 51.

Inokuchi K, and cooperative study group of portal hypertension in Japan (1990) Improved survival after prophylactic portal nondecompressive surgery for esophageal varices: a randomized controlled trial. *Hepatology* **12:** 1.

Iwatsuki S, Starzl TE, Todo S et al (1988) Liver transplantation in the treatment of bleeding esophageal varices. *Surgery* **104:** 697.

Jackson FC, Perrin EB, Smith AG et al (1968) A clinical investigation of the portacaval shunt. II. Survival analysis of the prophylactic operation. *American Journal of Surgery* **115:** 22.

Johansen K (1989) Partial portal decompression for variceal hemorrhage. *American Journal of Surgery* **157:** 479.

Johansen K & Helton WS (1992) Portal hypertension and bleeding esophageal varices. *Annals of Vascular Surgery* **6(6)**: 553.

Johnston GW & Rodgers HW (1973) A review of 15 years' experience in the use of sclerotherapy in the control of acute hemorrhage from oesophageal varices. *British Journal of Surgery* **60**: 797.

Knechtle SJ, Kalayoglu M, D'Alessandro AM et al (1994) Portal hypertension: surgical management in the 1990s. *Surgery* **116(4)**: 687.

LaBerge JM, Ring EJ, Gordon RL et al (1993) Creation of transjugular intrahepatic portosystemic shunt with wallstent endoprosthesis: results in 100 patients. *Radiology* **187**: 413.

Lebrec D (1994) Long-term management of variceal bleeding: the place of pharmacotherapy. *World Journal of Surgery* **18(2)**: 229.

Lebrec D, Wovel O, Corbic M et al (1980b) Propranolol: a medical treatment for portal hypertension. *Lancet* **ii**: 180.

Linton RR, Ellis DS & Geary JE (1961) Critical comparative analysis of early and late results of splenorenal and direct portacaval shunts performed in 169 patients with portal cirrhosis. *Annals of Surgery* **154**: 446.

Madden JL, Lore JM, Gerald FP et al (1954) The pathogenesis of ascites and a consideration of its treatment. *Surgery, Gynecology and Obstetrics* **99**: 585.

Maffei-Faccioli A, Gerunda G, Neri D et al (1990) Selective variceal decompression and its role relative to other therapies. *American Journal of Surgery* **211**: 178.

Mercado MA, Morales-Linares JC, Granados-Garcia J et al (1996) Distal splenorenal shunt versus 10 mm low-diameter mesocaval shunt for variceal hemorrhage. *American Journal of Surgery* **171**: 591.

Morillas RM, Planas R, Cabre E et al (1994) Propranolol plus isosorbide-5-mononitrate for portal hypertension in cirrhosis: long-term hemodynamic and renal effects. *Hepatology* **20(6)**: 1502.

Myberg JA (1990) Selective shunts: the Johannesburg experience. *American Journal of Surgery* **160**: 67.

North Italian Endoscopic Club for the Study and Treatment of Esophageal Varices (NIEC) (1988) Prediction of the first variceal hemorrhage in patients with cirrhosis of the liver and esophageal varices. *New England Journal of Medicine* **319**: 983.

Orloff MJ, Duguay LA & Kosta LD (1977) Criteria for selection of patients for emergency portacaval shunts. *American Journal of Surgery* **134**: 146.

Orloff MJ, Orloff MS, Orloff SL et al (1995) Three decades of experience with emergency portacaval shunt for acutely bleeding esophageal varices in 400 unselected patients with cirrhosis of the liver. *Journal of the American College of Surgeons* **180(3)**: 257.

Orozco H, Mercado HA, Takahashu T et al (1990) Role of the distal splenorenal shunt in management of variceal bleeding in Latin America. *American Journal of Surgery* **160**: 86.

Orozco H, Mercado MA, Takahashi T et al (1992) Elective treatment of bleeding varices with the Sugiura operation over 10 years. *American Journal of Surgery* **163**: 585.

Orozco H, Mercado MA, Takahashi T et al (1993) Selective splenocaval shunt for bleeding portal hypertension: fifteen-year evaluation period. *Surgery* **113(3)**: 260.

Pagliaro L, Burroughs AK, Sorensen T et al (1989) Therapeutic controversies and randomized controlled trials (RCTs): prevention of bleeding and re-bleeding in cirrhosis. *Gastroenterology International* **2**: 71.

Potts JR, Henderson JM, Millikan WJ et al (1984) Emergency distal splenorenal shunts for variceal hemorrhage refractory to nonoperative control. *American Journal of Surgery* **148**: 813.

Reichen J (1990) Liver function and pharmacological considerations in pathogenesis and treatment of portal hypertension. *Hepatology* **11(6)**: 1066.

Resnick RH, Chalmers TC, Ishihara AM et al (1969) A controlled trial of the prophylactic portacaval shunt. A final report. *Annals of Internal Medicine* **70**: 675.

Rikkers LF & Jin G (1994) Surgical management of acute variceal hemorrhage. *World Journal of Surgery* **18(2)**: 193.

Ringe B, Lang H, Tusch G et al (1994) Role of liver transplantation in management of esophageal variceal hemorrhage. *World Journal of Surgery* **18(2)**: 233.

Roberts LR & Kamath PS (1996) Pathophysiology and treatment of variceal hemorrhage. *Mayo Clinical Proceedings* **71**: 973.

Rosemurgy AS, Goode SE & Camps M (1996a) The effect of small-diameter H-graft portacaval shunts on portal blood flow. *American Journal of Surgery* **171**: 154.

Rosemurgy AS, Goode SE & Zwiebel BR (1996b) A prospective trial of transjugular intrahepatic por-tasystemic stent shunts versus small-diameter prosthetic H-graft portacaval shunts in the treatment of bleeding varices. *Annals of Surgery* **224:** 378.

Rossle M, Haag K, Ochs A et al (1994) The transjugular intrahepatic portosystemic stent shunt procedure for variceal bleeding. *New England Journal of Medicine* **330:** 165.

Sarfeh IJ & Rypins EB (1986) Partial versus total portacaval H-graft diameters. *Annals of Surgery* **204:** 356.

Sarfeh IJ, Rypins EB & Mason GR (1986) A systematic appraisal of portacaval H-Graft diameters: clinical and hemodynamic perspectives. *Annals of Surgery* **204:** 356.

Spina GP, Henderson JM, Rikkers LF et al (1992a) Distal splenorenal shunt for long term management of variceal bleeding. *Journal of Hepatology* **16:** 338.

Spina GP, Henderson JM, Rikkers LF et al (1992b) Distal spleno-renal shunt versus endoscopic sclerotherapy in the prevention of variceal bleeding: a meta-analysis of four randomized clinical trials. *Journal of Hepatology* **16:** 338.

Starzl TE, Demetris AJ & Van Thiel DH (1989) Medical progress: liver transplantation. *New England Journal of Medicine* **321:** 1014–1022.

Steigmann G, Goff J, Michaletz-Grody P et al (1992) Endoscopic sclerotherapy as compared with endoscopic ligation for bleeding esophageal varices. *New England Journal of Medicine* **326:** 1527.

Stipa S, Balducci G, Ziparo V et al (1994) Total shunting and elective management of variceal bleeding. *World Journal of Surgery* **18(2):** 200.

Sugiura M & Futagawa S (1973) A new technique for treating esophageal varices. *Journal of Thoracic and Cardiovascular Surgery* **66:** 677.

Terblanche J, Steigmann GV, Krige JE et al (1994) Long-term management of variceal bleeding: the place of varix injection and ligation. *World Journal of Surgery* **18(2):** 185.

Vorobioff J, Picabea E, Gamen M et al (1994) Propranolol compared with propranolol plus isosorbide dinitrate in portal-hypertensive patients: long-term hemodynamic and renal effects. *Hepatology* **20(6):** 1502.

Warren WD, Zeppa R & Foman JS (1967) Selective transplenic decompression of gastroesophageal varices by distal splenorenal shunt. *Annals of Surgery* **166:** 437.

Warren WD, Millikan WJ, Henderson JM et al (1986) Splenopancreatic disconnection: improved selectivity of distal splenorenal shunt. *Annals of Surgery* **204:** 346.

Whipple AO (1945) The problem of portal hypertension in relation to the hepatosplenopathies. *Annals of Surgery* **122:** 449.

White S (1906) Discussion of surgical treatment of ascites secondary to vascular cirrhosis of the liver. *British Medical Journal* **2:** 1287.

Yammamoto S, Hidemura R, Sanada M et al (1976) The late results of terminal esophago-proximal gastrectomy (TEPG) with extensive devascularization and splenectomy for bleeding esphageal varices in cirrhosis. *Surgery* **80:** 106.

10

Ascites and renal functional abnormalities in cirrhosis. Pathogenesis and treatment

PERE GINÈS* MD

Faculty Member
Liver Unit, Hospital Clínic i Provincial, Villarroel 170, 08036 Barcelona, Spain

GLÒRIA FERNÁNDEZ-ESPARRACH MD

Research Fellow
Liver Unit, Hospital Clínic i Provincial, Villarroel 170, 08036 Barcelona, Spain

VICENTE ARROYO MD

Professor of Medicine
University of Barcelona School of Medicine, Liver Unit, Hospital Clínic i Provincial, Villarroel 170, 08036 Barcelona, Spain

In the past few years, there have been important advances in the field of pathogenesis and management of ascites and hepatorenal syndrome in cirrhosis. A new pathogenic theory of ascites and renal dysfunction in cirrhosis has been presented and previously ill-defined conditions, such as refractory ascites and hepatorenal syndrome, have been defined precisely. The link between the diseased liver and the disturbances in renal function and vasoactive systems is not completely known, but a large body of evidence indicates that it consists of a circulatory dysfunction that affects mainly the arterial circulation and is characterized by an inability to maintain an effective arterial blood volume within normal limits. The research on the mechanisms of this circulatory dysfunction will give valuable information in the design of more pathophysiologically oriented therapeutic approaches to the management of ascites.

Key words: cirrhosis; ascites; oedema; hepatorenal syndrome.

Patients with cirrhosis often accumulate large amounts of fluid in the peritoneal and/or pleural cavities and interstitial tissue as a consequence of an abnormal regulation of extracellular fluid volume (Arroyo et al, 1991; Ginès P et al, 1996). This is associated with alterations in renal function,

* Address for correspondence.
Funding support: Portions of the work reviewed in this article were supported by grants from the Comisión Interministerial de Ciencia y Tecnología (CICYT SAF 96/0131), Dirección General de Investigación Científica y Técnica (DGICYT PB 93/1018) and Fondo de Investigaciones Sanitarias (FIS 96/1723), Spain.

Baillière's Clinical Gastroenterology—
Vol. 11, No. 2, June 1997
ISBN 0–7020–2339–6
0950–3528/97/020365 + 21 $12.00/00

365

mainly sodium retention, and, less commonly, water retention and vaso-constriction of the renal circulation. The current chapter reviews the patho-genesis and treatment of ascites and renal functional abnormalities in cirrhosis.

FACTORS INVOLVED IN THE FORMATION OF ASCITES

The formation of ascites in cirrhosis is the final consequence of a combi-nation of abnormalities in renal function, overactivity of vasoconstrictor and anti-natriuretic systems, which are responsible for fluid retention, and alterations in portal and splanchnic circulation, and which facilitate the accumulation of retained fluid in the peritoneal cavity.

Functional renal abnormalities

The main pathogenic factor of ascites and oedema formation in cirrhosis is sodium retention. The retention of sodium causes expansion of the extra-cellular fluid volume and results eventually in ascites and/or oedema formation. Sodium retention in cirrhosis is mainly because of an increased reabsorption of sodium in the renal tubules. A number of extrarenal and intrarenal factors are involved in the increased sodium reabsorption, the most important being hyperaldosteronism and enhanced renal sympathetic nerve activity. A detailed review of the mechanisms involved in sodium retention in cirrhosis may be found elsewhere (Arroyo et al, 1991; Epstein, 1996a; Ginès P et al, 1996). The intensity of sodium retention in patients with ascites is not uniform. In some patients sodium retention is moderate and patients are still able to eliminate significant amounts of the ingested sodium in the urine, whereas in other patients sodium retention is severe and urine sodium is negligible.

An impairment in the renal capacity to excrete water occurs frequently in cirrhotic patients with ascites and usually follows sodium retention in the natural course of the disease (Papper and Saxon, 1959; Shear et al, 1965a; Vaamonde, 1996). The clinical consequences of this abnormality are an increased total body water and, in severe cases, dilutional hyponatraemia. The prevalence of spontaneous hyponatraemia (serum sodium < 130 mEq/l) in hospitalized cirrhotic patients with ascites is approximately 30% (Arroyo et al, 1976). The pathogenesis of water retention in cirrhosis is complex and involves several factors, including a reduced delivery of filtrate to the ascending limb of the loop of Henle and the diluting segment of the nephron, reduced renal synthesis of prostaglandins and increased secretion of antidiuretic hormone. Several lines of evidence indicate that the latter is the most important factor in the pathogenesis of water retention in cirrhosis (Arroyo et al, 1994a; Ginès et al, 1994; Vaamonde, 1996). In some patients, water retention is mild and can only be detected by measuring water excretion after a water load. These patients are usually able to eliminate water normally and maintain a normal serum sodium concentration as long as their intake of fluids is kept within normal limits, but hyponatraemia may occur when water intake is increased. In other patients, the severity of the disorder is such that they retain most of water taken in the diet, causing hyponatraemia and hypo-osmolality. Therefore, hyponatraemia in cirrhotic patients with ascites is almost always dilutional in origin as it occurs in the setting of an increased total body water.

A vasoconstriction of the renal circulation is also a common finding in patients with cirrhosis and ascites (Arroyo et al, 1991, Ginès P et al, 1996). This vasoconstriction is more intense in the renal cortex and may result in a reduction of renal blood flow and glomerular filtration rate (GFR). Because renal vasoconstriction in cirrhosis occurs in the absence of morphological changes in the kidney, it is currently believed that alterations in vasoactive factors acting on the renal circulation play a crucial role in the pathogenesis of this disorder. The status of the renal circulation is very variable among patients with ascites, ranging from normal or only slightly reduced renal perfusion to marked renal hypoperfusion with severe reductions in renal blood flow and GFR. This latter condition is known as hepatorenal syndrome (HRS) (see below) (Bataller et al, 1997). In clinical practice the existence of renal vasoconstriction is usually assessed by measuring markers of GFR, such as serum creatinine or creatinine clearance. However, recent studies have demonstrated that the measurement of resistive index of the arcuate arteries by duplex Doppler ultrasonography, an index of intrarenal vascular resistance, is more sensitive than conventional markers of GFR in the detection of renal vasoconstriction in cirrhosis (Platt et al, 1992; Maroto et al, 1994).

Overactivity of vasoconstrictor systems

Extrarenal systems

Several neurohumoral systems with vasoactive properties and marked effects on renal function have been implicated as potential mediators of renal dysfunction in cirrhosis.

The activity of the two major vasoconstrictor and anti-natriuretic systems, the renin–angiotensin–aldosterone system and the sympathetic nervous system, is increased in a large proportion of cirrhotic patients with ascites (Arroyo et al, 1991). A large body of evidence indicates that the activation of these systems plays a major role in the increased tubular reabsorption of sodium in cirrhosis (Bernardi et al, 1990; Henriksen et al, 1990; Epstein, 1996b). However, other anti-natriuretic mechanisms may be also involved because some cirrhotic patients with ascites develop sodium retention in the setting of a normal activity of these anti-natriuretic systems (Wilkinson et al, 1979; Saló et al, 1995a). The activation of the renin–angiotensin–aldosterone system and the sympathetic nervous system is particularly noteworthy in patients with HRS, supporting a role for these systems in the vasoconstriction of the renal circulation (Arroyo et al, 1990). Another important vasoconstrictor factor that is frequently activated in cirrhosis with ascites is antidiuretic hormone (Arroyo et al, 1994a). The pharmacological interruption or blockade of these three major vasoconstrictor systems in human and/or experimental cirrhosis results in marked arterial hypotension, which suggests that these systems are activated as a homeostatic response to maintain arterial pressure (Schroeder et al, 1976; Arroyo et al, 1981; Pariente et al; 1985; Clària et al, 1991).

The circulating levels of endothelin, an endothelial-derived peptide with marked vasoconstrictor activity, are also increased in cirrhosis (Asbert et al, 1993; Moller et al, 1993). These increased levels are probably because of an enhanced release of endothelin from the hepatic and/or splanchnic circulation (Leivas et al, 1995; Moller et al, 1995). Several studies have demonstrated that hepatic stellate cells, which are strategically located in the space of Disse surrounding the sinusoids, produce endothelin, which may act as an autocrine factor contributing to the increased intrahepatic vascular resistance characteristic of cirrhosis (Housset et al, 1993; Pinzani et al, 1996; Rockey and Weisiger, 1996). It has been suggested that endothelin synthesis is also increased within the kidney and contributes to renal vasocontriction in patients with HRS (Moore et al, 1992). However, this assumption has not been proved definitely.

Though it may look paradoxical in a clinical condition characterized by marked sodium retention, the plasma concentration of major natriuretic hormones, namely atrial natriuretic peptide and brain natriuretic peptide, is markedly increased in cirrhosis with ascites (Ginès et al, 1988a; La Villa et al, 1992; Warner et al, 1993). The acute administration of HS-142-1, a selective antagonist of natriuretic peptide A and B receptors, to rats with cirrhosis and ascites causes renal vasoconstriction and a marked increase in plasma renin activity and plasma aldosterone concentration (Angeli et al, 1994), which supports the role of natriuretic peptides in maintaining renal perfusion and limiting the activation of the renin–angiotensin–aldosterone system in cirrhosis. By contrast, antagonism of natriuretic peptide action has no effect on arterial pressure, cardiac index or systemic vascular resistance, which argues against a role of natriuretic peptides as mediators of arterial vasodilation in cirrhosis.

Intrarenal factors

Besides extrarenal systems, there are a number of intrarenal factors with effects on the tubular transport of sodium and water and/or vasoactive properties that may be involved in functional renal abnormalities of cirrhosis (González-Campoy and Knox, 1992).

Arachidonic acid metabolites (prostaglandins and leukotrienes) are the intrarenal systems most extensively studied in cirrhosis. The renal prostaglandins (PGs) probably play little or no role in the regulation of renal function under physiological conditions, but have a protective effect on renal circulation and sodium and water transport in conditions characterized by an activation of the renin–angiotensin system, sympathetic nervous system and/or antidiuretic hormone. Cirrhotic patients with ascites without renal failure show increased renal production of vasodilator PGs, especially PGE_2 and PGI_2, as estimated by their urinary excretion, compared with healthy subjects or patients without ascites (Laffi et al, 1996). This increased production contributes to the maintenance of renal haemo-dynamics because PGs synthesis inhibition by non-steroidal anti-inflammatory drugs causes profound renal hypoperfusion, particularly in patients with marked overactivity of vasoconstrictor systems (Boyer et al, 1979; Arroyo et al, 1983; Quintero et al, 1986). By contrast, cirrhotic patients with ascites with HRS have a renal production of PGs below normal levels (Arroyo et al, 1990; Ginès P et al, 1996; Laffi et al, 1996). It has been suggested that renal circulation in cirrhosis with ascites depends on an adequate balance between vasoconstrictor systems and intrarenal production of PGs. An imbalance between these vasoconstrictor systems and PGs could result in unrelenting renal vasoconstriction. Eicosanoids with vasoconstrictor effects may also participate in the reduced renal perfusion in cirrhosis. Two studies have reported an increased renal production of cysteinyl leukotrienes, especially leukotriene E4, in cirrhotic patients with HRS (Huber et al, 1989; Moore et al, 1990).

Nitric oxide (NO), locally synthesized in different structures within the kidney, also participates in the regulation of renal function (Raij, 1993). Under normal circumstances, NO plays a role in the regulation of glomerular microcirculation by modulating arteriolar tone and mesangial cells contractility. Moreover, NO facilitates natriuresis in response to changes in renal perfusion pressure, and regulates renin release. There is still very limited information, derived only from studies in experimental animals, on the role of NO in the regulation of renal function in cirrhosis. Kidneys from cirrhotic rats show enhanced endothelium-dependent vasodilator response as compared with control animals, which suggests that in cirrhosis there is an increased renal production of NO (García-Estañ et al, 1994). The inhibition of NO synthesis in rats with cirrhosis and ascites does not result in renal vasoconstriction but induces a marked rise in urinary prostaglandin excretion (Clària et al, 1992). However, the simul-taneous inhibition of NO and PGs synthesis results in a marked renal vaso-constriction suggesting that NO interacts with PGs to maintain renal haemodynamics in cirrhosis (Ros et al, 1995a).

Other local vasoactive factors that may be involved in renal functional abnormalities in cirrhosis are the intrarenal kallikrein–kinin and renin–angiotensin systems and adenosine (Bataller et al, 1997).

Alterations in splanchnic and systemic haemodynamics

The existence of cirrhosis causes marked structural abnormalities in the liver, which result in a severe disturbance of the hepatic and splanchnic circulation. The deposition of fibrous tissue and the formation of nodules alter the normal vascular architecture, and result in increased resistance to portal flow. The increased intrahepatic vascular resistance causes marked effects not only in the portal venous system but also in arterial side of the splanchnic circulation (Benoit and Granger, 1986; Bosch et al, 1992). In the venous side, the main changes consist of the development of portal hyper-tension and formation/opening of portocollateral veins with shunting of blood from portal to systemic circulation. In the arterial side, there is marked arterial vasodilation, which increases portal venous inflow and contributes to the increased pressure in the portal venous system. All these changes in the splanchnic microcirculation predispose to ascites formation by increasing the filtration of fluid (Benoit and Granger, 1988; Korthuis et al, 1988).

Besides these changes in splanchnic haemodynamics, in human cirrhosis with ascites there is a hyperdynamic circulation, which consists of reduced systemic vascular resistance and arterial pressure, increased cardiac index, activation of vasoconstrictor and anti-natriuretic systems (renin–angiotensin and sympathetic nervous systems and antidiuretic hormone) and increased plasma volume. However, the increased plasma volume is distributed abnormally with a reduced central and arterial blood volume and an increased non-central blood volume (Henriksen and Moller, 1996). The hyperdynamic circulation starts before the formation of ascites and is more marked as the disease progresses (Arroyo et al, 1991; Groszmann, 1994) The main vascular territory responsible for the reduced vascular resistance in cirrhosis is the splanchnic circulation. Several humoral vasodilator factors, the concentration of which is increased in cirrhosis with ascites, including NO, glucagon, eicosanoids, adenosine, bile salts, platelet activating factor, substance P and calcitonin gene-related peptide, have been proposed as mediators of the hyperdynamic circulation (Groszmann, 1994; Ginès P et al, 1996). Several lines of evidence obtained over the last few years suggest that NO is a major contributor to the hyperdynamic circulation in cirrhosis (Clària et al, 1992; Sieber and Groszmann, 1992; Castro et al, 1993; Guarner et al, 1993; Clària et al, 1994; Albillos et al, 1995; Campillo et al, 1995, Laffi et al, 1995; Matsumoto et al, 1995; Niederberger et al, 1995a,b; Ros et al, 1995b; Sogni et al, 1995; Weigert et al, 1995; Martin et al, 1996; Mathie et al, 1996; Morales et al, 1996; Battista et al, 1997) (Table 1).

Table 1. Evidence for an increased synthesis of nitric oxide (NO) in cirrhosis.

1. Restoration of the impaired pressor response to vasoconstrictors either in experimental cirrhosis (isolated aortic rings and splanchnic vascular preparations) or human cirrhosis by NO synthesis inhibition.
2. Enhanced vasodilator response to endothelium-dependent vasodilators in experimental and human cirrhosis.
3. Normalization of arterial vasodilation and hyperdynamic circulation by chronic NO synthesis inhibition in rats with cirrhosis and ascites.
4. Increased NO synthase activity and expression in vascular tissue from rats with cirrhosis.
5. Increased plasma levels of NO and NO metabolites (nitrites and nitrates) in cirrhotic patients.
6. Increased concentration of NO in the exhaled air of cirrhotic patients.
7. Increased NO synthase activity in polymorphonuclear cells and monocytes from cirrhotic patients with ascites.

Theories of ascites formation

Two different mechanisms have been proposed to account for sodium and water retention and ascites and oedema formation in cirrhosis. The first mechanism suggests that there is a primary renal defect in sodium excretion that results in hypervolaemia. The reduction in systemic vascular resistance and increase in cardiac output would be adaptive responses of the systemic circulation to the increased fluid retention (Lieberman et al, 1970). When the retained fluid can no longer be maintained within the intravascular compartment, there is increased filtration of fluid to the interstitial space with ascites and oedema formation (overflow theory). The second mechanism proposes that sodium retention is not a primary event but rather the homeostatic response of the kidney to an underfilling of the arterial circulation secondary to arterial vasodilation (arterial vasodilation theory) (Schrier et al, 1988, 1994). The underfilling of the arterial circulation causes a reduction in effective arterial blood volume (the volume sensed by arterial and cardiopulmonary receptors) with a subsequent increase in vasoconstrictor and anti-natriuretic factors to compensate for the relative arterial underfilling. The retained fluid, however, cannot fill adequately the intravascular compartment and suppress the sodium-retaining signals, because fluid is continuously leaking in the peritoneal cavity, thus creating a vicious cycle (Figure 1). Most of the currently available data in human and experimental cirrhosis support this latter mechanism of formation of ascites (Schrier et al, 1988; Arroyo et al, 1991; Schrier et al, 1994; Ginès P et al, 1996).

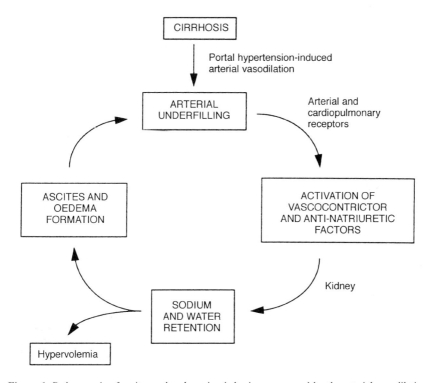

Figure 1. Pathogenesis of ascites and oedema in cirrhosis as proposed by the arterial vasodilation theory.

MANAGEMENT OF PATIENTS WITH ASCITES

The main clinical symptom of patients with ascites and oedema is discomfort because of abdominal and leg swelling. In some cases the accumulation of fluid is so important that respiratory function and physical activity may be impaired. Therefore, the objective of the treatment of ascites and oedema in cirrhosis is to reduce the patient's discomfort. In addition, the decrease in the amount of fluid in the peritoneal cavity reduces the risk of complications related to abdominal hernias, such as incarceration or rupture. Therapeutic measures should be oriented to reduce the amount of ascites and oedema and prevent their reaccumulation after therapy.

Treatment of ascites

Sodium restriction

The first step in the management of cirrhotic patients with ascites is sodium restriction, as the amount of fluid retained in the body depends on the balance between sodium ingested in the diet and sodium excreted in the urine. If the sodium excreted is lower than that ingested, patients accumulate ascites and/or oedema. Conversely, if sodium excretion is greater than intake, ascites and/or oedema decrease. The reduction of sodium content in the diet to 40–60 mEq/day (1 to 1.5 g of salt), without any other therapeutic intervention, causes a negative sodium balance and loss of ascites and oedema in patients with mild sodium retention (about 10% of patients with ascites). In patients with moderate or marked sodium retention, such sodium restriction is not sufficient by itself to achieve a negative sodium balance, but it may slow the accumulation of fluid. These patients would theoretically require a more severe restriction of sodium (less than 20 mEq/day). However, such intense sodium restriction is difficult to accomplish and may impair nutritional status.

Diuretic therapy

The pharmacological treatment of ascites has been based for many years in the administration of diuretics, drugs that increase urinary sodium excretion by reducing the tubular reabsorption of sodium. However, the reintroduction of therapeutic paracentesis has modified markedly the treatment of ascites in cirrhosis. Current indications for use of diuretics in cirrhotic patients include: (i) treatment of patients who are not eligible for paracentesis because of low ascites volume; (ii) prevention of ascites reaccumulation after paracentesis; (iii) treatment of patients with oedema without ascites; and (iv) prevention of fluid accumulation in patients who show a positive response to low-sodium diet alone but do not tolerate a prolonged sodium restriction. No major advances in the field of diuretic agents have been made in recent years. Diuretic therapy in cirrhosis is based on the administration of spironolactone (50–400 mg/day), a drug that competes with aldosterone for the binding to the mineralocorticoid receptor in the collecting tubular epithelial cells, alone or in combination with loop diuretics, especially furosemide (20–160 mg/day) or torasemide (10–40 mg/day), that act by inhibiting the Na^+-K^+-$2Cl^-$ co-transporter in the loop of Henle (Ginès et al, 1992). The response to diuretic therapy in cirrhotic patients should be evaluated by measuring body weight, urine volume and sodium excretion regularly. An inadequate sodium restriction is a common cause of failure to diuretic therapy. This situation should be suspected in patients in whom body weight and ascites do not decrease despite high urine volume and increased sodium excretion. Approximately 10 to 20% of patients with ascites either do not respond to diuretic therapy or develop diuretic-induced complications that prevent the use of high doses of these drugs. This condition is known as refractory ascites and should prompt the use of other therapeutic methods. The definition and diagnostic criteria of refractory ascites have been reviewed recently and are shown in Table 2 (Arroyo et al, 1996a). Common complications of diuretic therapy in patients with cirrhosis include electrolyte disturbances (hyponatraemia and hypo/hyperkalaemia), hepatic encephalopathy, renal impairment, gyneco-mastia and muscle cramps (Ginès et al, 1992). The impairment of renal failure during diuretic therapy is because of volume depletion, it occurs in patients with positive response to diuretics and is usually rapidly reversible after discontinuation of therapy (Forns et al, 1994).

Table 2. Definition and diagnostic criteria of refractory ascites as proposed by the International Ascites Club.

Definitions

Refractory ascites. Ascites that cannot be mobilized or the early recurrence of which (i.e. after therapeutic paracentesis) cannot be satisfactorily prevented by medical therapy. The term 'refractory ascites' includes two different subtypes: 'diuretic-resistant ascites' and 'diuretic-intractable ascites'.

Diuretic-resistant ascites. Ascites that cannot be mobilized or the early recurrence of which cannot be prevented because of a lack of response to sodium restriction (50 mEq/day sodium diet) and diuretic treatment (mean loss of weight less than 200 g/day during the last 4 days of intensive diuretic therapy—spironolactone 400 mg/day and furosemide 160 mg/day, and urinary sodium excretion of less than 50 mEq/day).

Diuretic-intractable ascites. Ascites that cannot be mobilized or the early recurrence of which cannot be prevented because of the development of diuretic-induced complications* that preclude the use of an effective diuretic dosage.

* Diuretic-induced complications: diuretic-induced hepatic encephalopathy: development of hepatic encephalopathy in the absence of other precipitating factors. Diuretic-induced renal failure: increase in serum creatinine by greater than 100% to a value above 2 mg/dl in patients with ascites respond-ing to diuretic treatment. Diuretic-induced hyponatraemia: decrease in serum sodium concentration by greater than 10 mEq/litre to a level lower than 125 mEq/litre. Diuretic-induced hypo- or hyper-kalaemia: decrease of serum potassium concentration to less than 3 mEq/litre or increase to more than 6 mEq/litre despite appropriate measures to normalize potassium levels.

Paracentesis

In the last 10 years, therapeutic paracentesis has progressively replaced diuretics as the treatment of choice in the management of large ascites in patients with cirrhosis (Arroyo et al, 1994b). This change in treatment strategy is based on the results of several randomized studies comparing paracentesis (either total removal of all ascitic fluid in a single tap or repeated taps of 4–6 litres/day) associated with plasma volume expansion and diuretics in cirrhotic patients with large ascites (Quintero et al, 1985; Ginès et al, 1987; Salerno et al, 1987; Hagège et al, 1992). The results of these studies indicate that paracentesis is more rapid and effective and is associated with a lower number of complications than conventional diuretic therapy. Because paracentesis does not modify the pre-existing renal functional abnormalities of cirrhosis, patients should be given diuretics after paracentesis to avoid reformation of ascites (Fernández-Esparrach et al, 1997).

The effects of paracentesis on systemic haemodynamics have been delineated in several recent studies. Immediately after paracentesis there are haemodynamic changes consistent with an improvement of effective blood volume, with a rise in cardiac output, deactivation of vasoconstrictor and anti-natriuretic systems (renin–angiotensin–aldosterone system and sympathetic nervous system) and an increase in the plasma concentration of atrial natriuretic peptide. However, this early phase is rapidly followed by opposite circulatory changes consistent with a decrease in effective blood volume with a reduction in cardiac output, activation of anti-natriuretic systems and reduced plasma atrial natriuretic peptide levels (Simon et al, 1987; Ginès et al, 1988b; Panos et al, 1990, Pozzi et al, 1994; Luca et al, 1995). A recent study has shown that these haemodynamic changes are not reversible and have a negative impact on the evolution of the disease, because patients who develop post-paracentesis circulatory dysfunction require higher doses of diuretics to prevent ascites formation, have a greater risk of ascites reaccumulation and, most importantly, a shorter survival than patients who do not develop this abnormality (Ginès A et al, 1996) (Table 3 and Figure 2). At present, the only effective method to prevent this complication is the administration of plasma expanders. Albumin is more effective than dextran-70 and hemaccel. In patients treated with albumin the risk of post-paracentesis circulatory dysfunction is low and independent of the volume of ascites removed. By contrast, in patients treated with non-albumin plasma expanders the risk of post-paracentesis circulatory dysfunction is higher than in those treated with albumin and increases with the volume of ascitic fluid removed. The patho-

Table 3. Characteristics of post-paracentesis circulatory dysfunction.

1. Occurs in up to 80% of cirrhotic patients with ascites treated by large-volume paracentesis without plasma volume expansion.
2. Is characterized by marked activation of vasoconstrictor and anti-natriuretic systems (renin–angiotensin and sympathetic nervous systems) and reduction in atrial natriuretic peptide levels.
3. Appears 1 to 6 days following paracentesis and is not spontaneously reversible.
4. Clinically silent. Only 20% of patients develop renal impairment and/or hyponatraemia.
5. Is associated with a greater risk of ascites reaccumulation and shorter survival.
6. Albumin (8 g/litre of ascites removed) is the most effective method in the prevention of this complication. Dextran-70 or hemaccel are less effective.

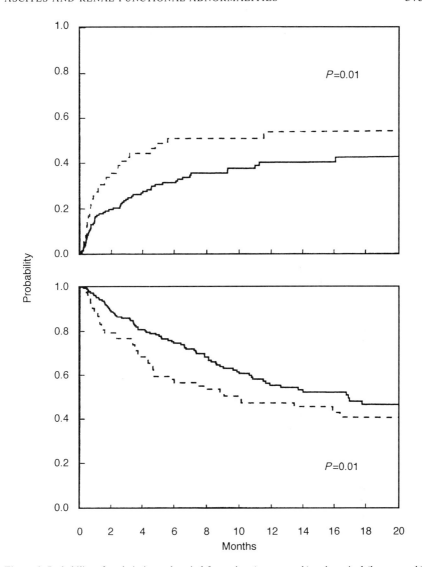

Figure 2. Probability of readmission to hospital for ascites (upper graph) and survival (lower graph) in cirrhotic patients with ascites who did (dotted line) and did not develop (continuous line) post-paracentesis circulatory dysfunction. Reproduced with permission from Ginès A et al, 1996.

genesis of post-paracentesis circulatory dysfunction is not completely understood, but it is not because of a paracentesis-induced hypovolaema, as plasma volume does not decrease in patients developing this complication (Saló et al, 1995b). More probably, this abnormality is because of an arterial vasodilatation that would cause a further impairment in the circulatory function of cirrhotic patients (Vila et al, 1995).

Other therapeutic methods

Peritoneovenous shunting was used frequently in the past in the treatment of ascites in cirrhosis, especially in patients with refractory ascites. However, its use has declined markedly because of the side effects (shunt occlusion, vena cava thrombosis, peritoneal fibrosis) and the introduction of alternative therapies such as paracentesis (Ginès et al, 1991; Arroyo et al, 1992).

A number of studies have been published recently on the use of transjugular intrahepatic portosystemic shunts (TIPS) in patients with refractory ascites (Ochs et al, 1995; Quiroga et al, 1995; Somberg et al, 1995, 1996). As with surgical portasystemic shunts, the reduction in portal pressure obtained with TIPS is associated with favourable effects on renal function (Table 4). The main advantage of TIPS over surgical shunts is the reduction of the operative mortality and the main disadvantage the frequent obstruction of the prosthesis, which results in increased portal pressure and reaccumulation of ascites. Potential problems of TIPS are the development of hepatic encephalopathy and impairment in liver function because of the shunting of blood from the liver to the systemic circulation. A recent comparative study in a small series of patients with refractory ascites showed an increased mortality in patients treated with TIPS, especially in those patients with poor liver function, compared with patients treated with paracentesis plus albumin (Lebrec et al, 1996). Larger controlled studies are required to define whether TIPS has a role in the management of cirrhotic patients with refractory ascites (Arroyo and Ginès, 1996).

Table 4. Pros and cons of transjugular portosystemic shunt in the management of cirrhotic patients with refractory ascites.

Pros
1. Improves sodium excretion and glomerular filtration rate.
2. Reduces the activity of the renin–angiotensin–aldosterone system.
3. Reduces ascites volume and diuretic requirements.

Cons
1. High incidence of obstruction.
2. May precipitate hepatic encephalopathy.
3. Impairs liver function?

Liver transplantation has become a standard therapy for patients with advanced cirrhosis as the 5-year survival rate for adult cirrhotic patients submitted to liver transplantation is greater than 70%. Earlier recommendations suggested that the main indications for liver transplantation in patients with ascites were refractory ascites, recovery from spontaneous bacterial peritonitis and HRS. However, with these guidelines a significant proportion of patients do not reach the transplantation because of the short survival expectancy associated with these conditions. A number of predictive factors of survival have been described in patients with cirrhosis and ascites, which may help in the identification of candidates for liver transplantation (Llach et al, 1988; Ginès et al, 1997). The most valuable factors associated with a poor prognosis in these patients are related to abnormalities in renal function and systemic haemodynamics and include an impaired ability to excrete a water load, dilutional hyponatraemia, arterial hypotension, reduced GFR, marked sodium retention, and increased plasma renin activity and norepinephrine concentration. Of interest, in patients with ascites these parameters are better predictors of prognosis than liver function tests.

Treatment of dilutional hyponatraemia

At present, no pharmacological therapy exists for dilutional hyponatraemia and the only therapeutic measure that improves or stops the progressive decrease in serum sodium concentration is water restriction. The administration of hypertonic saline solutions is not recommended because it invariably leads to further expansion of extracellular fluid volume and accumulation of ascites and oedema. Recently, two types of drugs have been developed that selectively increase water excretion: antagonists of the V2 receptor of antidiuretic hormone and selective kappa opioid agonists (Ginès and Jiménez, 1996). The former group of drugs antagonize selectively the water-retaining effect of antidiuretic hormone in the cortical collecting duct whereas the latter inhibit antidiuretic hormone release from the neurohypophysis and have also a direct tubular effect. Both groups of drugs induce a dose-dependent increase in urine flow and free water excretion in normal animals as well as in healthy subjects. These renal effects are different from those of classical diuretic agents because the increase in urine volume is associated with only mild or no increase in sodium excretion. Two recent investigations using single doses of non-peptide V2 receptor antagonists or the selective κ-opioid agonist niravoline showed that both agents selectively increase water excretion in rats with cirrhosis ascites and water retention (Tsuboi et al, 1994; Bosch-Marcé et al, 1995). Preliminary studies in cirrhotic patients with ascites have also shown that both drugs selectively increased water excretion (Gadano et al, 1996; Inoue et al, 1996). Therefore, these compounds offer a novel therapeutic approach for the treatment of water retention and dilutional hyponatraemia in cirrhotic patients with ascites.

HEPATORENAL SYNDROME

Hepatorenal syndrome (HRS) is a common and serious complication of cirrhosis characterized by impaired renal function and marked disturbances in the arterial circulation and activity of vasoactive systems. In the renal circulation there is a marked increase in vascular resistance, while total systemic vascular resistance is reduced. This reduction in systemic vascular resistance is mainly because of a vasodilation of the splanchnic circulation, as non-splanchnic vascular beds are vasoconstricted.

Pathogenesis

The pathophysiological hallmark of HRS is a vasoconstriction of the renal circulation (Epstein et al, 1970). The kidneys are structurally intact. The mechanism of this vasoconstriction is not completely known and probably involves both increased vasoconstrictor and reduced vasodilator factors acting on the renal circulation. The most accepted theory on the pathogenesis of HRS (arterial vasodilation theory) proposes the renal hypoperfusion represents the extreme manifestation of the underfilling of the arterial circulation present in cirrhotic patients (Schrier et al, 1988) (Figure 3). This arterial underfilling would result in a progressive baroreceptor-mediated activation of vasoconstrictor systems (i.e. renin–angiotensin and sympathetic nervous systems), which would cause vasoconstriction not only in the renal circulation but also in other vascular beds (lower and upper extremities). The splanchnic area would escape the effect of vasoconstrictors and a marked vasodilation would persist, probably because of the existence of very potent local vasodilator stimuli. In early phases following the development of ascites, renal perfusion would be maintained within normal or near normal levels despite the overactivity of vasoconstrictor systems by an increased synthesis/activity of renal vasodilator factors. The development of renal hypoperfusion leading to HRS would occur either as a result of a maximal activation of vasoconstrictor systems that could not be counteracted by vasodilator factors, a decreased activity of vasodilator factors and/or an increased production of

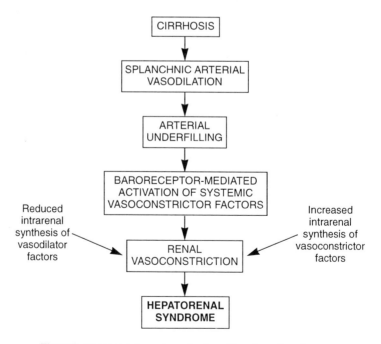

Figure 3. Proposed pathogenic mechanism of hepatorenal syndrome.

intrarenal vasoconstrictors. The recent observation that the improvement of effective arterial blood volume by the prolonged administration of the vasoconstrictor drug, ornipressin, and that plasma volume expansion with albumin is associated with suppression of activity of vasoconstrictor systems and marked improvement in renal perfusion, supports the proposed sequence of events in the pathogenesis of HRS (Guevara et al, 1996, 1997). An alternative theory proposes that renal vasoconstriction is the result of a direct relationship between the liver and the kidney without any relationship with disturbances in systemic haemodynamics. The link between the liver and the kidney would be either a liver vasodilator factor, the synthesis of which would be reduced as a consequence of liver failure or a hepatorenal reflex causing renal vasoconstriction (Kostreva et al, 1980; Alvestrand and Bergstrom, 1984).

Clinical features and diagnosis

The incidence of HRS in patients with cirrhosis hospitalized for the treatment of ascites is approximately 10% (Rodés et al, 1975). Two different types of HRS, which represent distinct expressions of the same pathogenic mechanism, exist. Type I HRS is characterized by rapid and progressive impairment of renal function as defined by a doubling of the initial serum creatine to a level greater than 2.5 mg/dl or a 50% reduction of the initial 24 hour creatinine clearance to a level lower than 20 ml/minute in less than 2 weeks (Arroyo et al, 1996). Renal failure in these patients is often associated with progressive oliguria, marked sodium retention and hyponatraemia. Patients with type I HRS are usually in a very severe clinical condition with signs of advanced liver failure. In approximately half of the cases, this type of HRS develops spontaneously without any identifiable precipitating factor, while in the remaining patients it occurs in close chronological relationship with some complications or therapeutic interventions (bacterial infection, particularly spontaneous bacterial peritonitis, paracentesis without plasma expansion) (Shear et al, 1965b; Rodés et al, 1975; Ginès et al, 1993). Type II HRS is characterized by moderate and stable reduction of GFR that does not meet the criteria proposed for type I. Unlike type I HRS, type II HRS usually occurs in patients with relatively preserved hepatic function. The main clinical consequence of this type of HRS is diuretic-resistant ascites (Arroyo and Rodés, 1975).

There is no specific test for the diagnosis of HRS. The diagnosis of HRS is based on the exclusion of other common causes of renal failure that may occur in patients with cirrhosis, such as pre-renal failure, acute tubular necrosis, administration of nephrotoxic agents (particularly non-steroidal anti-inflammatory drugs) and glomerulonephritis, and demonstration of low GFR. Criteria for the diagnosis of HRS are shown in Table 5 (Arroyo et al, 1996). Although a cut-off value of serum creatine of 1.5 mg/dl may seem low, cirrhotic patients with ascites with serum creatinine above 1.5 mg/dl have a GFR below 30 ml/minute, which represents only one-fourth of the normal GFR for healthy subjects of the same age. The low serum creatine values relative to the reduction in GFR are probably related

Table 5. International Ascites Club's diagnostic criteria of hepatorenal syndrome*.

Major criteria

1. Low glomerular filtration rate, as indicated by serum creatinine greater than 1.5 mg/dl or 24-h creatinine clearance lower than 40 ml/minute.
2. Absence of shock, ongoing bacterial infection, fluid losses and current treatment with nephrotoxic drugs.
3. No sustained improvement in renal function (decrease in serum creatinine to 1.5 mg/dl or less, or increase in creatinine clearance to 40 ml/minute or more) following diuretic withdrawal and expansion of plasma volume with 1.5 litre of a plasma expander.
4. Proteinuria lower than 500 mg/day and no ultrasonographic evidence of obstructive uropathy or parenchymal renal disease.

Additional criteria

1. Urine volume lower than 500 ml/day.
2. Urine sodium lower than 10 mEq/litre.
3. Urine osmolality greater than plasma osmolality.
4. Urine red blood cells less than 50 per high power field.
5. Serum sodium concentration lower than 130 mEq/litre.

* All major criteria must be present for the diagnosis of hepatorenal syndrome. Additional criteria are not necessary for the diagnosis, but provide supportive evidence. Reproduced from Arroyo et al, 1996, with permission.

to a reduced endogenous production of creatinine because of the poor nutritional status of cirrhotic patients. Most cases of HRS have urine sodium below 10 mEq/litre and urine osmolality above plasma osmolality because of the preservation of tubular function. Nevertheless, some patients may have high urine sodium and low urine osmolality, similar to what occurs in acute tubular necrosis. Conversely, cirrhotic patients with acute tubular necrosis may have low urine sodium and high osmolality. For these reasons, urinary indices are not considered major criteria for the diagnosis of HRS.

Treatment and prognosis

A variety of therapeutic modalities has been used in patients with HRS, with only minor or no beneficial effects. Recent reports suggest that the administration of systemic vasoconstrictors, particularly ornipressin combined with plasma expansion with albumin, or the insertion of TIPS may be useful (Ochs et al, 1995; Guevara et al, 1997). However, the efficacy of these methods should be evaluated in controlled investigations. The only effective treatment for HRS at present is liver transplantation. However, a significant proportion of patients died before transplantation can be made because of their extremely short survival rate. Therefore, liver transplantation should be indicated before the development of HRS. Patients more likely to develop HRS are those with markedly reduced urine sodium, dilutional hyponatraemia, arterial hypotension and marked activation of renin–angiotensin and sympathetic nervous systems (Ginès et al, 1993).

The prognosis of patients with HRS is very poor. Type I HRS is the complication with the worst prognosis of cirrhotic patients (Shear et al, 1965b; Ginès et al, 1993). The median survival time of these patients is less than 2 weeks, a survival shorter than that of patients with acute renal failure of other aetiologies (Kleinknecht, 1992). The combination of several factors, including renal failure, liver failure and, in some cases, associated conditions, accounts probably for this extremely poor outcome. Median survival of patients with type II HRS is usually of several months, a longer survival than those with type I, but shorter than patients with ascites without renal failure.

REFERENCES

Albillos A, Rossi I, Cacho G et al (1995) Enhanced endothelium-dependent vasodilation in patients with cirrhosis. *American Journal of Physiology* **268:** G459–464.

Alvestrand A & Bergstrom J (1984) Glomerular hyperfiltration after protein ingestion, during glucagon infusion, and in insulin-dependent diabetes is induced by a liver hormone: deficient production of this hormone in hepatic failure causes hepatorenal syndrome. *Lancet* **i:** 195–197.

Angeli P, Jiménez W, Arroyo V et al (1994) Renal effects of natriuretic peptide receptor blockade in cirrhotic rats with ascites. *Hepatology* **20:** 948–954.

Arroyo V & Rodés J (1975) A rational approach to the treatment of ascites. *Postgraduate Medical Journal* **51:** 558–562.

Arroyo V & Ginès P (1996) TIPS and refractory ascites. Lessons from recent history of ascites therapy. *Journal of Hepatology* **25:** 221–223.

Arroyo V, Rodés J, Gutiérrez-Lizarraga MA & Revert L (1976) Prognostic value of spontaneous hyponatremia in cirrhosis with ascites. *American Journal of Digestive Diseases* **21:** 249–256.

Arroyo V, Bosch J, Mauri M et al (1981) Effect of angiotensin-II blockade on systemic and hepatic haemodynamics and on the renin–angiotensin–aldosterone system in cirrhosis with ascites. *European Journal of Clinical Investigation* **11:** 221–229.

Arroyo V, Planas R, Gaya J et al (1983) Sympathetic nervous activity, renin–angiotensin system and renal excretion of prostaglandin E2 in cirrhosis. Relationship to functional renal failure and sodium and water excretion. *European Journal of Clinical Investigation* **13:** 271–278.

Arroyo V, Ginès P & Jiménez W (1990) Renal circulation and pathogenesis of functional renal failure in cirrhosis. In Bomzon A & Blendis LM (eds) *Cardiovascular Complications of Liver Disease*, pp 125–149. Boca Raton: CRC Press.

Arroyo V, Ginès P, Jiménez W & Rodés J (1991) Ascites, renal failure, and electrolyte disorders in cirrhosis. Pathogenesis, diagnosis, and treatment. In McIntyre N, Benhamou JP, Bircher J, Rizetto M, Rodés J (eds) *Textbook of Clinical Hepatology*, 1st edn, pp 429–470. Oxford: Oxford Medical Press.

Arroyo V, Ginès P & Planas R (1992) Treatment of ascites in cirrhosis. Diuretics, peritoneovenous shunt, and large-volume paracentesis. In Groszmann RJ & Grace N (eds) *Gastroenterology Clinics of North America*, pp 237–256. Philadelphia: WB Saunders Company.

Arroyo V, Clària J, Saló J & Jiménez W (1994a) Antidiuretic hormone and the pathogenesis of water retention in cirrhosis with ascites. *Seminars in Liver Disease* **14:** 44–58.

Arroyo V, Ginès A & Saló J (1994b) A European survey on the treatment of ascites in cirrhosis. *Journal of Hepatology* **21:** 667–672.

*Arroyo V, Ginès P, Gerbes A et al (1996) Definition and diagnostic criteria of refractory ascites and hepatorenal syndrome in cirrhosis. *Hepatology* **23:** 164–176.

Asbert M, Ginès A, Ginès P et al (1993) Circulating levels of endothelin in cirrhosis. *Gastroenterology* **104:** 1485–1491.

Bataller R, Ginès P, Guevara M & Arroyo V (1997) Hepatorenal syndrome. *Seminars in Liver Disease* (in press).

Battista S, Bar F, Mengozzi G et al (1997) Hyperdynamic circulation in patients with cirrhosis: direct measurement of nitric oxide levels in hepatic and portal veins. *Journal of Hepatology* **26:** 75–80.

Benoit JN & Granger DN (1986) Splanchnic hemodynamics in chronic portal hypertension. *Seminars in Liver Disease* **6:** 287–298.

Benoit JN & Granger DN (1988) Intestinal microvascular adaptation to chronic portal hypertension in the rat. *Gastroenterology* **94:** 471–476.

Bernardi M, Trevisani F & Gasbarrini G (1990) The renin–angiotensin–aldosterone system in liver disease. In Bomzon A & Blendis LM (eds) *Cardiovascular Complications of Liver Disease*, pp 29–62. Boca Raton: CRC Press.

Bosch J, Garcia-Pagán JC, Feu F & Pizcueta MP (1992) Portal hypertension. In Prieto J, Rodés J & Shafritz DA (eds) *Hepatobiliary Diseases*, pp 429–463. Berlin: Springer-Verlag.

Bosch-Marcé M, Jiménez W, Angeli P et al (1995) Aquaretic effects of the κ-opioid agonist RU-51599 in cirrhotic rats with ascites and water retention. *Gastroenterology* 109: 217–224.

Boyer TD, Zia P & Reynolds TB (1979) Effect of indomethacin and prostaglandin A1 on renal function and plasma renin activity in alcoholic liver disease. *Gastroenterology* 77: 215–222.

Campillo B, Chabrier PE, Pelle G et al (1995) Inhibition of nitric oxide synthesis in the forearm arterial bed of patients with advanced cirrhosis. *Hepatology* 22: 1423–1429.

Castro A, Jiménez W, Clària J et al (1993) Impaired responsiveness to angiotensin II in experimental cirrhosis: role of nitric oxide. *Hepatology* 18: 367–372.

Clària J, Jiménez W, Arroyo V et al (1991) Effect of V1-vasopressin receptor blockade on arterial pressure in conscious rats with cirrhosis and ascites. *Gastroenterology* 100: 494–501.

Clària J, Jiménez W, Ros J et al (1992) Pathogenesis of arterial hypotension in cirrhotic rats with ascites: role of endogenous nitric oxide. *Hepatology* 15: 343–349.

Clària J, Jiménez W, Ros J, et al (1994) Increased nitric oxide-dependent vasorelaxation in aortic rings of cirrhotic rats with ascites. *Hepatology* 20: 1615–1621.

Epstein M (1996a) Renal sodium handling in liver disease. In Epstein M (ed.) *The Kidney in Liver Disease*, 4th edn pp 1–31. Philadelphia: Hanley and Belfus.

Epstein M (1996b) Renin-angiotensin system in liver disease. In Epstein M (ed.) *The Kidney in Liver Disease*, 4th edn, pp 267–289. Philadelphia: Hanley and Belfus.

Epstein M, Berck DP, Hollemberg NK et al (1970) Renal failure in the patient with cirrhosis. The role of active vasoconstriction. *American Journal of Medicine* 49: 175–185.

Fernández-Esparrach G, Guevara M, Sort P et al (1997) Diuretic requirements after therapeutic paracentesis in non-azotemic patients with cirrhosis. A randomized double-blind trial of spironolactone versus placebo. *Journal of Hepatology* 26: 614–620.

Forns X, Ginès A, Ginès P et al (1994) The management of ascites and renal failure in cirrhosis. *Seminars in Liver Disease* 14: 82–96.

Gadano A, Moreau R, Trombino C et al (1996) Aquaretic effects of niravoline in patients with cirrhosis. *Hepatology* 24 (**Supplement**): A448 (Abstract).

Garcia-Estañ J, Atucha N, Mario J et al (1994) Increased endothelium-dependent renal vasodilation in cirrhotic rats. *American Journal of Physiology* 267: R549–R553.

Ginès A, Escorsell A, Ginès P et al (1993) Incidence, predictive factors, and prognosis of the hepatorenal syndrome in cirrhosis with ascites. *Gastroenterology* 105: 229–236.

*Ginès A, Fernández-Esparrach G, Monescillo A et al (1996) Randomized trial comparing albumin, dextran-70 and polygelin in cirrhotic patients with ascites treated by paracentesis. *Gastroenterology* 111: 1002–1010.

*Ginès P & Jiménez W (1996) Aquaretic agents: a new potential treatment of dilutional hyponatremia in cirrhosis. *Journal of Hepatology* 24: 506–512.

*Ginès P, Arroyo V, Quintero E et al (1987) Comparison of paracentesis and diuretics in the treatment of cirrhotics with tense ascites. Results of a randomized study. *Gastroenterology* 93: 234–241.

Ginès P, Jiménez W, Arroyo V et al (1988a) Atrial natriuretic factor in cirrhosis with ascites: plasma levels, cardiac release and splanchnic extraction. *Hepatology* 8: 636–642.

*Ginès P, Tító LI, Arroyo V et al (1988b) Randomized comparative study of therapeutic paracentesis with and without intravenous albumin in cirrhosis. *Gastroenterology* 94: 1493–1502.

*Ginès P, Arroyo V, Vargas V et al (1991) Paracentesis with intravenous infusion of albumin as compared with peritoneovenous shunting in cirrhosis with refractory ascites. *New England Journal of Medicine* 325: 829–835.

Ginès P, Arroyo V & Rodés J (1992) Current guidelines for pharmacotherapy of ascites associated with cirrhosis. *Drugs* 43: 316–332.

Ginès P, Abraham W & Schrier RW (1994) Vasopressin in pathophysiological states. *Seminars in Nephrology* 14: 384–397.

Ginès P, Arroyo V & Rodés J (1996) Disorders of renal function in cirrhosis: pathophysiology and clinical aspects. In Zakim D & Boyer TD (eds) *Hepatology: A Textbook of Liver Disease*, 3rd edn, pp 650–675. Philadelphia: WB Saunders Company.

Ginès P, Martin PY & Niederberger M (1997) Prognostic significance of renal dysfunction in cirrhosis. *Kidney International* (in press).

González-Campoy JM & Knox FG (1992) Integrated responses of the kidney to alterations in extracellular fluid volume. In Seldin DW & Giebisch G (eds) *The Kidney: Physiology and Pathophysiology*, 2nd edn, pp 2041–2098. New York: Raven Press.

Groszmann RJ (1994) Hyperdynamic circulation of liver disease 40 years later: pathophysiology and clinical consequences. *Hepatology* **20:** 1359–1363.

Guarner C, Soriano G, Tomas A et al (1993) Increased serum nitrite and nitrate levels in patients with cirrhosis: relationship with endotoxemia. *Hepatology* **18:** 1139–1143.

Guevara M, Ginès P, Fernández-Esparrach G et al (1996) Effects of normalization of vasoconstrictor systems on renal function in cirrhotic patients with hepatorenal syndrome (HRS) (abstract). *Journal of Hepatology* **25 (Supplement 1):** S71.

*Guevara M, Ginès P, Fernández-Esparach G et al (1997) Reversal of hepatorenal syndrome by prolonged administration of ornipressin and plasma volume expansion (abstract). *Journal of Hepatology* **26 (Supplement 1):** S104.

Hagège H, Ink O, Ducreux M et al (1992) Traitement de l'ascite chez les malades atteints de cirrhose sans hyponatrémie ni insuffisance rénale. Résultats d'une étude randomisée comparant les diurétiques et les ponctions compensées par l'albumine. *Gastroenterologie Clinique et Biologique* **16:** 751–755.

*Henriksen JH & Moller MD (1996) Hemodynamics, distribution of blood volume, and kinetics of vasoactive substances in cirrhosis. In Epstein M (ed.) *The Kidney in Liver Disease*, 4th edn, pp 241–258. Philadelphia: Hanley and Belfus Inc.

Henriksen JH, Ring-Larsen H & Christensen NJ (1990) Autonomic nervous function in liver disease. In Bomzon A & Blendis LM (eds) *Cardiovascular Complications of Liver Disease*, pp 63–79. Boca Raton: CRC Press.

Housset C, Rockey DC & Bissell DM (1993) Endothelin receptors in rat liver: lipocytes as a contractile target for endothelin 1. *Procedures of the National Academy of Sciences USA* **90:** 9266–9270.

Huber M, Kastner S, Scholmerich J et al (1989) Analysis of cysteinyl leukotrienes in human urine: enhanced excretion in patients with liver cirrhosis and hepatorenal syndrome. *European Journal of Clinical Investigation* **19:** 53–60.

Inoue T, Ohnishi A, Matsuo A et al (1996) Aquaretic effect of a potent, orally active, nonpeptide V2 antagonist in cirrhosis. *Hepatology* **23:** 1–23 (Abstract).

Kleinknecht D (1992) Management of acute renal failure. In Cameron S, Davison AM, Grunfeld JP et al (eds) *Oxford Textbook of Clinical Nephrology*, 1st edn, pp 1015–1025. Oxford: Oxford University Press.

Korthuis RJ, Kinden DA, Brimer GE et al (1988) Intestinal capillary filtration in acute and chronic portal hypertension. *American Journal of Physiology* **254:** G339–G345.

Kostreva DR, Castaner A & Kampine JP (1980) Reflex effects of hepatic baroreceptors on renal and cardiac sympathetic nervous activity. *American Journal of Physiology* **238:** R390–R394.

Laffi G, La Villa G, Pinzani M & Gentilini P (1996) Lipid-derived autacoids and renal function in liver cirrhosis. In Epstein M (ed.) *The Kidney in Liver Disease*, 4th edn, pp 307–337. Philadelphia: Hanley and Belfus.

Laffi G, Foschi M, Masinin E et al (1995) Increased production of nitric oxide by neutrophils and monocytes from cirrhotic patients with ascites and hyperdynamic circulation. *Hepatology* **22:** 1666–1673.

Lebrec D, Giuily N, Hadengue A et al (1996) Transjugular intrahepatic portosystemic shunts: comparison with paracentesis in patients with cirrhosis and refractory ascites: a randomized trial. *Journal of Hepatology* **25:** 135–144.

Leivas A, Jiménez W, Lamas S et al (1995) Endothelin-1 does not play a major role in the homeostasis of arterial pressure in cirrhotic rats with ascites. *Gastroenterology* **108:** 1842–1848.

Lieberman FL, Denison EK & Reynolds TB (1970) The relationship of plasma volume, portal hypertension, ascites, and renal sodium retention in cirrhosis: the overflow theory of ascites formation. *Annals of New, York Academy of Sciences* **170:** 202–212.

*Llach J, Ginès P, Arroyo V et al (1988) Prognostic value of arterial pressure, endogenous vasoactive systems, and renal function in cirrhotic patients admitted to the hospital for the treatment of ascites. *Gastroenterology* **94:** 482–487.

Luca A, Garcia-Pagan JC, Bosch J et al (1995) Beneficial effects of intravenous albumin infusion on the hemodynamic and humoral changes after total paracentesis. *Hepatology* **22:** 753–758.

Maroto A, Ginès A, Saló J et al (1994) Diagnosis of functional renal failure of cirrhosis by Doppler sonography. Prognostic value of resistive index. *Hepatology* **20:** 839–844.

Martin PY, Xu DL, Niederberger M et al (1996) Upregulation of the endothelial constitutive NOS: a major role in the increased NO production in cirrhotic rats. *American Journal of Physiology* **39**: F494–F499.

Mathie RT, Ralevic V, Moore KP et al (1996) Mesenteric vasodilator responses in cirrhotic rats: a role for nitric oxide? *Hepatology* **23**: 130–136.

Matsumoto A, Ogura K, Hirata Y et al (1995) Increased nitric oxide in the exhaled air of patients with decompensated liver cirrhosis. *Annals of Internal Medicine* **123**: 110–113.

Moller S, Emmeluth C & Henriksen JH (1993) Elevated circulating plasma endothelin-1 concentrations in cirrhosis. *Journal of Hepatology* **19**: 285–290.

Moller S, Gülberg V, Henriksen JH & Gerbes AL (1995) Endothelin-1 and endothelin-3 in cirrhosis: relations to systemic and splanchnic hemodynamics. *Journal of Hepatology* **23**: 135–144.

Moore K, Taylos GW, Maltby NH et al (1990) Increased production of cysteinyl leukotrienes in hepatorenal syndrome. *Journal of Hepatology* **11**: 263–271.

Moore K, Wendon J, Frazer M et al (1992) Plasma endothelin immunoreactivity in liver disease and the hepatorenal syndrome. *New England Journal of Medicine* **327**: 1774–1778.

Morales M, Jiménez W, Pérez-Sala D et al (1996) Increased nitric oxide synthase expression in arterial vessels of cirrhotic rats with ascites. *Hepatology* **24**: 1481–1486.

*Niederberger M, Martin PY, Ginès P et al (1995a) Normalization of nitric oxide production corrects arterial vasodilation and hyperdynamic circulation in rats with cirrhosis and ascites. *Gastroenterology* **109**: 1624–1630.

Niederberger M, Ginès P, Tsai P et al (1995b) Increased aortic cyclic guanosine monophosphate concentration in experimental cirrhosis in rats: evidence for a role of nitric oxide in the pathogenesis of arterial vasodilation in cirrhosis. *Hepatology* **21**: 1625–1631.

Ochs A, Rössle M, Haag K et al (1995) The transjugular intrahepatic portosystemic stent-shunt procedure for refractory ascites. *New England Journal of Medicine* **332**: 1192–1197.

Panos MZ, Moore K, Vlavianos P et al (1990) Single, total paracentesis for tense ascites: sequential hemodynamic changes and right atrial size. *Hepatology* **11**: 662–667.

Papper S & Saxon L (1959) The diuretic response to administered water in patients with liver disease. II. Laennec's cirrhosis of the liver. *Archives of Internal Medicine* **103**: 750–757.

Pariente EA, Bataille C, Bercoff E et al (1985) Acute effects of captopril on systemic and renal hemodynamics and on renal function in cirrhotic patients with ascites. *Gastroenterology* **88**: 1255–1259.

Pinzani M, Milani S, De Franco R et al (1996) Endothelin 1 is overexpressed in human cirrhotic liver and exerts multiple effects on activated hepatic stellate cells. *Gastroenterology* **110**: 534–548.

Platt JF, Marn CS, Baliga PK et al (1992) Renal dysfunction in hepatic disease: early identification with renal Duplex Doppler US in patients who undergo liver transplantation. *Radiology* **183**: 801–806.

*Pozzi M, Osculati G, Boari G et al (1994) Time course of circulatory and humoral effects of rapid total paracentesis in cirrhotic patients with tense, refractory ascites. *Gastroenterology* **106**: 709–719.

Quintero E, Ginès P, Arroyo V et al (1985) Paracentesis versus diuretics in the treatment of cirrhotics with tense ascites. *Lancet* **i**: 611–612.

Quintero E, Ginès P, Arroyo V et al (1986) Sulindac reduces the urinary excretion of prostaglandins and impairs renal function in cirrhosis with ascites. *Nephron* **42**: 298–303.

Quiroga J, Sangro B, Nuñez M et al (1995) Transjugular intrahepatic portal-systemic shunt in the management of refractory ascites: effect on clinical, renal, humoral and hemodynamic parameters. *Hepatology* **21**: 986–994.

Raij L (1993) Nitric oxide and the kidney. *Circulation* **87 (Supplement V)**: S26–S29.

Rockey DC & Weisiger R (1996) Endothelin induced contractility of stellate cells from normal and cirrhotic rat liver: implications for regulation of portal pressure and resistance. *Hepatology* **24**: 233–240.

Rodès J, Bosch J & Arroyo V (1975) Clinical types and drug therapy of renal impairment in cirrhosis. *Postgraduate Medical Journal* **55**: 492–497.

Ros J, Clária J, Jiménez W et al (1995a) Role of nitric acid and prostaglandin in the control of renal perfusion in experimental cirrhosis. *Hepatology* **22**: 915–920.

Ros J, Jiménez W, Lamas S et al (1995b) Nitric oxide production in arterial vessels of cirrhotic rats. *Hepatology* **21**: 554–560.

Salerno F, Badalamenti S, Incerti P et al (1987) Repeated paracentesis and iv albumin infusion to treat 'tense' ascites in cirrhotic patients: a safe alternative therapy. *Journal of Hepatology* **5**: 102–108.

Saló J, Ginès A, Anibarro L et al (1995a) Effect of upright posture and physical exercise on endogenous neurohormonal systems in cirrhotic patients with sodium retention and normal supine plasma renin, aldosterone, and norepinephrine levels. *Hepatology* **22:** 479–487.

Saló J, Ginès A, Ginès P et al (1995b) The impairment in effective intravascular volume after paracentesis is not due to a reduction of plasma volume. *Journal of Hepatology* **23 (Supplement 1):** S117.

*Schrier RW, Arroyo V, Bernardi M et al (1988) Peripheral arterial vasodilation hypothesis: a proposal for the initation of renal sodium and water retention in cirrhosis. *Hepatology* **8:** 1151–1157.

Schrier RW, Niederberger M, Weigert A et al (1994) Peripheral arterial vasodilation: determinant of functional spectrum of cirrhosis. *Seminars in Liver Disease* **14:** 14–22.

Schroeder ET, Anderson GH, Goldman SH & Streeten DHP (1976) Effect of blockade of angiotensin II on blood pressure, renin and aldosterone in cirrhosis. *Kidney International* **9:** 511–519.

Shear L, Hall PW & Gabuzda GJ (1965a) Renal failure in patients with cirrhosis of the liver. II. Factors influencing maximal urinary flow rate. *American Journal of Medicine* **39:** 199–209.

Shear L, Kleinerman J & Gabuzda GJ (1965b) Renal failure in patients with cirrhosis of the liver. I. Clinical and pathologic characteristics. *American Journal of Medicine* **39:** 184–192.

Sieber CC & Groszmann RJ (1992) Nitric oxide mediates hyporeactivity to vasopressors in mesenteric vessels of portal hypertensive rats. *Gastroenterology* **103:** 235–239.

Simon DM, McCain JR, Bonkovsky HL et al (1987) Effects of therapeutic paracentesis on systemic and hepatic hemodynamics and on renal and hormonal function. *Hepatology* **7:** 423–429.

Sogni P, Garnier P, Gadano A et al (1995) Endogenous pulmonary nitric oxide production measured from exhaled air is increased in patients with severe cirrhosis. *Journal of Hepatology* **23:** 471–473.

*Somberg KA (1996) Transjugular intrahepatic portosystemic shunt in the treatment of refractory ascites and hepatorenal syndrome. In Epstein M (ed.) *The Kidney in Liver Disease* 4th edn, pp 507–516. Philadelphia: Hanley and Belfus Inc.

Somberg KA, Lake JR, Tomlanovich SJ et al (1995) Transjugular intrahepatic portosystemic shunt for refractory ascites: assessment of clinical and humoral response and renal function. *Hepatology* **21:** 709–716.

Tsuboi Y, Ishikawa SE, Fujisawa G et al (1994) Therapeutic efficacy of the non-peptide AVP antagonist OPC-31260 in cirrhotic rats. *Kidney International* **46:** 237–243.

Vaamonde CA (1996) Renal water handling in liver disease. In Epstein M (ed.) *The Kidney in Liver Disease*, 4th edn, pp 33–74. Philadelphia: Hanley and Belfus.

Vila MC, Solà R, Molina L et al (1995) Hemodynamic changes in patients with effective hypovolemia after total paracentesis of ascites. *Hepatology* **22:** A163.

La Villa G, Romanelli RG, Raggi VC et al (1992) Plasma levels of brain natriuretic peptide in patients with cirrhosis. *Hepatology* **16:** 156–161.

Warner L, Skorecki K, Blendis LM & Epstein M (1993) Atrial natriuretic factor and liver disease. *Hepatology* **17:** 500–513.

Weigert AL, Martin PY, Niederberger M et al (1995) Endothelium-dependent vascular hyporesponsiveness without detection of nitric oxide synthase induction in aortas of cirrhotic rats. *Hepatology* **22:** 1856–1862.

Wilkinson SP, Smith IK & Williams R (1979) Changes in plasma renin activity in cirrhosis: a reappraisal based on studies in 67 patients and 'low-renin' cirrhosis. *Hypertension* **1:** 125–129.

11

Hepatopulmonary syndrome: the paradigm of liver-induced hypoxaemia

ROBERT RODRIGUEZ-ROISIN MD, FRCPE

Professor of Medicine, Chief of Service, Senior Consultant

JOSEP ROCA MD

Associate Professor of Medicine; Chief of Section; Consultant

Servei de Pneumologia i Al·lèrgia Respiratòria, Departament de Medicina, Hospital Clínic, Universitat de Barcelona, Barcelona, Spain

The current chapter deals with the concept, clinical manifestations and diagnostic tools of the hepatopulmonary syndrome (HPS) and highlights its most salient pathophysiological, mechanistic and therapeutic aspects. Defined as a clinical triad, including a chronic liver disorder, pulmonary gas exchange abnormalities and generalized pulmonary vascular dilatations, in the absence of intrinsic cardiopulmonary disease, this entity is currently growing in interest with both clinicians and surgeons. The combination of arterial hypoxaemia, high cardiac output with normal or low pulmonary artery pressure, and finger clubbing in a patient with advanced liver disease should strongly suggest the diagnosis of HPS. Its potential high prevalence together with failure of numerous therapeutic approaches depicts a life-threatening unique clinical condition that may dramatically benefit with an elective indication of liver transplantation (LT). A better orchestration of the concepts of the pathophysiology of this lung–liver interplay may foster our knowledge and improve the clinical management and indications of LT.

Key words: gas exchange abnormalities; liver failure; liver transplantation; nitric oxide; pulmonary circulation; ventilation–perfusion relationships.

Since the first liver transplantation more than 30 years ago, this unique surgical procedure has become a widely accepted therapeutical approach for patients with a large spectrum of end-stage liver disorders. For many years, severe gas exchange abnormalities were regarded as an absolute contraindication for liver transplantation (LT). Later, as experience with patients with extremely low arterial oxygen pressure (PaO_2) suffering from hepatopulmonary syndrome (HPS) became available, showing complete or

Supported by Grants from the Comissionat per a Universitats i Recerca (1995 SGR 00446) de la Generalitat de Catalunya and the Fondo de Investigación Sanitaria (FIS) 97/0126.

partial resolution of the disorder following LT, HPS began to be viewed as an elective indication (Rodriguez-Roisin and Krowka 1994).

Mild levels of arterial hypoxaemia (60 mmHg $<PaO_2 <$ 80 mmHg) are relatively common in the setting of chronic liver diseases; yet, severe hypoxaemia is less frequent in the absence of cardiopulmonary disease. The prevalence of arterial hypoxaemia in a population of more than 1100 patients with end-stage liver disease assembled over the last 5 years ranged between 9 and 29% (Table 1). Hence, the presence of severe hypoxaemia associated with a chronic liver disorder alone should be strongly suggestive of HPS. However, because patients with advanced liver disorders characteristically hyperventilate, which results in hypocapnia, the alveolar–arterial PO_2 difference ($AaPO_2$), that incorporates in its calculation the levels of arterial carbon dioxide pressure ($PaCO_2$), emerges as a more accurate functional outcome measure of gas exchange abnormalities in these patients. Using the $AaPO_2$, the prevalence of abnormal pulmonary gas exchange in patients with advanced liver disease increases substantially up to 69% (Table 1).

Table 1. Arterial hypoxaemia and end-stage liver disease.

	N	Low $PaO_2(\%)$	Increased $AaPO_2(\%)$
Hourani et al (1991)	116	NR	45
Fahy et al (1991)	190	22	69
Krowka et al (1992)	95	13	47
Castro et al (1994)	368	NR	55
Marks et al (1996)	319	9	NR
Martínez-Pallí et al (1996)	45	29	40

PaO_2, arterial PO_2; $AaPO_2$, alveolar-arterial PO_2; NR, not reported.

CONCEPT AND PATHOLOGY

Flückiger (1984) was the first to identify in 1884, the case of a woman with severe hepatic cirrhosis, cyanosis and finger clubbing. Since then, numerous reports have described similar patients in an effort to clarify, firstly, the pathophysiology and, secondly, the pathogenesis of this tantalizing entity. In 1977, Kennedy and Knudson (1977) originally, although unsuccessfully, coined the term HPS as the concept of hepatorenal syndrome, to define a disorder of chronic renal failure with normal kidneys that resulted from the abnormal circulatory dynamics of liver cirrhosis was introduced at that time. By HPS they meant an end-stage lung dysfunction produced by a hyperkinetic status associated with liver cirrhosis. The term was then abandoned until the late 1980s when Sherlock (1989), in the last edition of her classic textbook on hepatic diseases, quoted it again. Subsequently, we (Rodriguez-Roisin et al, 1992; Rodriguez-Roisin, 1995) and others (Eriksson et al, 1988; Krowka and Cortese, 1990) have supported this nomenclature and contributed to its dissemination, although not always with identical meaning.

Thus, Sherlock revised the term to encompass any condition of arterial hypoxaemia ($PaO_2 < 80$ mmHg), which was supposed to occur in approximately one-third of patients with liver cirrhosis in the absence of detectable cardiorespiratory disease (Sherlock, 1989). Notwithstanding, Raffy et al (1996) have accurately pointed out that HPS should not be used as an equivalent to hypoxaemia because the latter can be related to other respiratory conditions, such as portal hypertension-associated primary pulmonary hypertension with secondary intracardiac shunt. Because different outcomes appear to exist, it is essential to discriminate between HPS and pulmonary hypertension (Rodriguez-Roisin and Krowka, 1994), as the latter finding is conspicuously absent in the context of HPS.

We suggest a definition of HPS as a syndrome that is characterized by a clinical triad, including an advanced, chronic liver disorder, pulmonary gas exchange abnormalities leading ultimately to life-threatening arterial hypoxaemia, and widespread pulmonary vascular dilatations, in the absence of intrinsic cardiopulmonary disease (Rodriguez-Roisin et al, 1992; Rodriguez-Roisin, 1995). This notion is challenged in part by Krowka and Cortese (1994) who support the concept that HPS can still coexist with other pulmonary conditions, such as pleural effusion or cigarette smoking-induced airflow obstruction, which is relatively common in patients with chronic liver disorders. In principle, our view is to endorse a more restrictive conceptualization of the syndrome as its pathophysiology still remains unsettled. Although more prevalent in patients with all types of liver cirrhosis and in other common chronic liver diseases, such as chronic active hepatitis, HPS has also been reported in the context of more bizarre hepatic conditions, namely non-specific hepatitis, non-cirrhotic portal hypertension, alpha$_1$-antitrypsin deficiency and Wilson's disease (Krowka and Cortese, 1989). It is not intended, however, that HPS includes all cardiorespiratory disorders that may coexist with chronic liver disease states. The prevailing clinical interest in HPS is based on four aspects: a high prevalence according to some ongoing studies; a life-threatening condition with a poor prognosis; failure of numerous medical therapeutic strategies to minimize or antagonize it; and, a spectacular improvement or complete resolution after LT.

Pathologically, although Rydell and Hoffbauer (1956) were the first to demonstrate numerous post-mortem intrapulmonary arteriovenous anastomoses in a young patient with juvenile cirrhosis, Berthelot and co-workers (1966) had the credit for showing in a seminal study, the structural changes in lung specimens from patients with liver cirrhosis and different degrees of hypoxaemia, by using micro-opaque gelatin injections into the pulmonary vascular tree as a gold-standard method. However, the most salient finding was a remarkable dilatation involving the fine peripheral branches of the pulmonary artery at both the pre-capillary and capillary levels of the lung, and this basically affected arterial vessels up to 160 μm in diameter. In addition, spider naevi were apparent on the pleura in half of the patients. Obvious peripheral arteriovenous communications were demonstrated in only one such patient. These vascular abnormalities contrasted with an otherwise intact pulmonary architecture. Similarly,

Williams et al (1979) found, in fatal hypoxic patients with fulminant hepatic failure, diffuse dilatation affecting all intra-acinar vessels, although this was not as severe as in cirrhosis, and pleural spiders. Other post-mortem studies (Rodman et al, 1959; Georg et al, 1960) have failed to identify definite anatomical arteriovenous communications for intra-pulmonary shunt and, an extrapulmonary site, namely portopulmonary communications (Calabresi and Abelmann, 1957) was postulated.

Collectively, these studies strongly indicate a considerable structural dis-organization of the pulmonary circulation, which is sufficient to allow mixed venous blood to pass either very rapidly or directly into the pulmonary veins, hence jeopardizing partially or completely arterial oxygenation. Thus, the most common structural finding is widespread vasodilatation of the pulmonary vascular bed at the pre-capillary and capillary levels, 15–150 µm in diameter, near the gas exchange area (Figure 1.) However, larger arteriovenous anastomoses not necessarily near the gas exchange units may be also seen. This may develop through dilatation of normal capillaries to pre-capillary diameter or, alternatively, by the opening either by recruitment or distensibility, or both, of anatomic pre-capillary pulmonary arteriovenous communications. In addition, a few pleural spiders have been observed. This constellation of extensive pulmonary vascular deformities in patients with liver diseases lends further support to the research of Krowka and Cortese (1989) who preferentially use the term intrapulmonary vascular dilatations.

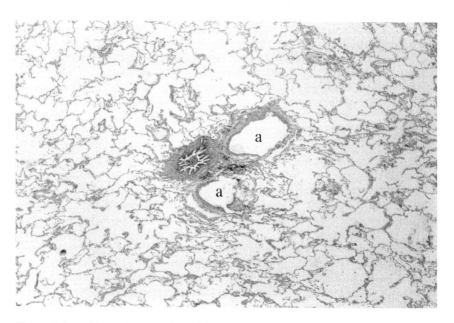

Figure 1. Lung biopsy from a patient with HPS. Note the presence of two dilated pulmonary capillaries (a) surrounding a normal terminal bronchiole. The rest of the pulmonary architecture is strictly preserved.

CLINICAL MANIFESTATIONS, PREVALENCE AND DIAGNOSTIC IMAGING

We have proposed a set of four diagnostic criteria for HPS (Rodriguez-Roisin et al, 1992): (i) the presence of a chronic liver disease without intrinsic cardiopulmonary disease; (ii) normal chest radiograph or with nodular basal shadowing; (iii) gas exchange disturbances including an elevated AaPO$_2$ (≥ 15 mmHg) with or without arterial hypoxaemia; and (iv) a positive contrast-enhanced (CE) echocardiogram or, alternatively, demonstration of intravenous radiolabelled microspheres in extrapulmonary sites (kidneys, liver, spleen, brain). We also have suggested that other additional features can be helpful to further establish the diagnosis of HPS, such as abnormal diffusing capacity or low transfer factor (T$_{LCO}$), dyspnoea with or without platypnoea (increased shortness of breath in the upright position relieved by recumbency) and orthodeoxia (enhanced arterial hypoxaemia in the upright position), a hyperkinetic status (i.e. high cardiac output and low systemic arterial pressures) with a normal or low pulmonary artery pressure, and a poor hypoxic pulmonary vascular response.

Two-dimensional CE echocardiography seems to be the most sensitive non-invasive approach, as it identifies echoes (microbubbles of air or indocyanine green) in the left atrium within three to six beats of their visualization in the right heart cavities (Krowka and Cortese, 1989) (Figure 2). In normal conditions echogenicity in the left heart chambers is not detected since microbubbles (as large as 60–90 µm in diameter) are trapped in the pulmonary capillary. Although CE echocardiography cannot differentiate between the different types of vascular malformations, i.e. precapillary, capillary and pleural dilatations versus direct arteriovenous communications, it can distinguish clearly between any type of intrapulmonary vascular deformities (widespread dilatation, arteriovenous connections) and intracardiac malformations (i.e. opening of the foramen ovale). Similarly, the presence of extrapulmonary radionuclide ^{99m}Tc-MAA activity over other organs (kidneys, brain) indicates the presence of a right-to-left intrapulmonary shunting. Under normal conditions, the albumin macroaggregates (20–60 µm in diameter) should be trapped in the normal pulmonary capillary bed (8–15 µm in diameter).

From a clinical viewpoint, the vast majority of patients with HPS are cyanosed, clubbed and have a hyperkinetic circulation. They may complain of shortness of breath and platypnea. Although most of the patients exhibit the typical stigmata of severe liver dysfunction and abnormal liver function tests, including portal hypertension, in a few cases severe gas exchange abnormalities may precede manifestations of liver failure. We have suggested that the presence of cutaneous spiders could be a clinical marker of the severity of abnormal systemic and pulmonary haemodynamics as well as of the gas exchange alterations reported in patients with HPS (Rodriguez-Roisin et al, 1987). At first glance, the more severe the hepatic failure, the greater the severity of HPS. Yet, no correlations have been shown between the severity of portal hypertension, on the one hand, or that of liver failure, as assessed by the Child–Pugh

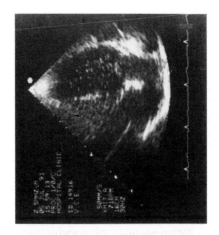
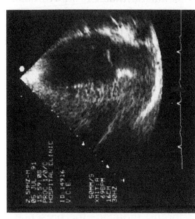
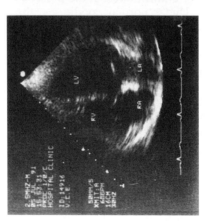

Figure 2. Contrast-enhanced echocardiogram in a patient with HPS showing (left) normal four-chamber view (RA, right atrium; RV, right ventricle; LV, left ventricle; LA, left atrium). Note opacification of RA and RV with microbubbles (centre) and also delayed opacification of RV and LV (right). The echogenic presence of microbubbles in the left heart chambers is strongly suggestive of intrapulmonary vascular dilatations with or without the presence of anatomic arteriovenous communications.

classification, and that of the clinical and pulmonary functional outcomes of HPS, on the other.

The actual prevalence of clinical manifestations of HPS still remains uncertain as the diagnostic criteria have been used heterogeneously and most of the series are retrospective. To date, only two studies have assessed more detailed information (Table 2). The first is retrospective, from the Mayo Clinic (USA) (Krowka et al, 1993), including 22 patients with end-stage liver disease whose diagnosis was based on the presence of vascular abnormalities identified non-invasively (positive echocardiography or extrapulmonary location of macroaggregated particles); the second, still in progress (Martínez-Pallí et al, 1996), includes nine patients out of a population of 45 candidates for LT, who were prospectively screened for the diagnosis of HPS over a 1-year period, and all showed the diagnostic criteria alluded to (Rodriguez-Roisin et al, 1992). Both populations include middle-aged patients without gender differences. Interestingly, while the prevalence of signs and symptoms that relate to liver problems and finger clubbing is substantially elevated, that of shortness of breath and of platypnoea and orthodeoxia differ substantially. In our experience, the latter two findings are less common in relation to what has been quoted in the current literature. As for gas exchange abnormalities, both series show predominantly basal severe hypoxaemia, which is conventionally measured under conditions of breathing room air in the upright position, low $PaCO_2$ and increased $AaPO_2$ (only in Martínez-Pallí et al's series, 1996), and includes a low transfer factor (T_{LW}). By contrast, there were no or very few spirometric alterations, and lung volumes were within normal limits.

Table 2. Clinical manifestations in hepatopulmonary syndrome.

	Krowka et al (1993)	Martínez-Pallí et al (1996)
Age (years)	49	52
Platypnoea and orthodeoxia	88%	22%
Dyspnoea	18%	67%
Finger clubbing	83%	77%
Symptoms/signs of liver disease	82%	89%

The prevalence of HPS is unknown so far. Using CE echocardiogram as the gold-standard to identify intrapulmonary vascular dilatations, the prevalence of a positive CE echocardiography varies between 5 and 46% of the series (Table 3) (Castro and Krowka, 1996). In our experience, the prevalence is 20% (Table 2). Yet, if we look at those patients who also have associated arterial hypoxaemia, then the prevalence decreases sharply to 29%. In addition, the relative opacification of the left ventricle in patients with positive CE echocardiograms has been quantitatively assessed on a scale of 1+ to 4+: the PaO_2 of those with at least 2+ opacification being significantly lower (Hopkins et al, 1992). The relevance of a positive CE echocardiogram without gas exchange abnormalities, including a normal $AaPO_2$, remains unsettled as yet. These patients could be considered a *forme fruste* of HPS in that they have a diagnostic imaging suggestive of

Table 3. Screening contrast-enhanced echocardiography in end-stage liver disease.

	N	Positive (%)	Positive and hypoxaemia (%)
Park et al	73	5	NR
Krowka et al	37	13	5
Stoller et al	34	38	29
Hopkins et al (1992)	53	47	15
Jensen et al	47	23	13
Martínez-Pallí et al (1996)	45	20	16

NR, not reported. Adapted from Castro and Krowka (1996) (with permission). Except for Hopkins et al and Martínez-Pallí et al, the other references are quoted in Castro and Krowka (1996).

HPS without fitting one of the cardinal criteria that form the diagnosis of this disorder (Castro and Krowka, 1996).

In a retrospective study that includes 10 patients with HPS diagnosed by radiological evidence of intrapulmonary shunting, either using a CE echo-cardiogram or ^{99m}Tc-MAA perfusion lung scans, McAdams et al (1996) showed medium-sized nodular or reticulonodular opacities in all chest radiographs. The opacities were always located in the lung bases and bilaterally in all but one patient. No purely linear opacities were identified, lung volumes were always normal and lung vessels were equally engorged in both the apices and bases. In a few cases there was also mild enlargement of the central pulmonary arteries. Of more interest were the thoracic computer tomography (CT) findings that showed distal vascular dilatations in all cases; these always coexisted with an abnormally large number of visible terminal branches that did not taper normally and therefore extended to the pleural surface (Figure 3). The degree of CT scan abnor-malities roughly correlated with the degree of hypoxaemia and severity of dyspnoea. Yet, no macroscopic arteriovenous malformations, nor evidence of pulmonary fibrosis as the cause of abnormal opacities, were visible on CT scans. In the experience of the authors (McAdams et al, 1996), these vascular opacities sometimes resemble irregular linear opacities of pulmonary fibrosis on CT scans. The absence of other classical CT images that relate to lung fibrosis, such as honeycombing, architectural distortion, traction bronchiectasis, septal lines and/or ground-glass deformities, excludes this diagnosis. All these findings are better shown by conventional CT scans than by high-resolution CT scans. Moreover, it is of note that the use of CT scans in this clinical setting helps to soundly exclude other more common causes of arterial hypoxaemia, such as the features of chronic obstructive pulmonary disease or pulmonary fibrosis.

Cardiac catheterization may reveal normal or low pulmonary pressures whilst intracardiac shunts are absent. Similarly, pulmonary hypertension is absent in HPS. Pulmonary angiography may show three different patterns (Krowka et al, 1993). The most common, Type 1, corresponds to a 'spongy' appearance of a distal arterial tree with multiple vessels (Type 1-moderate). These patients have normal or nearly normal PaO_2 that increases abruptly during 100% O_2 breathing; yet the Type 1 pattern can be also more

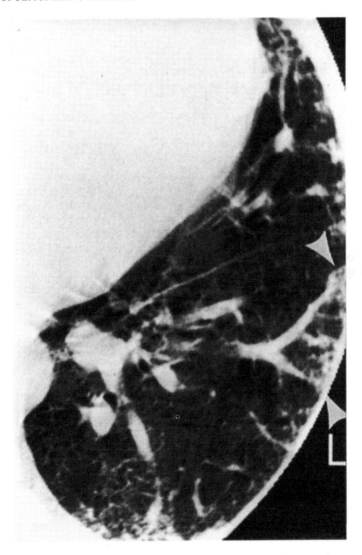

Figure 3. High-resolution CT (lung window) coned to left lung showing vascular dilatations of the lung extending to pleura and an abnormally large number of visible branches. The arrows indicate subpleural vascular opacities resembling telangiectasias (taken with permision from McAdams et al, 1996).

developed (Type 1-advanced). In Type 2 pattern, individual arteriovenous communications are notorious and the patients are hypoxaemic and severely dyspnoeic at rest, and show a poor response to 100% O_2 breathing. Angiography is not necessary for the diagnosis of HPS. Although these vascular deformities are indistinguishable, from an imaging diagnostic viewpoint, from those seen in hereditary haemorrhagic telangiectasia

(Rendu–Osler syndrome), the former never bleed and are not a cause of haemoptysis. Systemic hypotension, a low pulmonary artery pressure, an inordinately high cardiac output and a reduced pulmonary vascular reactivity are the four haemodynamic hallmarks of HPS. Furthermore, the combination of arterial hypoxaemia, with normal or low pulmonary artery pressure, and the presence of finger clubbing in a patient with advanced liver disease should strongly suggest the diagnosis of HPS. In a rat model of biliary cirhosis (Chang and Ohara, 1992), it was observed that hepatic cirrhosis-induced gas exchange abnormalities were related to a reversible ablation of hypoxic pulmonary vasoconstriction. This experimental attenuated pulmonary vascular reactivity, which was restored following angiotensin II, was interpreted as partial reversibility of the depressed hypoxic vascular response. It was postulated therefore that circulating vasodilating substances in liver cirrhosis may lead to accumulation of intracellular cGMP and/or cAMP, hence resulting in generalized vaso-dilatation with abolished hypoxic pulmonary vasocontriction (see below, Pathogenesis).

Although data describing the natural history of HPS are scarce, it appears that HPS can have a progressive and life-threatening evolution. In a small study followed at the Mayo Clinic, four out of seven patients with HPS died within 4 years after initial diagnosis (Krowka et al, 1993).

PATHOPHYSIOLOGY

For many years, low arterial oxygenation in patients with cirrhosis had been imputed to one or more of the following mechanisms (Agustí et al, 1990): changes in the affinity of oxyhaemoglobin, both intrapulmonary and portopulmonary shuntings, limitation of alveolar-capillary diffusion for O_2 and ventilation-perfusion ($\dot{V}_A/\dot{Q}$) imbalance, the latter being caused by an increased closing volume (Ruff et al, 1971) and/or failure of hypoxic pulmonary vasoconstriction to develop (Daoud et al, 1972; Naeije et al, 1981). By contrast, the fourth well-known intrapulmonary determinant of hypoxaemia, alveolar hypoventilation, is always absent. In fact, patients with liver cirrhosis characteristically hyperventilate such that $PaCO_2$ always tends to be, or is, decreased.

The rightward shift in the O_2 dissociation curve, namely decreased affinity of oxyhaemoglobin, appears to be related to an increased concen-tration of 2,3-diphosphoglycerate within the red blood cell. Notwith-standing, this right-shift of the O_2 dissociation curve cannot explain by itself the levels observed of arterial hypoxaemia (Agustí et al, 1990). Yet, the relevance of the three other intrapulmonary mechanisms has remained unsettled. Cigarette smoking, a common feature in patients with alcoholic cirrhosis, enhances closing volume and produces a dysfunction of the small airways resulting in airflow obstruction, hence leading to both a mild decrease of diffusing capacity and a slight ventilation-perfusion ($\dot{V}_A/\dot{Q}$) heterogeneity. The use of the multiple inert gas elimination technique (MIGET), a state-of-the-art, robust tool with the ability to estimate the functional distribution of $\dot{V}_A/\dot{Q}$ ratios in the lung and also to unravel the interaction between the intrapulmonary (see above) and extrapulmonary (more specifically, overall ventilation, O_2 consumption and cardiac output) factors influencing arterial blood gases, represents a major breakthrough in our understanding of pulmonary gas exchange in HPS (Rodriguez-Roisin et al, 1987). Using MIGET the role of $\dot{V}_A/\dot{Q}$ distributions and intrapulmonary shunting on pulmonary gas exchange has been investigated extensively, and includes a wide spectrum of patients with liver cirrhosis and different degrees of abnormal hypoxaemia.

In a seminal study, the role of $\dot{V}_A/\dot{Q}$ mismatch in patients with cirrhosis with mild-to-moderate hepatocellular dysfunction was investigated (Rodriguez-Roisin et al, 1987). Under baseline conditions, there was mild systemic and pulmonary vasodilatation, a normal PaO_2, mild hypocapnia, a small shift to the right of the oxyhaemoglobin dissociation curve and normal diffusing capacity. Yet, the underlying $\dot{V}_A/\dot{Q}$ distributions displayed mild $\dot{V}_A/\dot{Q}$ imbalance, namely a small proportion of blood flow perfused areas with low $\dot{V}_A/\dot{Q}$ ratios; by contrast, intrapulmonary shunting was conspicuously trivial, neither was diffusion limited for O_2. When patients breathed 11% O_2, both pulmonary artery pressure and vascular resistance increased but $\dot{V}_A/\dot{Q}$ distributions remained unvaried; yet, when patients breathed 100% O_2 a small degree of shunt (< 2% of cardiac output) became ostensible and there was some deterioration of $\dot{V}_A/\dot{Q}$ inequalities without haemodynamic changes. This study confirmed not only a reduced pulmonary vasopressor tone as previously shown (Daoud et al, 1972; Naeije et al, 1981), but also the presence of some pulmonary vasoconstriction and that these were consistent with the insufficient pulmonary vascular tone that enhanced the development of alveolar units with low $\dot{V}_A/\dot{Q}$ ratios. From a pathophysiological viewpoint, it is of note that when the hypoxic vascular response is enhanced $\dot{V}_A/\dot{Q}$ mismatch is ameliorated; and, vice versa, when the pulmonary vasomotor tone is minimized or abolished the matching between ventilation and perfusion deteriorates (Wagner and Rodriguez-Roisin, 1991). If the site of hypoxic pulmonary vasoconstriction is in small arteries (in vessels less than 500 µm in diameter), as it supposedly is, then it is clear that all the structural vascular derangement will disrupt the ability of the pulmonary circulation to constrict in response to alveolar hypoxia.

Mélot et al (1989) further studied the contribution of both intra-pulmonary and extrapulmonary determinants of PaO_2 in patients with liver cirrhosis, a majority of whom had mild-to-moderate hypoxaemia that was essentially caused by $\dot{V}_A/\dot{Q}$ disturbances. In patients with non-alcoholic liver cirrhosis, most of whom were non-smokers, with mild degrees of hypoxaemia, hypoxaemia could be accounted for by a combination of intrapulmonary shunting and $\dot{V}_A/\dot{Q}$ mismatch (Hedenstierna et al, 1991) (Figure 4). Based on the principles of MIGET it was also suggested that O_2 diffusion limitation could coexist in these patients. In another study conducted on patients with cirrhosis and severe hypoxaemia, there were high levels of intrapulmonary shunting (above 15–20% of cardiac output) along with an increased $\dot{V}_A/\dot{Q}$ heterogeneity, which was essentially related to low $\dot{V}_A/\dot{Q}$ ratios and each contributed nearly half to the underlying hypoxaemia (Edell et al, 1989); likewise, a component of mild diffusion impairment was shown.

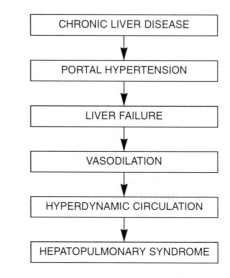

Figure 4. Suggestive scheme of the pathogenesis of HPS (for further explanation, see text).

Castaing and Manier (1989) confirmed even larger shunts and mild $\dot{V}_A/\dot{Q}$ mismatch in a small series of patients with cirrhosis and severe hypoxaemia, as well as the coexistence of diffusion limitation for O_2, which was probably related to post-pulmonary (bronchial and thebesian veins) and/or extrapulmonary (i.e. portopulmonary communications) shunting. However, based on the relatively high PO_2 in the portal circulation and the relatively small percentage of cardiac output contributing to splanchnic blood flow, it is questionable whether the mechanism of portopulmonary shunts could contribute significantly to hypoxaemia. Agustí et al (1989) investigated normoxaemic patients with cirrhosis before and during exercise, and showed that exercise did not alter the efficiency of the lung as a gas exchanger. During exercise, $\dot{V}_A/\dot{Q}$ mismatching remained unchanged and there was no diffusion limitation for O_2. They observed that $\dot{V}_A/\dot{Q}$ heterogeneity at rest did not result in arterial hypoxaemia, because both the high minute ventilation and cardiac output values maintained PaO_2 within the normal range by their respective well-known effects on alveolar PO_2 and mixed venous PO_2, respectively (West, 1969). The high cardiac output in these patients, a common haemodynamic finding of patients with liver cirrhosis (Martini et al, 1972), is one of the principal mechanisms of adjustment of gas exchange in pulmonary medicine (Rodriguez-Roisin and Wagner, 1989), the most influential one being through the O_2 content of the mixed venous blood (Dantzker, 1983).

Both Andrivet et al (1993) and our group (Martínez-Pallí et al, 1996) have confirmed the $\dot{V}_A/\dot{Q}$ findings alluded to, including the influence of a major component of intrapulmonay shunting in hepatic patients with extreme hypoxaemia; by contrast, no role for diffusion impairment was observed. Recently, using two complementary techniques, MIGET and intravenous radiolabelled particles, Crawford et al (1995) have interpreted the findings of a single anecdotal case report as convincing evidence that alveolar-capillary diffusion disequilibrium for O_2 related to intrapulmonary vascular dilatations contributes critically to the development of arterial hypoxaemia.

One of the most intriguing questions in HPS is the reduction of diffusing capacity (transfer factor), whose mechanism still remains elusive. At first glance, the combination of a widespread pulmonary vasodilatation with low or even absent pulmonary vascular tone, as a hallmark of the disorder, and, second, an inordinately elevated cardiac output, should both facilitate an increased diffusing capacity, other things being equal. A 'diffusion-perfusion defect' has also been implicated for explaining a diffusion gradient for O_2 in dilated pulmonary vessels (Genovesi et al, 1976; Thorens and Junod, 1992). It was postulated that the widespread pulmonary vaso-dilatation at the capillary or precapillary level in cirrhosis would cause not only substantial $\dot{V}_A/\dot{Q}$ inequality, characterized by low $\dot{V}_A/\dot{Q}$ ratios, but also that there may be inadequate diffusion of O_2 to the centre of the enlarged capillaries in the lung, which would result in partially deoxygenated blood and hence in alveolar–capillary disequilibrium for O_2. The coexistence of a high cardiac output commonly found in patients with liver cirrhosis, thus resulting in a shorter transit time, would exaggerate further this functional abnormality. However, we visualize this 'diffusion-perfusion defect' as possibly reflecting an example of $\dot{V}_A/\dot{Q}$ inequality with some degree of diffusion limitation rather than a diffusion impairment for O_2 by itself.

Thus, the intriguing question of whether blood flow through the dilated pulmonary capillary vessels constitutes intrapulmonary shunting, $\dot{V}_A/\dot{Q}$ mismatch or diffusion disequilibrium for O_2, may be ultimately answered by saying that it is probably a combination of all three, at least in those patients with more severe hypoxaemia (Rodriguez-Roisin et al, 1992). When HPS is mild, the predominant mechanism is $\dot{V}_A/\dot{Q}$ imbalance, whereas intrapulmonary shunting emerges as the capital factor when the severity of HPS is extreme, a situation in which diffusion limitation for O_2 can also coexist. Furthermore, HPS is the only clinical condition in pulmonary medicine in which a high intrapulmonary shunt, resulting in severe hypoxaemia, is associated with a normal or low pulmonary artery pressure. In the other two disorders in which similar high levels of intra-pulmonary shunting are detected, namely acute respiratory distress syndrome (ARDS) and life-threatening pneumonia, pulmonary hyper-tension is a hallmark of the disorder. The response of PaO_2 to 100% O_2 breathing may be also of help to the clinician to predict the principal intra-pulmonary mechanism of hypoxaemia in HPS. If PaO_2 remains essentially unchanged while breathing 100% O_2, then the predominant underlying determinant should be intrapulmonary shunting because of the presence of truly arteriovenous communications, although with more moderate increases of PaO$_2$, i.e. less than 500 mmHg, this still cannot be ruled out. On the contrary, a substantial rise of PaO_2, above 600 mmHg, eliminates the existence of intrapulmonary shunt such that $\dot{V}_A/\dot{Q}$ heterogeneity arises as the major factor influencing abnormal PaO_2.

PATHOGENESIS

Irrespective of the specific pathogenesis of HPS, it can be postulated that chronic liver disease together with portal hypertension and perhaps portosystemic shunting will induce hepatic failure, and thereby a wide-spread vasodilatation with a hyperkinetic status results ultimately in HPS (Figure 4). However, the precise mechanism underlying HPS still remains unsettled despite numerous investigations. Whether the precise mechanism underlying the vascular systemic and pulmonary disturbances in HPS is related to failure of metabolism or insufficiency of production of one or several circulating vasoactive substances by the damaged liver cells, or to altered metabolism of some of the recently discovered paracrine factors synthetized by endothelial cells (Vanhoutte, 1988), remains to be determined. A large body of potential circulating humoral vasodilating agents, including glucagon and prostacyclin, have been detected. The latter probably contributes to vascular disturbances in patients with chronic liver diseases, including a blunted hypoxic pulmonary vasoconstriction. Notwithstanding, clear evidence of their involvement is yet needed (Rodriguez-Roisin et al, 1992).

Glucagon has been shown to be increased experimentally in a rat model of pre-hepatic portal hypertension, and clinically in patients with portal hypertension and portosystemic shunting (Groszmann, 1994). Other studies have failed to show a closer relationship between the degree of vaso-dilatation and circulating levels of glucagon both in animals (Sikuler and Groszmann, 1986) and in patients with HPS (Krowka et al, 1993). The infusion of somatostatin, an inhibitor of glucagon release, which induces vasoconstriction of the splanchnic and systemic circulations, did not influence pulmonary gas exchange abnormalities in patients with HPS (Krowka et al, 1993), hence suggesting that somatostatin may be mediated by other peptides in addition to glucagon release. Other endogenous vasodilators have also been investigated as potential humoral mediators of the hyperdynamic circulatory hallmarks of HPS. Prostacyclin (PGI$_2$) also could play a role in mediating the haemodynamic status of HPS.

Another endothelium-derived vasodilator in which recent interest has been also placed is nitric oxide (NO), a ubiquitous biological agent considered to be a fine tuner of vascular tone and now identified to be a key signalling molecule that is potentially involved in the pathophysiology of many diseases (Moncada and Higgs, 1993). Because NO behaves as a selective vasodilator within the lung, it has been implicated in the cardio-vascular changes associated with HPS (Vallance and Moncada, 1991). Based on the observation that animal studies indicate that bacterial endotoxin and cytokines induce NO synthase expression within the vessel walls, with sustained NO release and subsequent hypotension, and that endotoxaemia is a common finding in patients with liver cirrhosis, Vallance and Moncada (1991) postulated that persistent induction of NO synthase may account for the hyperkinetic features of HPS. NO is synthesized from the natural amino acid L-arginine by the action of a family of enzymes, also known as NO synthases (NOS) with varying subtypes in different tissues, possibly encoded by the same gene, such that three different isoforms of NOS have been identified. Constitutive isoforms (cNOS) are expressed in neurones (nNOS or Type I NOS) and endothelial cells (eNOS or Type III NOS) of the airways (Kobzik et al, 1993). The third isoform of NOS is not expressed in normal cells, but is induced by pro-inflammatory cytokines and endotoxin (iNOS or Type II NOS). Inducible NOS is expressed in target tissues after exposure to pro-inflammatory cytokines, such as human bronchial epithelial cells, and is expressed in the airway epithelium of patients with asthma but not in normal individuals.

Synthesis of NO by the iNOS pathway in the walls of the vessels is responsible of the vasodilatation that occurs in septic shock (Thiemerman and Vane, 1990). Endotoxins activate cytokine production, hence inducing NO synthesis with subsequent vasodilatation. Among the repertoire of cytokines, tumour necrosis factor (TNF) has been shown to mimic the clinical spectrum of septic shock both in animals and humans. This cytokine, derived from macrophages and/or lymphocytes, is known to induce a hyperkinetic status in mammals by activating NO synthesis (Kilbourn et al, 1990). It has been hypothesized that in the endotoxaemia of cirrhosis, high levels of circulating endotoxin are observed even in patients with cirrhosis who do not have clinical evidence of infection, and who directly induce NO synthase in peripheral blood vessels or indirectly, through cytokines release (Fong et al, 1990). This increased NO synthesis and release could therefore account for the hyperdynamic situation of HPS (Vallance and Moncada, 1991; Jiménez, 1995).

Consistent with this hypothesis, we have found that the levels of exhaled NO in patients with HPS have a trend to be greater compared with patients without HPS, and are significantly increased compared with controls (Martínez-Pallí et al, 1996). Cremona et al (1995) showed that three patients with HPS had increased exhaled NO levels compared with patients with liver cirrhosis without HPS and with normal controls, who were either breathing room air or a hypoxic mixture. Furthermore, the increased levels of exhaled NO decreased sharply after LT in one patient, while arterial O_2 saturation returned to normal values, thereby suggesting that increased NO within the lung may contribute to the development of HPS. In another report, methylene blue increased systemic arterial pressure and reversed arterial hypoxaemia in a patient with HPS (Rolla et al, 1994). Methylene blue is an oxidizing agent that blocks the stimulation of soluble guanylate cyclase by NO. This inhibitory effect of methylene blue has been attributed to a direct effect on guanylate cyclase or the generation of superoxide or both. Matsumoto et al (1995) showed that patients with clinically unstable liver cirrhosis had greater levels of exhaled NO than those with stable disease or controls; cardiac index, more elevated in patients with liver disturbances, was correlated linearly with exhaled NO. Similarly, Sogni et al (1995) also showed increased levels of exhaled NO in patients with severe liver cirrhosis that were negatively correlated with pulmonary vascular resistance. All these findings point to a main role for NO, in that increased exhaled NO is associated with, and even may contribute to, systemic haemodynamic abnormalities in patients with advanced liver disease. Of equal importance is that enhanced pulmonary production of endogenous NO could contribute to the development of HPS.

THERAPEUTIC APPROACH

Except for a few anecdotal cases, including patients with HPS who recover spontaneously, a variety of medical agents including garlic preparations have been used in the treatment of HPS without substantial improvement in outcome (Table 4). Theoretically, these agents hold promise because of their effect on enhancing generalized widespread pulmonary vasoconstriction, this would be the case of bismesilate almitrine; or for blocking vasodilatation with, for example propranolol. Alternatively, invasive therapeutic procedures, such as embolization of peripheral small vessel arteriovenous fistulae or plasma exchange, have also been disappointing (Krowka and Cortese, 1994). Slightly more encouraging has been the experience of portal decompression after transjugular intrahepatic portosystemic shunting (TIPS) as a palliative approach in a patient with HPS awaiting for LT (Riegler et al, 1995).

By contrast, LT has been shown to be a much more promising therapeutic approach for HPS (Rodriguez-Roisin and Krowka, 1994). The contention is that the replacement of the injured liver antagonizes or minimizes all the systemic and pulmonary haemodynamic consequences induced by HPS, thereby improving gas exchange abnormalities. The experience with LT in the setting for HPS still remains unsettled. A review of the literature shows that there were 41 cases with reversal or improvement of arterial

Table 4. Medical treatments used in hepatopulmonary syndrome.

Agent	N	Improvement
Almitrine	11	1 Patient
Prostaglandin	1	Yes
Indomethacin	6	None
Plasma exchange	5	None
Somatostatin	18	1 Patient
Cyclophosphamide	1	Yes
Propranolol	8	None
Garlic preparation	1	Yes
Methylene blue	1	Yes

Except for methylene blue, (Rolla et al, 1994) the other data are taken from Rodriguez-Roisin and Krowka (1994) and Rodriguez-Roisin et al (1992).

hypoxaemia related to HPS over the last 25 years, but also 13 failures (Lange and Stoller, 1996). Recently we reviewed 22 reports of end-stage liver disease with severe resting hypoxaemia (PaO_2 <65 mmHg) and found that all but two patients showed a complete or partial resolution of all gas exchange disturbances after LT (Rodriguez-Roisin and Krowka, 1994).

The predictors of reversibility of LT in HPS are still elusive (Lange and Stoller, 1996). Firstly, it is shown that youth may favour responsiveness of HPS, possibly because better cardiorespiratory reserve and/or intrinsic differences in the underlying intrapulmonary vascular dilatations facilitate better closure of arteriovenous communications after LT. Secondly, the response of PaO_2 to 100% O_2 breathing and the degree of severity of pre-operative arterial hypoxaemia may also need to be taken into account. The greater the response of PaO_2 to 100% O_2 and the greater the basal pre-operative PaO_2, suggesting less intrapulmonary shunting and a greater $\dot{V}_A/\dot{Q}$ mismatch as the main component of abnormal gas exchange, the greater and the faster the improvement of HPS after LT. Current experience suggests that restoration of arterial oxygenation takes several months after LT if the prime mechanism of hypoxaemia is intrapulmonary shunting, whereas abnormal gas exchange is improved quickly, within a few weeks, when the principal determinant is $\dot{V}_A/\dot{Q}$ heterogeneity (Eriksson, 1991). This would indicate that while $\dot{V}_A/\dot{Q}$ mismatch is an early, reversible, component of abnormal gas exchange, the development of intrapulmonary shunting gives evidence of a more severe, advanced pulmonary vascular involvement.

Two years ago we would have answered the question as to whether or not severe arterial hypoxaemia, caused by hepatic disease, was an indication for LT (Rodriguez-Roisin and Krowka, 1994), with the term of hypoxaemia being synonymous with HPS; now we could ask *when* LT is indicated for HPS. Possibly, any clinical condition in which hypoxaemia or related manifestations in a patient with advanced liver disease is life-threatening can be the right answer. However, several challenging questions about the natural history, pathogenesis and role of LT HPS are as yet concealed. Conceivably, these issues will be the target for future research.

REFERENCES

Agustí AGN, Roca J, Rodriguez-Roisin R et al (1989) Pulmonary hemodynamics and gas exchange during exercise in liver cirrhosis. *American Review of Respiratory Disease* **139:** 485–491.

Agustí AGN, Roca J, Bosch J & Rodriguez-Roisin R (1990) The lung in patients with cirrhosis. *Journal of Hepatology* **10:** 251–257.

Andrivet P, Cadranel J, Housset B et al (1993) Mechanisms for impaired arterial oxygenation in patients with liver cirrhosis and severe respiratory insufficiency: effects of indomethacin. *Chest* **103:** 500–507.

*Berthelot P, Walker JG, Sherlock S & Reid L (1966) Arterial changes in the lungs in cirrhosis of the liver-lung spider nevi. *New England Journal of Medicine* **274:** 291–298.

Calabresi P & Abelmann WH (1957) Portocaval and porto-pulmonary anastomoses in Laennec's cirrhosis and in heart failure. *Journal of Clinical Investigation* **36:** 1257–1265.

Castaing Y & Manier G (1989) Hemodynamic disturbances and $\dot{V}_A/\dot{Q}$ matching in hypoxemic cirrhotic patients. *Chest* **96:** 1064–1069.

Castro M & Krowka MJ (1996) Hepatopulmonary syndrome: a pulmonary vascular complication of liver disease. *Clinics in Chest Medicine* **17**: 35–48.

Castro M, Krowka MJ, Beck KC et al (1994) Survival in liver transplant patients with pulmonary hypertension—correlation with pulmonary function (abstract). *American Journal of Respiratory and Critical Care Medicine* **149**: A734.

*Chang S & Ohara N (1992) Pulmonary circulatory dysfunction in rats with biliary cirrhosis. An animal model of the hepatopulmonary syndrome. *American Review of Respiratory Disease* **145**: 798–805.

Crawford ABH, Regnis J, Laks L et al (1995) Pulmonary vascular dilatation and diffusion-dependent impairment of gas exchange in liver cirrhosis. *European Respiratory Journal* **8**: 2015–2021.

*Cremona G, Higenbottam T, Mayoral V et al (1995) Elevated exhaled nitric oxide in patients with hepatopulmonary syndrome. *European Respiratory Journal* **8**: 1883–1885.

Dantzker DR (1983) The influence of cardiovascular function on gas exchange. *Clinics in Chest Medicine* **4**: 149–159.

Daoud FS, Reeves JT & Schaefer JW (1972) Failure of hypoxic pulmonary vasoconstriction in patients with liver cirrhosis. *Journal of Clinical Investigation* **51**: 1076–1080.

Edell ES, Cortese DE, Krowka MJ & Rehder K (1989) Severe hypoxemia and liver disease. *American Review of Respiratory Disease* **140**: 1631–1635.

Eriksson LS (1991) Is intrapulmonary arteriovenous shunting and hypoxemia a contraindication for liver transplantation? *Hepatology* **14**: 575–576.

Eriksson LS, Söderman C, Wahren J et al (1988) Is hypoxemia in cirrhotic patients due to a functional 'hepato-pulmonal syndrome'? (abstract). *Journal of Hepatology* **1 (Supplement 1)**: S29.

Fahy JV, Kerr KM, Lake JR et al (1991) Pulmonary function before and after liver transplantation (abstract). *American Review of Respiratory Disease* **145**: A303.

Flückiger M (1884) Vorkommen von trommelschägerformigen Fingerendphalangen ohne chronische Veränderungen der Lungen oder am Herzen. *Wiener Medizinische Wochenschrift* **49**: 1457–1458.

Fong Y, Marano MA, Moldawer LL et al (1990) The acute splanchnic and peripheral tissue metabolic response to endotoxin in humans. *Journal of Clinical Investigation* **85**: 1896–1904.

Genovesi MG, Tierney DF, Taplin GV & Eisenberg H (1976) An intravenous radionuclide method to evaluate hypoxemia caused by abnormal alveolar vessels. *American Review of Respiratory Disease* **114**: 59–65.

Georg J, Mellemgaard K, Tysgrup N & Winkler K (1960) Venoarterial shunts in cirrhosis of the liver. *Lancet* **i**: 852–854.

Groszmann RJ (1994) Vasodilatation and hyperdynamic circulatory state in chronic liver disease. In Bosch J & Groszmann RJ (eds) *Portal Hypertension. Pathophysiology and Treatment*, pp 17–26. Oxford: Blackwell Scientific Publications.

Hedenstierna G, Söderman C, Eriksson LS & Wahren J (1991) Ventilation-perfusion inequality in patients with non-alcoholic liver cirrhosis. *European Respiratory Journal* **4**: 711–717.

Hopkins WE, Waggoner AD & Barzilai B (1992) Frequency and significance of intrapulmonary right-to-left shunting in end-stage hepatic disease. *American Journal of Cardiology* **70**: 516–519.

Hourani JM, Bellamy PE, Tashkin DP et al, (1991) Pulmonary dysfunction in advanced liver disease: frequent occurrence of an abnormal diffusing capacity. *American Journal of Medicine* **90**: 693–700.

Jiménez W (1995) Endotelina, óxido nítrico y control de tono vascular: importancia fisiopatológica en la cirrosis hepática. *Medicina Clinica* (Barc) **104**: 671–675.

Kennedy TC & Knudson RJ (1977) Exercise-aggravated hypoxemia and orthodeoxia in cirrhosis. *Chest* **72**: 305–309.

Kilbourn RG, Gross SS, Jubran A et al (1990) N^G-methyl-L-arginine inhibits tumor necrosis factor induced hypotension: implications for the involvement of nitric oxide. *Proceedings of the National Academy of Science USA* **87**: 3629–3632.

Kobzik L, Bredt DS, Lowenstein CJ et al (1993) Nitric oxide synthase in human and rat lung: immunocytochemical and histochemical localization. *American Journal of Respiratory and Cell Molecular Biology* **9**: 371–377.

*Krowka MJ & Cortese DA (1989) Pulmonary aspects of liver disease and liver transplantation. *Clinics in Chest Medicine* **10**: 593–616.

Krowka MJ & Cortese DA (1990) Hepatopulmonary syndrome. *Chest* **98**: 1053–1054.

Krowka MJ & Cortese DA (1994) Hepatopulmonary syndrome. Current concepts in diagnostic and therapeutic considerations. *Chest* **105**: 1528–1537.

*Krowka MJ, Dickson ER & Cortese DA (1993) Hepatopulmonary syndrome: clinical observations and lack of therapeutic response to somatostatin analogue. *Chest* **104**: 515–521.

Krowka MJ, Dickson ER, Wiesner RH et al (1992) A prospective study of pulmonary function and gas exchange following liver transplantation. *Chest* **102**: 1161–1166.

*Lange PA & Stoller JK (1996) The hepatopulmonary syndrome: effect of liver transplantation. *Clinics in Chest Medicine* **17**: 115–124.

McAdams P, Erasmus J, Crokett R et al (1996) The hepatopulmonary syndrome: radiologic findings in 10 patients. *American Journal of Radiology* **166**: 1379–1385.

Marks SA, Krowka MJ & Plevak DJ (1996) Prevalence of preperative hypoxemia in liver transplant (LT) patients, and relation to post transplant course. *American Journal of Respiratory and Critical Care Medicine* **153**: A827.

Martínez-Pallí G, Barberà JA, Visa J et al (1996) Hepatopulmonary syndrome: prevalence and clinical markers (abstract). *European Respiratory Journal* **9**: 179s.

Martini GA, Baltzer G & Arndt H (1972) Some aspects of circulatory disturbances in cirrhosis of the liver. *Progress in Liver Disease* **4**: 231–250.

*Matsumoto A, Ogura K, Hirata Y et al (1995) Increased nitric oxide in the exhaled air of patients with decompensated liver cirrhosis. *Annals of Internal Medicine* **123**: 110–113.

Mélot C, Naeije R, Dechamps P et al (1989) Pulmonary and extrapulmonary factors to hypoxemia in liver cirrhosis. *American Review of Respiratory Disease* **139**: 632–640.

Moncada S & Higgs A (1993) The L-arginine–nitric oxide pathway. *New England Journal of Medicine* **329**: 2002–2012.

Naeije R, Hallemans R, Mols P & Mélot C (1981) Hypoxic pulmonary vasoconstriction in liver cirrhosis. *Chest* **80**: 570–574.

Raffy O, Sleiman C, Vachiery F et al (1996) Refractory hypoxemia during liver cirrhosis. Hepatopulmonary syndrome or 'primary' pulmonary hypertension? *American Journal of Respiratory and Critical Care Medicine* **153**: 1169–1171.

Riegler JL, Lang KA, Johnson SP & Westerman JH (1995) Transjugular intrahepatic portosystemic shunt improves oxygenation in hepatopulmonary syndrome. *Gastroenterology* **109**: 978–983.

Rodman T, Hurwitz JK, Pastor BH & Close HP (1959) Cyanosis, clubbing and arterial oxygen unsaturation associated with Laennec's cirrhosis. *American Journal of Medical Science* **238**: 534–541.

Rodriguez-Roisin R (1995) Síndrome hepatopulmonar: un nuevo concepto. Un tratamiento nuevo? *Medicina Clínica* (Barc) **105**: 269–274.

Rodriguez-Roisin R & Wagner PD (1989) Clinical relevance of ventilation-perfusion inequality determined by inert gas elimination. *European Respiratory Journal* **3**: 469–482.

Rodriguez-Roisin R & Krowka MJ (1994) Is arterial hypoxaemia due to hepatic disease an indication for liver transplantation? A new therapeutic approach. *European Respiration Journal* **7**: 839–842.

*Rodriguez-Roisin R, Agustí AGN & Roca J (1992) The hepatopulmonary syndrome: new name, old complexities. *Thorax* **47**: 897–902.

*Rodriguez-Roisin R, Roca J, Agustí AGN et al (1987) Gas exchange and pulmonary vascular reactivity in patients with liver cirrhosis. *American Review of Respiratory Disease* **135**: 1085–1092.

Rolla G, Bucca C & Brussino L (1994) Methylene blue in the hepatopulmonary syndrome (letters to editor). *New England Journal of Medicine* **331**: 1098.

Ruff F, Hughes JMB, Stanley NN et al (1971) Regional lung function in patients with hepatic cirrhosis. *Journal of Clinical Investigation* **50**: 2403–2413.

Rydell R & Hoffbauer FW (1956) Multiple pulmonary arteriovenous fistulas in juvenile cirrhosis. *American Journal of Medicine* **21**: 450–460.

Sherlock S (1989) *Disorders of the Liver and the Biliary System*. 8th edn, pp 82–86. Oxford: Blackwell Scientific.

Sikuler E & Groszmann RJ (1986) Hemodynamic studies in long and short term portal hypertensive rats: the relation to systemic glucagon levels. *Hepatology* **6**: 414–418.

Sogni P, Garnier P, Adano A et al (1995) Endogenous pulmonary nitric oxide production measured from exhaled air is increased in patients with hepatic cirrhosis. *Journal of Hepatology* **23**: 471–473.

Thiemerman C & Vane J (1990) Inhibition of nitric oxide synthesis reduces the hypotension induced by bacterial lipopolysaccharides in the rat *in vivo*. *European Journal of Pharmacology* **182**: 591–595.

Thorens JB & Junod AF (1992) Hypoxaemia and liver cirrhosis: a new argument in favour of a 'diffusion-perfusion defect'. *European Respiratory Journal* **5:** 754–756.

*Vallance P & Moncada S (1991) Hyperdynamic circulation in cirrhosis: a role for nitric oxide? *Lancet* **337:** 776–778.

Vanhoutte PM (1988) The endothelium-moderator of vascular smooth muscle tone. *New England Journal of Medicine* **319:** 512–513.

Wagner PD & Rodriguez-Roisin R (1991) Clinical advances in pulmonary gas exchange. *American Review of Respiratory Disease* **143:** 883–888.

West JB (1969) Ventilation–perfusion inequality and overall gas exchange in computer lung models of the lung. *Respiratory Physiology* **7:** 88–110.

Williams A, Trewby P, Williams R & Reid L (1979) Structural alterations to the pulmonary circulation in fulminant hepatic failure. *Thorax* **34:** 447–453.

Index

Note: Page numbers of article titles are in **bold** type.

Abdominal collateral circulation, 222–223
Acetylcholine, 210, 214
Acrylates, for variceal obturation, 293
Acute variceal bleeding, 248–249, 296–300, 331–332
  duration of, 248
  mortality and, 248–249
  and TIPS, 331–332
  see also Portal hypertension *and also* Variceal bleeding
Adult respiratory distress syndrome (AARDS), 340, 399
Albumin, 368
Alcoholism, 206, 245, 250
Aldosterone, 367–368
Almitrine, 402–403
Amyloidosis, 206
Anaemia, 264
Angiotensin, 211, 367–368
Antibiotics, *see* Bacterial infections
Antinatriuresis, *see* Ascites
α_1-Antitrypsin deficiency, 389
Arginine vasopressin, *see* Vasopressin
Arterial oxygen, *see* Hepatopulmonary syndrome
Ascites, 251–252, **365–385**
  diuretics in, 372–373
  extrarenal factors in, 367–368
  formation of, theories of, 370–371
  intrarenal factors in, 368–369
  paracentesis and, 373–375
  refractory, and TIPS, 333–334
  renal dysfunction and, 366–367
  sodium restriction and, 372, 377
  splanchnic haemodynamics, 369–370
  treatment of, 372–377
Atenolol, 273–275
  see also Beta-blockers
Azygous blood flow, 226–227

Bacterial infections, 260, 292, 318
  and TIPS, 339–340
Bacterial peritonitis, 252
Balloon tamponade, 297–298, 316–317

Banding ligation, 293–296
  complications with, 295–296
  technique of, 295
Beta-blockers, 247–248, 251, 264–266, 273–275, 300–304
  with isosorbide-5-mononitrate, 281–282
  in prophylaxis, 280–282
  see also Propranolol
Bile acids, 208
Bleeding, acute, and surgery, 357–358
  see also Acute variceal bleeding *and also* Variceal bleeding
Bucrylate, 293, 304
Budd–Chiari syndrome, 209–210, 335–336

Calcium-channel blockers, 278
Caput medusae, 223
'Cherry red' spots, 246, 251
Child–Pugh score, 231, 247, 250, 253, 334
Cholestyramine, 208
Chylous fistula, 335
Cirrhosis, *see* Ascites, Portal hypertension *and also* Portal hypertensive gastropathy; *see also* Variceal bleeding *and* Alcoholism
Clonidine, 212–213, 276–277
Collateral circulation, *see* Portosystemic collateral resistance
Colour Doppler, 233
  see also Doppler sonography
Computed tomography, 236, 394–395
Congestion index, 232
'Congestive gastropathy', *see* Portal hypertensive gastropathy
Coronary-caval shunt, 355
Coronary vein, 228–229
Creatininaemia, 252
Cruveilhier–Baumgarten syndrome, 223
Cyclophosphamide, 402–403
Cyclosporin, 345
Cytokines, 401
  see also Endothelins *and also specific names of incl.* Prostaglandins

Devascularization, 356, 358, 361

Diffuse gastric lesions, *see* Portal hypertensive
    gastropathy
Dilutional hyponatraemia, 377
Distal splenorenal shunt, 355, 360
Diuretic-intractable ascites, 373
    see also Ascites
Diuretic-resistant ascites, 373
    see also Ascites
Diuretics, 277–278
Domperidome, 312
Doppler sonography, 228–236, 358
    collaterals, 229–231
    congestion index, 232
    of hepatic arteries, 232
    of hepatic veins, 233
    limitations of, 232
    mean portal velocity and, 231–232
    portal blood flow and, 232
    portal vein and, 228–232
    splanchnic arteries, 232
    splanchnic veins, 228–229
    and TIPS, 331
Drug therapy, for acute variceal haemorrhage,
    311–326
    see also Variceal bleeding
Duplex Doppler, 233
    see also Doppler sonography

Echocardiography, 391–396
Electyrolyte imbalances, *see under* Ascites
Encephalography, 343
Endoluminal sonography, 247
    see also Doppler sonography
Endoscopy, 223–224, **289–309**, 319–320
    banding ligation and, 293–296
    injection sclerotherapy, 290–292
    oesophagogastro-, 223
    of portal hypertensive gastropathy, 258–259
    sonography, 223–224
    variceal bleeding, 246
    variceal obturation, 293
Endothelial factors, 262–263
Endothelin receptors, 320
Endothelins, 320, 400–402
Endothelium, 207, 368
    nitric oxide and, 209–211
    prostaglandins and, 210–211
Erosion theory, 214–216
Ethanolamine oleate, 291, 304
Extrahepatic portal hypertension, 233–234

Furosemide, 373

Gallbladder varices, 229–230
Garlic, 402–403
Gastric antral vascular ectasia (GAVE), 258
Gastric varices, therapy of, 304
Gastrin, 262
Gastrointestinal bleeding, 236

see also Variceal bleeding
Glomerular filtration rate, 367
    and hepatorenal syndrome, 379–380
    see also Kidney
Glucagon, 208–209, 262, 400
Glucose-water solution, 304
Glypressin, 248, 266, 313, 316

'Haemorrhagic gastritis', *see* Portal hypertensive
    gastropathy
Helicobacter pylori, 260
Hepatic blood flow, 227
Hepatic encephalopathy, *see* Encephalopathy
Hepatic hydrothorax, 335–336
Hepatic vein obturation, 233, 235
Hepatic vein pressure, 224–225
    gradient (HVPG), *see under* Inferior vena
    cava pressure
Hepatitis, 206
Hepatopulmonary syndrome, 337, **387–406**
    cardiac catheterization in, 394–396
    computed tomography of, 394
    diagnosis of, 391–396
    diffusion–perfusion defect, 399
    echocardiography of, 391–396
    pathogenesis of, 400–402
    pathophysiology of, 396–400
    therapy of, 402–403
    ventilation–perfusion imbalance in, 396–
    400
Hepatorenal syndrome, 252, 377–381
    arterial vasodilatation theory, 378
    diagnosis of, 379–380
    glomerular filtration rate in, 379–380
    treatment of, 380–381
    type I, 379–381
    type II, 379–381
Histoacryl, 293
Hypersplenism, 222
Hyponatraemia, 377
    see also Ascites
Hypoxaemia, *see* Hepatopulmonary syndrome

Indomethacin, 210–211, 402–403
Infections, 252, 292
    in portal hypertensive gastropathy, 260
    and TIPS, 339–340
Inferior vena cava pressure, 245–248, 263, 278–
    279, 282, 283
Injection sclerotherapy, 290–293
    agents for, 291
    complications in, 291–292
    site of, 291
    technique of, 290
    timing of, 291
Intestinal varices, 335
Intrahepatic portal hypertension, 233
Intrahepatic resistance, 205–207
Intraperitoneal haemorrhage, 339

IPS, *see* Transjugular intrahepatic postsystemic shunt
Iron deficiency, 251, 263
Isoprenaline, 214
Isosorbide dinitrate, 275–279
Isosorbide-5-mononitrate, 275–279, 302
    with propranolol, 281–283

Ketanserin, 276
Kidney, 227, 366–369, 377–381
    and cirrhosis, **365–385**
    see also Hepatorenal syndrome

Laplace's law, 215, 225–226
Large volume paracentesis, 334
Leukotrienes, 368–369
    see also Endothelins
Liver—
    histology of, 206–207
    intrahepatic resistance of, 205–207
    see also Portal hypertension *and also* Hepatic *aspects*
Liver transplants, 227–228, 264, 356, 359, 376–377
    and TIPS, 334–335
Lungs, **387–406**
    haemodynamics of, 226
    and TIPS, 340

Mean portal velocity, 231
Methoxamine, 211
Metoclopramide, 314
MIGET, 396–397
Molsidomine, 276
Mosaic portal hypertensive gastropathy, 258–259
MRI, 236–238
Myofibroblasts, 207

Nadolol, 273–275, 302
    see also Beta-blockers
L-NAME, 210–211
Natriuresis, *see under* Ascites
Nicardepine, 278
Nifedipine, 278
Nipradilol, 279
Niravoline, 377
Nitrates, 302
    transdermal, 248
Nitric oxide, 207, 209–210, 262, 320, 369–370, 400–402
Nitroglycerin, 278, 318–320, 357
Nitrovasodilators, 275–276
Noradrenaline, 211, 214, 262
Norepinephrine, *see* Noradrenaline
Norfloxacin, 252
North Italian Endoscopic Club (NIEC), 247, 292

Octreotide, 212, 297–299, 301, 313–314, 316–320

in variceal bleeding prevention programmes, 300–302
Oedema, and ascites, 370–371
Oesophageal perforation, 292
Oesophageal varices, 212–214
    see also Portal hypertension *and also* Variceal bleeding
Oesophagogastro-endoscopy, 223
Ohm's law, 204
Omeprazole, 292
Omipressin, 379–380
κ-Opioid agonists, 377
Orthotopic liver transplantation, *see* Liver transplants
Oxygen, arterial, *see* Hepatopulmonary syndrome

Paracentesis, 373–375
Paraumbilical vein, 229–230
Partial shunts, 354–355
    see also Shunts
Patency, of shunts (TIPS), 341
    see also Shunts
Pericytes, 206–207
Peritoneovenous shunts, 376
    see also Shunts
Peritonitis, 252, 292
Physical laws, and portal hypertension—
    Laplace, 215, 225–226
    Ohm, 204
    Pouseuille, 204
Piperacillin, 340
Plasma volume, 211–212
Polidocanol, 291
Portal blood flow, 232
Portal hypertension—
    abdominal collateral circulation, 222–223
    acute, **311–326**
    aetiology of, by Doppler sonography, 233–235
    ascites in, **365–385**
    azygous blood flow, 226–227
    bleeding risk in, **243–256**
    clinical-haemodynamic correlations in, **243–256**
    collaterals, 229–231
    complications in, 236
    computed tomography in, 236
    diagnosis of, by Doppler sonography, 228–233
    Doppler sonography in, 228–236
    drug therapy, basis of, 216
    endoscopy in, *see under* Endoscopy
    evaluation of, **221–241**
        methods in, 222
    extrahepatic, 233
    factors involved in, 204–205
    gastrointestinal bleeding in, 236
    gastropathy, *see* Portal hypertensive gastropathy
    hepatic arteries, 232

Portal hypertension—(*cont.*)
  hepatic blood flow, 227
  hepatic veins, 233
  hepatic venous pressure, 224–225
  hepatodynamic circulation, 208–212
    plasma volume, 211–212
    systemic vasodilatation, 208–211
  intrahepatic, 233
  kidney function in, **365–385**; *see also* Hepato-
    renal syndrome
  lungs and, 226; *see also* Hepatopulmonary
    syndrome
  MRI of, 236–238
  natural history of, **243–256**
  Ohm's law and, 204
  outcome in, 252–254
  paraumbilical vein and, 229–230
  pathophysiology of, **203–219**
  portal vein and, 228–232
  portal venous pressure, 224–225
  and Pouseuille's law, 204
  splanchnic arteries and, 232
  splanchnic veins and, 228–229
  splenomegaly, 222
  suprahepatic, 233, 235
  surgery for, **351–364**
  TIPS and, **327–349**
  variceal pressure and, 225–226
Portal hypertensive gastropathy, 250–251, **257–
    270**
  anaemia in, 264
  classification of, 258
  clinical manifestations of, 263–264
  diagnosis of, 259
  endoscopy of, 258–259
  gastric mucosa in, 263
  Helicobacter pylori, 260
  histology of, 258–259
  mosaic, 258–259
  pathogenesis, 260–263
  prevalence of, 259–260
  red speckling in, 258–259
  scarlatina form of, 258–259
  snake skin pattern form of, 258–259
  therapy of, 264–266
  watermelon stomach in, 258–259
Portal pressure gradient, *see under* Inferior vena
    cava pressure
Portal vein thrombosis, 233–234
  and TIPS, 335–336
Portal venous pressure, 224–225
Portosystemic collateral resistance, 207–208
Portosystemic shunt, *see* Transjugular intra-
    hepatic portosystemic shunt
Pouseuille's law, 204
Prazosin, 277, 279
Pressure, *see* Portal hypertension
Prophylactic rubber band ligation, 296
Prophylactic sclerotherapy, 296

Propranolol, 212–214, 264–266, 273–275, 278–
    282, 402
  see also Beta-blockers
Prostacyclin (PGI₂), 210–211, 400
Prostaglandin E₂, 210
Prostaglandin I₂, *see* Prostacyclin
Prostaglandins, 210–211, 262, 368–369, 400
Pulmonary haemodynamics, 226
  see also under Lungs *and also* Hepato-
    pulmonary syndrome

Rebleeding, prevention by surgery, 358–361
Recurrent variceal bleeding, 249–250, 332–333
  see also Portal hypertension *and also* variceal
    bleeding
Red speckling, in portal hypertensive gastropathy,
    258–259
Refractory ascites, 373
  see also Ascites
Renal haemodynamics, 227
  see also Hepatorenal syndrome *and also*
    Kidney
Rendu–Osler syndrome, 396
Renin, 367–368
Renin–angiotensin system, 212
Resistance, in portal hypertension, 204–208
  intrahepatic, 205–207
  portosystemic collateral, 207–208
Ritanserin, 276
Rubber band ligation, 296, 297–298, 302–304

Salt restriction, 372
Scarlatina rash, 258–259
Schistosomiasis, 206
Sclerotherapy, 319–320
  emergency, 297–300
  injection, 290–292
  long-term, 300–304
  prophylactic, 296
  transplantation, *see* Liver transplants; *see also*
    Shunts
Secretin, 262
Selective shunts, 355
  see also Shunts
Serotonin S2-receptor blockers, 276
Shunts, 359–361
  coronary-caval, 355
  dislodgement of, 339
  distal splenorenal, 355, 360
  partial, 354–355, 360
  peritoneovenous, 376
  selective, 355
  stenosis and, 341–342
    causes of, 341–342
    detection of, 342
    treatment of, 342
  thrombosis, 339
  total, 353–354, 360–361
  see also Surgery

Snake skin pattern, in portal hypertensive gastropathy, 258–259
Sodium ions, 252
  salt restriction, 372
Sodium morrhuate, 291
Sodium retention, *see under* Ascites
Sodium tetradecilsulphate, 291, 304
Somatostatin, 209, 266, 298–299, 313, 316–317, 318–320, 402–403
Sonography—
  Doppler, *see* Doppler sonography
  endoscopy, 223
  see also under Endoscopy; *see also* Echocardiography
Spironolactone, 277, 372–373
Splanchnic circulation, in ascites, 359–370
Splanchnic vasodilatation, in portal hypertensive gastropathy, 261–262
Spleen, 222
Splenomegaly, 222
Spontaneous bacterial peritonitis, 252
  see also Bacterial infections
Staphylococcus aureus, 340
Stellate cells, 206–207, 320, 368
Streptococcal infections, 252
  see also Bacterial infections
Sucralfate, 292
Suprahepatic portal hypertension, 233, 235
Surgery, for portal hypertension, **351–364**
  devascularization, 356; *see also* Devascularization
  historical aspects of, 351–353
  and non-surgical procedures, *see* Devascularization
  partial shunts and, 354–355
  selective shunts and, 355
  timing of, 357–361
  total portal systemic shunts, 353–354
  see also Shunts
Systemic vasodilatation, 208–211
  vasoconstrictors and, 211
  vasodilators, circulating, 208–209
  endothelium and, 209–211

Terlipressin, 281, 304, 312–313, 315–316, 318–320
Thalidomide, 210
Ticarcillin, 340
Timolol, 273–275
  see also Beta-blockers
Torasemide, 373
Total portal systemic shunts, 353–354
Transfer factor, 399
TIPPS, *see* Transjugular intrahepatic portosystemic shunt
Transjugular intrahepatic portosystemic shunt (TIPS), 249, 266, **327–349**, 353, 359, 361, 376
  cardiopulmonary changes and, 340

complications after, 337–338
  in the long term, 339–343
complications during, 339–340
contraindications for, 336–337
encephalopathy and, 343
history of, 328
indications for, 331–336
  acute varices, 331–332
  liver transplant, 334–335
  miscellaneous, 335–336
  recurrent varices, 332–333
  refractory varices, 333–334
and infection, 339–340
intraperitoneal haemorrhage, 339
mortality and, 338
post-, 331
pre-, 328–329
shunt patency in, 341
shunt problems, 339, 341–342
technique of, 329–331
terminology for, 328
see also Surgery
Transmural pressure, 215, 225–226
  see also Wall tension
Transplantation, *see* Liver transplants
Triglycyl lysine vasopressin, *see* Terlipressin
Tumour necrosis factor-α, 210

Ulceration, 292
Ultrasound, *see* Doppler sonography
Urea nitrogen (BUN), 249

Variceal bleeding, 214–216
  acute, 248–249; *see also under* Acute variceal bleeding
    surgery for, 357–358
  and ascites, 251–252; *see also* Ascites
  chronic, recurrent, 249–250
  epidemiology of, 244
  indicators of, 246–248
    endoscopic, 246
    haemodynamic, 246–248
  and portal hypertensive gastropathy, *see under* Portal hypertensive gastropathy
  prevention, **271–287**, 296
    of rebleeding, 300–304
  recurrent, and TIPS, 331–333
  treatment, 296–300
  see also Portal hypertension
Variceal obturation, 293, 298–300
  complications of, 293
  technique of, 293
Variceal pressure, 225–226
Varices, development of, 244–245
Vascular endothelium, *see* Endothelium
  see also Endothelins *and specific forms of*
Vasoconstrictors, 211
Vasodilatation, *see* Systemic vasodilatation
Vasodilator drugs, 275

Vasodilators, circulating, 208–211
   endothelium and, 209–211
      nitric oxide, 209–210; *see also* Nitric oxide
      prostaglandins, 210–211; *see also* Prosta-
         glandins
Vasopressin, 211, 248, 278, 312, 314–315, 318–
      320, 357
   side effects of, 312

Ventilation-perfusion imbalance, 396–400, 403
Verapamil, 278
Viscosity, 204
V2-receptors, 377

Wall tension, 215, 225–226, 247
Water retention, *see under* Ascites
Wilson's disease, 389